T0227176

Pediatric Orthopedics

Editor

PAUL T. HAYNES

PEDIATRIC CLINICS OF NORTH AMERICA

www.pediatric.theclinics.com

Consulting Editor
BONITA F. STANTON

February 2020 • Volume 67 • Number 1

ELSEVIER

1600 John F. Kennedy Boulevard • Suite 1800 • Philadelphia, Pennsylvania, 19103-2899

http://www.theclinics.com

THE PEDIATRIC CLINICS OF NORTH AMERICA Volume 67, Number 1
February 2020 ISSN 0031-3955, ISBN-13: 978-0-323-71042-8

Editor: Kerry Holland
Developmental Editor: Casey Potter

The Pediatric Clinics of North America (ISSN 0031-3955) is published bimonthly by Elsevier Inc., 360 Park Avenue South, New York, NY 10010-1710. Months of issue are February, April, June, August, October, and December. Periodicals postage paid at New York, NY and additional mailing offices. Subscription prices are $240.00 per year (US individuals), $695.00 per year (US institutions), $315.00 per year (Canadian individuals), $924.00 per year (Canadian institutions), $362.00 per year (international individuals), $924.00 per year (international institutions), $100.00 per year (US students and residents), $100.00 per year (Canadian students and residents), and $165.00 per year (international residents and students). To receive students/resident rare, orders must be accompanied by name of affiliated institution, date of term, and the signature of program/residency coordinator on institution letterhead. Orders will be billed at individual rate until proof of status is received. Foreign air speed delivery is included in all *Clinics* subscription prices. All prices are subject to change without notice. **POSTMASTER:** Send address changes to *The Pediatric Clinics of North America*, Elsevier Health Sciences Division, Subscription Customer Service, 3251 Riverport Lane, Maryland Heights, MO 63043. **Customer Service: 1-800-654-2452 (US and Canada). From outside of the US and Canada: 1-314-447-8871. Fax: 1-314-447-8029. For print support, E-mail: JournalsCustomerService-usa@elsevier.com. For online support, E-mail: JournalsOnlineSupport-usa@elsevier.com.**

Reprints. For copies of 100 or more, of articles in this publication, please contact the Commercial Reprints Department, Elsevier Inc., 360 Park Avenue South, New York, NY 10010-1710. Tel.: 212-633-3874; Fax: 212-633-3820; E-mail: reprints@elsevier.com.

The Pediatric Clinics of North America is also published in Spanish by McGraw-Hill Inter-americana Editores S.A., Mexico City, Mexico; in Portuguese by Riechmann and Affonso Editores, Rua Comandante Coelho 1085, CEP 21250, Rio de Janeiro, Brazil; and in Greek by Althayia SA, Athens, Greece.

The Pediatric Clinics of North America is covered in *MEDLINE/PubMed (Index Medicus)*, *Excerpta Medica*, *Current Contents*, *Current Contents/Clinical Medicine*, *Science Citation Index*, *ASCA*, *ISI/BIOMED*, and *BIOSIS*.

PROGRAM OBJECTIVE
The goal of the *Pediatric Clinics of North America* is to keep practicing physicians and residents up to date with current clinical practice in pediatrics by providing timely articles reviewing the state-of-the-art in patient care.

TARGET AUDIENCE
All practicing pediatricians, physicians and healthcare professionals who provide patient care to pediatric patients.

LEARNING OBJECTIVES
Upon completion of this activity, participants will be able to:
1. Review the clinical manifestations and orthopedic management of common neuromuscular disorders.
2. Discuss the general approach to performing a pediatric orthopaedic physical examination for newborn, children and adolescents.
3. Recognize which pediatric musculoskeletal infections should be referred for specialist evaluation.

ACCREDITATIONS
Physician Credit

The Elsevier Office of Continuing Medical Education (EOCME) is accredited by the Accreditation Council for Continuing Medical Education (ACCME) to provide continuing medical education for physicians.

The EOCME designates this journal-based activity for a maximum of 14 *AMA PRA Category 1 Credit*(s)™. Physicians should claim only the credit commensurate with the extent of their participation in the activity.

All other healthcare professionals requesting continuing education credit for this this journal-based activity will be issued a certificate of participation.

ABP Maintenance of Certification Credit

Successful completion of this CME activity, which includes participation in the activity and individual assessment of and feedback to the learner, enables the learner to earn up to 14 MOC points in the American Board of Pediatrics' (ABP) Maintenance of Certification (MOC) program. It is the CME activity provider's responsibility to submit learner completion information to ACCME for the purpose of granting ABP MOC credit.

DISCLOSURE OF CONFLICTS OF INTEREST
The EOCME assesses conflict of interest with its instructors, faculty, planners, and other individuals who are in a position to control the content of CME activities. All relevant conflicts of interest that are identified are thoroughly vetted by EOCME for fair balance, scientific objectivity, and patient care recommendations. EOCME is committed to providing its learners with CME activities that promote improvements or quality in healthcare and not a specific proprietary business or a commercial interest.

The planning committee, staff, authors and editors listed below have identified no financial relationships or relationships to products or devices they or their spouse/life partner have with commercial interest related to the content of this CME activity:
Alice Chu, MD; Christopher Collins, MD; Laury A. Cuddihy, MD; Evan Curatolo, MD; Kristen DePaola, MS; Robert Dolitsky, MD; Joel P. Fechisin, MD; Justin Fernicola, MD; David S. Geller, MD; Benjamin Giliberti, MD; Aron Green, MD; Jamie Grossman, MD, MS; Paul T. Haynes, MD; Kerry Holland; Alison Kemp; Bum Kim, BA; Kamen Kutzarov, MD; Alexander H. Lopyan, MD, MS; Rajkumar Mayakrishnan Christopher Michel, MD; Bertrand W. Parcells, MD; Gregory Parker, MD; Monica Payares-Lizano, MD, FAAOS, FAAP; Cassandra Pino, MS, MPH; Casey Potter; Amit Singla, MD; Lawrence M. Stankovits, MD; Bonita F. Stanton, MD; Natasha Trentacosta, MD; Mark Woernle, MD; Jeffrey P. Wu, MD.

UNAPPROVED/OFF-LABEL USE DISCLOSURE
The EOCME requires CME faculty to disclose to the participants:
1. When products or procedures being discussed are off-label, unlabelled, experimental, and/or investigational (not US Food and Drug Administration [FDA] approved); and
2. Any limitations on the information presented, such as data that are preliminary or that represent ongoing research, interim analyses, and/or unsupported opinions. Faculty may discuss information about pharmaceutical agents that is outside of FDA-approved labelling. This information is intended solely for CME and is not intended to promote off-label use of these medications. If you have any

questions, contact the medical affairs department of the manufacturer for the most recent prescribing information.

TO ENROLL
To enroll in the *Pediatric Clinics of North America* Continuing Medical Education program, call customer service at 1-800-654-2452 or sign up online at http://www.theclinics.com/home/cme. The CME program is available to subscribers for an additional annual fee of USD 301.60.

METHOD OF PARTICIPATION
In order to claim credit, participants must complete the following:
1. Complete enrolment as indicated above.
2. Read the activity.
3. Complete the CME Test and Evaluation. Participants must achieve a score of 70% on the test. All CME Tests and Evaluations must be completed online.

In order to claim MOC points, participants must complete the following:
1. Complete steps listed above for claiming CME credit
2. Provide your specialty board ID#, birth date (MM/DD), and attestation.
3. Online MOC submission is only available for the American Board of pediatrics' (ABP) Maintenance of Certification (MOC) program

CME INQUIRIES/SPECIAL NEEDS
For all CME inquiries or special needs, please contact elsevierCME@elsevier.com.

Contributors

CONSULTING EDITOR

BONITA F. STANTON, MD
Founding Dean, Hackensack Meridian School of Medicine at Seton Hall University,
President, Academic Enterprise, Hackensack Meridian Health Robert C. and Laura C.
Garrett Endowed Chair for the School of Medicine, Professor of Pediatrics, Nutley, New
Jersey

EDITOR

PAUL T. HAYNES, MD
Medical Director of Pediatric Orthopedics, Hackensack Meridian Health, Jersey Shore
University Medical Center, Neptune City, New Jersey; Pediatric Orthopedic Surgeon,
Seaview Orthopaedics & Medical Associates, Ocean, New Jersey

AUTHORS

OMKAR BAXI, MD
Hand Surgery Fellow, The Hand Center of San Antonio, San Antonio, Texas

JASON CHAN, MD
Resident, Orthopedic Surgery, Rutgers-New Jersey Medical School, Newark, New Jersey

ALICE CHU, MD
Associate Professor, Orthopedic Surgery, Rutgers-New Jersey Medical School, Newark,
New Jersey

CHRISTOPHER COLLINS, MD
Pediatric Orthopedic Surgery Attending, Seaview Orthopedic & Medical Associates,
Ocean, New Jersey

LAURY A. CUDDIHY, MD
Spine Surgery, Institute for Spine and Scoliosis, Lawrenceville, New Jersey; Assistant
Clinical Professor, Orthopedics, Mount Sinai Hospital, New York, New York; Assistant
Clinical Professor, Orthopedics, St Peters University Hospital, New Brunswick, New
Jersey

EVAN CURATOLO, MD
Attending Physician, Department of Orthopedics, Monmouth Medical Center, Long
Branch, New Jersey; Atlantic Pediatric Orthopedics, Shrewsbury, New Jersey

KRISTEN DePAOLA, MS
Medical Student, Rowan University School of Osteopathic Medicine, Stratford, New
Jersey

ROBERT DOLITSKY, MD
Orthopedic Resident, Department of Orthopedics, Monmouth Medical Center, Long Branch, New Jersey

JOEL P. FECHISIN, MD
Orthopaedic Surgeon, Seaview Orthopaedic & Medical Associates, Ocean, New Jersey

JUSTIN FERNICOLA, MD
Orthopedic Resident, Monmouth Medical Center, Long Branch, New Jersey

DAVID S. GELLER, MD, FAOA, FACS
Vice-Chairman of Strategy and Innovation, Department of Orthopedic Surgery, Montefiore Medical Center, Associate Professor of Orthopedic Surgery and Pediatrics, Albert Einstein College of Medicine, Bronx, New York

BENJAMIN GILIBERTI, MD
Orthopedic Resident, Department of Orthopedics, Monmouth Medical Center, Long Branch, New Jersey

ARON GREEN, MD
Seaview Orthopedic & Medical Associates, Ocean, New Jersey

JAMIE GROSSMAN, MD, MS
Orthopedic Resident, Department of Orthopedics, Monmouth Medical Center, Long Branch, New Jersey

BUM KIM, BA
Medical School Candidate, Manalapan, New Jersey

KAMEN KUTZAROV, MD
Orthopedic Resident, Department of Orthopedics, Monmouth Medical Center, Long Branch, New Jersey

ALEXANDER H. LOPYAN, MD, MS
Resident Physician, Orthopedic Surgery, Monmouth Medical Center, Long Branch, New Jersey

CHRISTOPHER MICHEL, MD
Orthopedic Surgery Resident, Monmouth Medical Center, Long Branch, New Jersey

BERTRAND W. PARCELLS, MD
Seaview Orthopaedic & Medical Associates, Ocean, New Jersey

GREGORY PARKER, MD
Orthopedic Resident, Department of Orthopedics, Monmouth Medical Center, Long Branch, New Jersey

MONICA PAYARES-LIZANO, MD, FAAOS, FAAP
Attending Surgeon, Orthopedic Surgery Program, Nicklaus Children's Hospital, Miami, Florida

CASSANDRA PINO, MS, MPH
Medical Student, Wayne State University School of Medicine, Detroit, Michigan

AMIT SINGLA, MD
Department of Orthopaedic Surgery, Montefiore Medical Center, Bronx, New York

LAWRENCE M. STANKOVITS, MD
Section Chief, Pediatric Orthopedic Surgery, Monmouth Medical Center, Long Branch, New Jersey

NATASHA TRENTACOSTA, MD
Cedars-Sinai Kerlan-Jobe Institute, Los Angeles, California

MARK WOERNLE, MD
Orthopedic Surgery Resident, Monmouth Medical Center, Long Branch, New Jersey

JEFFREY P. WU, MD
Department of Anesthesiology, Jersey Shore University Medical Center, Neptune, New Jersey

Contents

 Video content accompanies this article at http://www.pediatric.
theclinics.com.

> This article serves as a guide for the pediatric orthopedic physical exam-
> ination for newborn, children, and adolescents. The newborn physical ex-
> amination is very unique and therefore is classified separately from the
> children and adolescent examination. The following pages should be
> used as an overview of the pediatric orthopedic physical examination
> and to provide normal parameters, guide a more focused approach that
> will improve proper diagnoses, and aid in developing a proper manage-
> ment plan. The art of examining a pediatric patient comes with time, and
> some helpful hints (look for the ♠) can improve the experience.

> A wide of array of patients with genetic and metabolic conditions present
> with orthopedic manifestations. This article discusses the most common
> conditions seen in a typical pediatric orthopedic practice. A few pearls
> are highlighted for each condition to alert practitioners to some of the pit-
> falls encountered when treating these often highly challenged children.

> Neuromuscular disorders are pathologies that can severely affect the quality
> of life as well as longevity of patients. The most common disorders include ce-
> rebral palsy and myelodysplasia. The orthopedic manifestations of these dis-
> orders can be treated operatively or nonoperatively. Both focus on the
> prolongation of mobility and preservation of ambulatory capacity for patients.

> Pediatric populations are prone to infections and most can be managed
> appropriately in a primary care setting. There are, however, some infec-
> tious processes that require intervention or management from an orthope-
> dic surgeon. The most serious infectious processes in the pediatric

development of a differential diagnosis based on limp type, patient's age, and the anatomic site that is most likely affected, provides a selective approach to diagnostic testing. Laboratory tests are indicated when infection, inflammatory arthritis, or a malignancy is considered. Imaging usually begins with plain radiography. Ultrasonography is valuable in assessing irritable hips. Advanced imaging is done in select cases. Prompt referral to an orthopedist is essential, especially if septic joint, vascular or compartment issues, or open fractures are suspected.

Femoroacetabular Impingement (FAI) are two common and distinct forms of structural pathology in the pediatric hip. We will also discuss two of the more common, and often questioned, pediatric hip disorders — slipped capital femoral epiphysis and Leggs-Calves-Perthes disease. There is a wide spectrum to the natural variation in the shape of our hip and pelvis. Individual, subtle variation does not necessarily predispose children to future pathology such as arthritis or deformity. However, research is increasingly showing that some shapes of the hip joint can increase such risks. The correlation between anatomic variation and present or future symptoms is rarely straight forward. Thus, future investigations are aimed at identifying risk factors to provide pediatric orthopedists tools to risk stratify their patients and understand when conservative approaches such as close observation versus surgical interventions are more appropriate.

Pediatric knee disorders are various and range from trauma and sports injuries to chronic overuse injuries. Because pediatric patients are different from adults, management of pediatric injuries and general knee disorders is also often different. Primary treatment regimen goals focus on a return to the previous level of function, preservation of anatomy, and decreasing potential long-term effects. Long-term complications may include damage to the physis with resultant potential limb length discrepancy or deformity.

Foot and ankle pathology is common in the pediatric population. Common issues may be traumatic in nature, congenital, or age dependent. This article reviews common problems and pathology found in the pediatric foot and ankle.

Pediatric spine disorders are numerous and are quite different when compared with the adult population. This article focuses on some of the more common pediatric spine disorders. This article summarizes such disorders and discusses typical treatment options in the pediatric orthopedic armamentarium.

With increasing pediatric participation in organized sport and the early specialization of children in single sports, the number of injuries seen in the pediatric and adolescent athletic population continues to increase. Children experience acute traumatic injuries during practice and competition as well as chronic overuse injuries secondary to the repetitive stress on their developing bodies. The unique nature of the pediatric patient often requires a different diagnostic, prognostic, and treatment approach to sports injuries compared with their adult counterparts.

Pediatric musculoskeletal tumors can arise in both bone and soft tissues. The overwhelming majority of these are benign; however, rarely, malignant neoplasms do occur. These are collectively termed sarcomas, indicating their mesenchymal origin. Sarcoma treatment requires careful adherence to the well-described tenets of tumor management. This article summarizes the basic principles and a few of the recent advances in the management of soft tissue and bone tumors.

PEDIATRIC CLINICS OF NORTH AMERICA

SERIES OF RELATED INTEREST

Clinics in Perinatology
https://www.perinatology.theclinics.com/
Advances in Pediatrics
https://www.advancesinpediatrics.com/

THE CLINICS ARE AVAILABLE ONLINE!
Access your subscription at:
www.theclinics.com

Foreword

Creating a Strong Infrastructure for Healthy Growth

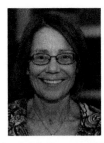

Bonita F. Stanton, MD
Consulting Editor

In this issue of *Pediatric Clinics of North America*, Dr Haynes and his colleagues have created a wonderful overview of current state-of-the-art approaches to a wide range of pediatric orthopedic issues. The primary emphasis of this issue is on surgical interventions, but the importance of judicious use of surgery informed by other less invasive approaches is emphasized throughout this issue.

In his preface, Dr Haynes underscores the importance of interdisciplinary collaboration and safety on improved musculoskeletal outcomes for children. Dr Haynes reflects his profession's focus on safety and patient outcomes in his remarks. Indeed, in 2011, the Pediatric Orthopedic Society of North America, seeking to improve outcomes in all these realms among children requiring musculoskeletal interventions, established the "Quality, Safety, and Value Initiative" (QSVI). The QSVI seeks to develop and identify clinical tools that will improve pediatric care, to conduct research collaboratively to create an outcomes base for assessing outcomes, and to identify best practices for all professionals involved in musculoskeletal care.[1] Substantial improvements in these 3 outcomes have been achieved in many areas of pediatric orthopedic surgery, including advances in casting (cast immobilization and removal), infection prevention and appropriate use of antibiotics, standardization of treatment to reduce variability and improve outcomes, reduction of blood loss, reduction of thromboembolic disease, and judicious use of radiographs to guide orthopedic care among children.[2] The simultaneous emphasis on utilizing advances in technology, safeguarding the lives and functioning of the children receiving such procedures, and continuously assessing the actual outcomes among children is reflected in the articles within this issue emphasizing advances in pediatric orthopedic care.

After reading this issue of *Pediatric Clinics of North America*, pediatric care providers should have an increased understanding of the range of musculoskeletal disorders that may or may not require a surgical approach to resolve and the process of determining

Pediatr Clin N Am 67 (2020) xv–xvi
https://doi.org/10.1016/j.pcl.2019.09.016
0031-3955/20/© 2019 Published by Elsevier Inc.

the best approach to maximize outcomes and reduce risk. For those requiring surgery, the readers will better understand the reasons for the surgery, what will occur in the surgery, and expected outcomes. The issue is both informative and practical, whether as a general update or to find information about a specific disorder.

Bonita F. Stanton, MD
Hackensack Meridian School of Medicine
at Seton Hall University
Academic Enterprise
340 Kingsland Street, Building 123
Nutley, NJ 07110, USA

E-mail address:
bonita.stanton@shu.edu

REFERENCES

1. Glotzbecker MP, Wang K, Waters PM, et al. Quality, safety and value in pediatric orthopedic surgery. J Pediatric Orthop 2016;36:549–57.
2. Miller DJ, Cahill PJ, Janicki JA, et al. What's new in pediatric orthopaedic quality, safety, and value? A systematic review with results of the 2016 POSNA Quality, Safety, and Value Initiative (QSVI) Challenge. J Pediatr Orthop 2018;38(10): e646–51.

Preface

Pediatric Orthopedics

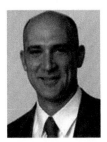

Paul T. Haynes, MD
Editor

As a practicing pediatric orthopedic surgeon and having the opportunity and honor to work with and teach pediatric residents, I find myself impressed by how these training physicians navigate the increasing demands placed upon them and the wealth of knowledge requiring mastery. This continues to hold true as trainee becomes trainer, resident becomes fellow, fellow becomes attending. Such increasing demands and wealth of knowledge requiring mastery coupled with tertiary care settings make practicing in a multidisciplinary team so important. Indeed, numerous studies evaluating care for patients from osteomyelitis, posttraumatic cervical spine clearance protocols, to decreasing infection rates after spine surgery all seem to conclude or infer care is improved with a multidisciplinary approach.[1–3] Whether it be the initiation of standardized protocols or simply improving interdisciplinary communication, improvement in overall care and likely patient outcomes and experiences can be improved as all services work together.

Pediatricians are truly on the "front lines." Navigating, deciphering, and treating the multitude of symptoms, physical exams, and potential treatment options is a gargantuan task particularly as the understanding of disease processes improves. Understanding when to refer and when to treat is equally challenging. The articles to follow have been written with the purpose of updating the pediatric orthopedic knowledge base of pediatricians and trainees. The majority of pediatric orthopedic conditions are encountered, diagnosed, and treated well by pediatricians; the following

Pediatr Clin N Am 67 (2020) xvii–xviii
https://doi.org/10.1016/j.pcl.2019.09.015
0031-3955/20/© 2019 Published by Elsevier Inc.

articles are intended additionally to add guidance as to when appropriate referral is suggested. The cornerstone of the pediatric multidisciplinary team is the pediatrician.

Paul T. Haynes, MD
Pediatric Orthopedics
Seaview Orthopaedics &
Medical Associates
1200 Eagle Avenue
Suite 100
Ocean, NJ 07712, USA

E-mail address:
haynespa2@yahoo.com

REFERENCES

1. Ballard M, Miller NH, Nyquist AC, et al. A multidisciplinary approach improves infection rates in pediatric spine surgery. J Pediatr Orthoped 2012;32(3).
2. Copley L, Kinsler MA, Gheen T, et al. The impact of evidence-based clinical practice guidelines applied by a multidisciplinary team for the care of children with osteomyelitis. J Bone Joint Surg 2013;95.
3. Lee SL. A multidisciplinary approach to the development of a cervical spine clearance protocol: process, rationale, and initial results. J Pediatr Surg 2003;38(3): 358–62.

Pediatric Orthopedic Examination

Monica Payares-Lizano, MD, FAAOS, FAAP[a],*, Cassandra Pino, MS, MPH[b]

KEYWORDS

- Pediatric orthopedic examination • Physical examination
- Musculoskeletal examination

KEY POINTS

- The pediatric examination can be challenging for the novice orthopedist.
- Knowing how to perform a comprehensive musculoskeletal and neuromuscular examination is important. However, it may not be possible or warranted in every patient, and thus, a focused examination guided by history is more common practice.
- Follow these 4 basic steps in every examined region: recognize deformities, recognize ranges-of-motion parameters, determine strength and neurologic assessment, and know the variance based on age.
- With an organized approach and the helpful hints provided, over time the art of examining a pediatric patient can be mastered.

 Video content accompanies this article at http://www.pediatric.theclinics.com.

INTRODUCTION

Because of the numerous possible musculoskeletal and neuromuscular conditions, the pediatric orthopedic examination equally varies based on chief complaints, the age of the child, the severity of the problem, and the concern of the parent or caregiver. Keep in mind that the musculoskeletal system is closely intertwined with the neurologic system for proper functioning, and thus, pediatric orthopedists must be familiar with the neurologic examination at different stages of development.[1]

♦ Start by making sure the *environment is welcoming* with a well-lit room, bright colors, and age-appropriate "distraction tools." These can range from books, stickers, and stuffed animals to dolls with different types of casts among other "distraction tools."

---

[a] Orthopedic Surgery Program, Nicklaus Children's Hospital, 3100 Southwest 62nd Avenue, Miami, FL 33155, USA; [b] Wayne State University School of Medicine, 540 E. Canfield St, Detroit, MI 48201, USA
* Corresponding author.
E-mail address: Monica.Payares-Lizano@nicklaushealth.org

Pediatr Clin N Am 67 (2020) 1–21
https://doi.org/10.1016/j.pcl.2019.09.004
0031-3955/20/© 2019 Elsevier Inc. All rights reserved.
pediatric.theclinics.com

- It is helpful and efficient to have the family *fill out an intake form* before seeing the physician. This can help focus the history-taking and examination while saving precious time. In the Appendix, a copy of the form used at Nicklaus Children's Hospital is available.
- *Do not use a white coat.* The changes in blood pressure and anxiety caused by the white coat are well described. Recent articles have confirmed the existence of white-coat hypertension in children and adolescents.[2,3]
- *Introduce yourself and all your staff and their purpose.* Acknowledge everyone in the room: siblings, grandparents, and so forth. Having everyone participating and involved promotes an environment of trust, familiarity, and comfort. Multiple studies have shown that good physician-patient communication results in improved outcomes by improving diagnostic accuracy fostering shared decision making and increasing the likelihood that a patient will follow through with the proposed treatment plan.[4]
- *Do not look rushed.* In this day and age of electronic medical records and demands for increased productivity, the physician is often pressed for time, but once the physician is with a patient, he or she must be engaged, must *make eye contact*, and must examine the patient himself or herself.
- *Every minute of the interaction is valuable.* The examination begins with observing the child even before coming into the room. This may be the only chance to see the patient ambulating "normally" and unaffected by the physician's presence (**Box 1**).

HISTORY

Depending on the age of the child, obtaining an accurate history can be difficult; thus, being able to interview the parents or primary caregiver is important. If suspecting nonaccidental trauma or possible sexually transmitted disease exposure, it may be beneficial to interview the patient child and parent or caregiver separately. When obtaining a history, always begin with the chief complaint. Get the history from the patient and the caregiver; they may have different views on what is bothering them the most. The history of present illness describes how and when the chief complaint began. Ask about details, such as onset, location, duration, and evolution of symptoms, and what alleviates or aggravates the symptoms should also be obtained. It

---

Box 1
Helpful hints for a successful pediatric examination

- Welcoming environment
- Age-appropriate "distraction tools"
- Use intake form
- Skip the white coat
- Introduce yourself to all members present
- Do not look rushed
- Make eye contact
- Take advantage of every minute of the interaction
- Test unaffected side first
- Perform painful range movements last

is also important to note whether any other treatments have been recommended or initiated and whether they were effective.

The past medical history includes information such as previous major illnesses, hospitalizations, surgeries, and any current medications the patient may be taking. Developmental history is also very important, because any pregnancy or delivery complications can clue the physician in on potential developmental delays. Ask about timing of the milestones. **Table 1** lists common milestones and average timing.[4] For a more comprehensive look at all milestones, The Centers for Disease Control and Prevention has a Web site with more comprehensive guidelines, which can be accessed at the following URL: https://www.cdc.gov/ncbddd/actearly/milestones/index.html.

Regarding the family history, the focus should mostly be on the immediate family, such as siblings, parents, grandparents, and close relatives.

The review of systems should include a general medical overview of all organ systems.

The social history should include the patient's living situation. The physician should also ask whether the child is involved in any sports or extracurricular activities and current grade at school.

The best musculoskeletal examinations always begin by listening; often the diagnosis can be made when obtaining the patient history and observing their disposition and attitude. When possible, include the patient; by allowing the child to have some control, the physician is effectively creating a rapport with the patient.

PHYSICAL EXAMINATION

The pediatric orthopedic physical examination varies based on age of the patient. Once the height and weight of the patient have been measured by the staff, the physician will begin the physical examination with a general assessment of the child's state. What is the general appearance? Is the child in distress? Is the child lethargic? Is the child well nourished, overweight, or cachectic? What is their affect or mood?

As a general process, these 4 steps should be examined per anatomic region: (1) inspect for deformities; (2) assess joint range of motion (ROM); (3) test muscular strength; and (4) perform neurologic assessment. Regarding the *deformity*, try to answer the following questions:

| Table 1 |
| Average developmental achievement by age |

Month	Achievement
1 mo	Partial head control in prone position
2 mo	Partial head control in supine position
4 mo	Rolls over prone to supine
5 mo	Rolls over supine to prone
6 mo	Lifts head and chest with weight on hands in prone position
8 mo	Sits independently
10 mo	Crawls
12 mo	Walks independently
2 y	Jumps and knows full name
3 y	Goes up stairs alternating feet; knows age and gender
4 y	Hops on 1 foot and throws ball overhead

- Where is the deformity? Is it found in the bones, the joints, or the soft tissues?
- How severe is the deformity? Is it correctible? Or is it fixed?
- What factors are causing the deformity?
- Is there associated muscle spasm, local tenderness, or pain with motion?[1]

Assessment of joint ROM will vary by age and sex. **Table 2** summarizes and describes the commonly tested motions. In general, children have more laxity than adults; with aging, the connective tissue becomes stiffer. Girls tend to have increased joint laxity[4] (**Fig. 1**).

Each joint will have different active and passive ROM based on each age group. It is important to recognize that if there is an increase in tone (otherwise known as spasticity), as it can affect the ROM. Spasticity is commonly seen in neurologic conditions, such as cerebral palsy. The degree of spasticity can vary within the time of a single evaluation, depending on the level of anxiety, temperature, and/or time of day.

Muscle strength testing is commonly graded from 0 to 5 based on contraction, gravity, and resistance (**Table 3**).[4]

Neurologic assessment is a key portion of the pediatric orthopedic examination owing to the functional relationship of the 2 systems. Oftentimes orthopedists are the initial physician to evaluate delays in motor milestones, muscle weakness, incoordination, or other disturbances In neuromuscular function. One must therefore assess developmental reflexes (**Table 4**), deep and superficial reflexes, sensory function, cranial nerves, and mental and emotional state.

Newborn

A focused musculoskeletal newborn examination can be done in a systematic way in very little time, checking key areas to not miss important abnormalities. Focused musculoskeletal examination of a newborn can be performed in less than 3 minutes (Video 1).

As opposed to older children, it is preferable to have a quieter, warm room with lower lighting so the infant may be more comfortable for the examination. Feeding the newborn just before the examination can help them be calmer.

Table 2
Description of joint motions

Motion	Description
Flexion	Bending the joint away from the zero-starting point
Extension	Bending the joint toward the zero-starting point
Hyperextension	The joint extends abnormally beyond the zero-starting point
Abduction	Movement of the limbs away from the midline
Adduction	Movement of the limbs toward the midline
Supination	Palms of hand turn face-upward or toward the anterior surface of the body
Pronation	Palms of hand turn face-downward or toward the posterior surface of the body
Inversion	Inward turning motion
Eversion	Outward turning motion
Internal rotation	Turning limb on an imaginary axis toward the midline
External rotation	Turning limb on an imaginary axis away from the midline

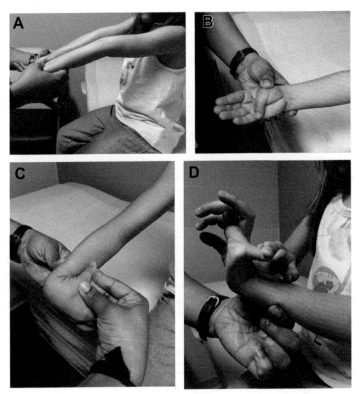

Fig. 1. A 4-year-old girl with signs of hypermobility. (*A*) Cubitus recurvatum greater than 10°. (*B*) Opposition of the thumb past the fifth MCP joint. (*C*) Opposition of the thumb to the volar aspect of the ipsilateral forearm. (*D*) Passive dorsiflexion of the fifth MCP joint to greater than 90°.

Skin

The newborn should be fully undressed while observing their general state. Assess the skin temperature. If the room is too cold, the patient's skin will look mottled.

The generalized appearance of the skin should be assessed. Is there jaundice? Is there depigmentation? Café-au-lait spots can indicate neurofibromatosis[5] or

Table 3 Grading of muscle strength	
Grade	Description
0	No muscular contraction detected
1	Trace of contraction barely detectable
2	Active movement with gravity eliminated
3	Active movement against gravity
4	Active movement against gravity and some resistance
5	Active movement against full resistance

Data from Medical Research Council. Aids to the examination of the peripheral nervous system, Memorandum no. 45, Her Majesty's Stationery Office, London, 1981.

Table 4
Primitive reflexes

Reflex	Age When It Disappears (mo)	Description
Moro	6	Sudden neck extension causes shoulder abduction, extension of limbs, spreading of fingers, and ends with an embrace
Grasp	3	Infant clasps onto physician's finger when placed in their palm
Neck righting	10	Positive if trunk and limbs spontaneously turn toward the same side when head is turned to 1 side
Symmetric tonic neck	6	Upper limbs flex, and lower limbs extend with flexion of the neck
Asymmetric tonic neck	6	Turning the neck to 1 side, upper and lower extremities extend on the side to which the head is turned and flexion of the upper and lower extremities on the opposite side
Walking or stepping	1–2	Elicited by supporting the trunk and holding the infant upright. The soles of the feet are positioned onto table, and the infant is gently inclined and moved forward. This automatically initiates alternating flexion and extension of the lower limbs, simulating walking (Video 2)

Reflex	Age When Appears	Description
Postural Reflexes		
Foot placement	Early infancy	Holding the infant under their arms, gently lift them so that the dorsum of the feet and anterior aspect of tibia touch the side of the table; if the infant lifts up the extremity and steps onto the table, it is positive
Parachute	12 mo	Holding the infant in the prone position, lower the infant toward the table (stimulating a fall). If positive, the infant will extend the upper extremities to break the fall

McCune-Albright syndrome. Are there birthmarks or hemangiomas? Palpation of the skin can also provide further information in regard to ligamentous laxity or other connective tissue disorders.

Face, Head, and Neck

Notice head size and measure the head circumference with a tape measure just above the eyebrows and the most prominent part of the occiput, then plot on the newborn head circumference chart when suspecting an abnormality. Note the shape of the head and place a hand around the occiput of skull; notice any plagiocephaly. Run fingers across the skin of the infant's scalp and notice the fontanel. A sunken fontanel can be a sign of dehydration, and too much fullness can be hydrocephalus.

After a general impression, look at each part of the face for any indications of potential congenital anomalies or syndromic features. Look at the parents and notice any similarities in the appearance. Evaluate the appearance, spacing, and function of the eyes. The ears should be at the level of the eyes. Notice the preference of side as seen in torticollis and evaluate for possible masses. Note if neck webbing or redundant skin is present, because this can be a sign of Turner syndrome. Assess ROM by rotating the infant's head toward either shoulder.

Clavicle and Shoulders

Next, run hands over the infant's clavicles; they should feel smooth without any crepitus or step-offs. Palpation of the clavicles can detect damage caused during traumatic delivery. If local tenderness is present after birth, a callus will soon form a bump, which will be readily palpable within a few days. Assess the overall symmetry and contour of the shoulders.

Assess the ROM of the shoulders by assessing shoulder flexion, abduction, and internal and external rotation of the joint. It is important to note that infants are expected to have decreased abduction of the shoulder (see **Table 3**). Excessive limited ROM, however, could indicate congenital dislocation of the shoulder, or deformity of the scapula.[5]

Hands and Upper Extremity

It is expected that infants have flexion contractures of the elbow, hips, and knees (**Box 2**). Watch for spontaneous movements and abnormal posturing. For instance, an arm held in adduction, internal rotation with elbow extended, pronated forearm, and flexed wrist and digits, known as a waiter tip, can be a sign of a brachial plexopathy (**Fig. 2**).

Examine the appearance of the hands as well as the number of fingers and thumbs. Note any syndactyly, webbing, or hypoplasia of any aspect of the hand, wrist, or forearm. Finally, check ROM of the wrist and fingers.

As the ROM is being checked, and starting proximal to distal, the muscle strength is also evaluated. In addition, notice perfusion of the extremities and check for pulses.

Chest and Abdomen

Observe the shape of the chest and placement and appearance of the nipples. Note the pectus excavatum or pectus carinatum. Check for asymmetry in abdominal reflexes. Also, note hypoplasia of the pectoralis, which can be related to Poland syndrome. In the abdomen, look for hernias or protrusions.

Hips, Knees, and Legs

Look at the overall aspect of the extremities and for deformities or asymmetries.

Box 2
Infant range of motion

Decreased abduction of the shoulder

Greater external rotation of the hip

Limited internal rotation of the hip

Greater dorsiflexion and limited plantar flexion of the ankle

Flexion contractures at elbow, hip, and knee

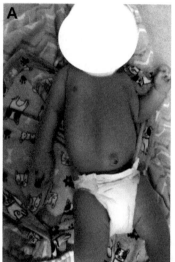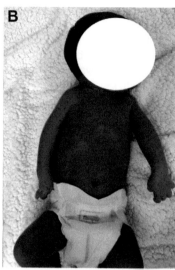

Fig. 2. (*A*) A 2-week-old infant with right brachial plexus injury. Waiter tip posturing consisting of the right arm held in adduction, internal rotation with elbow extended, pronated forearm, and flexed wrist and digits. This patient has normal contour of the shoulders and full passive ROM bilaterally as well as spontaneous movement and typical newborn posturing in the unaffected, left side. (*B*) One-week-old patient with symmetric bilateral deformities. Shoulders are narrow, and there is limitation to passive ROM at shoulders, elbows, wrists, and digits. Spontaneous movements only consisting of shoulder shrugging. This patient's findings are more consistent with arthrogryposis.

A discrepancy between leg lengths can indicate any of various abnormalities. To assess leg length, the child should be lying flat and straight with hip and knee joints extended; assess the heel soft tissue as well as the medial malleoli and compare both legs.

The appearance, symmetry, knee stability, and range of knee motion should be examined as well. The Galeazzi sign can help determine leg length discrepancy coming from femur versus developmental dysplasia of the hip (DDH). **Fig. 3** demonstrates how to check for the Galeazzi sign. Also assess flexion, extension, and internal and external rotation of the hip.

With the diaper removed, assess hip joint ROM. Because of the intrauterine posture of the neonate, all newborns are expected to have some degree of flexion contracture of hip and knee, at approximately 30°. Examine the stability of the hips; address each one individually: while holding the pelvis steady, flex the hips and knee to 90° while placing the index finger along the axis of the femur and thumb of each hand on the inner thigh. While stabilizing the opposite hip and pelvis, take the thigh into abduction. This maneuver, known as the Ortolani maneuver, demonstrates whether the femoral head reduces into the acetabulum; if you feel a "click" that is a sign the hip was in fact dislocated.[4] Next, apply pressure laterally and posteriorly with the thumb on the inner thigh as the hip is adducted. If a "click" is felt, this is a sign of exit. The femoral head dislocates from the acetabulum; this is called the Barlow maneuver. These tests detect hip instability but become negative by 3 months of age.[4] After 3 months, if the hip is dislocated or subluxates, the child will eventually develop contractures, manifesting as limited abduction of the hip. An important point regarding these 2 maneuvers is that one cannot elicit both the

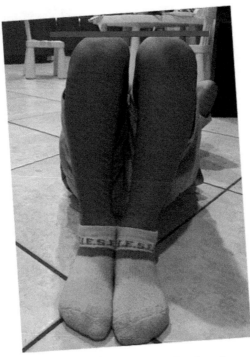

Fig. 3. Galeazzi test assesses leg length discrepancy coming from femur or a hip dislocation. This patient is a 5-year-old boy with no leg length discrepancy, negative Galeazzi sign.

Barlow and Ortolani signs from the same hip. Either the femoral head is sitting in the acetabulum and can be temporarily dislocated on examination (Barlow sign) or the head is dislocated and can be temporarily reduced on examination (Ortolani sign). If the physical examination findings are equivocal and the patient is considered to be at high risk for DDH, ultrasound studies should be ordered. The American Academy of Pediatrics strongly recommends against routine screening ultrasounds. Imaging can be performed in infants considered high risk from 6 weeks to 6 months of age who have normal findings on physical examination. Radiography can be an option for children older than 4 months who have normal findings on physical examination.[6] Please see the Bertrand W. Parcells's article, "Pediatric Hip and Pelvis," in this issue on developmental dysplasia of the hip for further information and guidelines.

Foot and Ankle

As always, start by inspecting for deformities followed by ROM of the ankle, and subtalar joints should be included. Limited dorsiflexion can indicate congenital anomalies, such as clubfoot.[5] Infants will often have greater dorsiflexion because of position in utero. Otherwise known as calcaneovalgus, which a relatively benign deformity and must be differentiated from posteromedial tibial bowing, or congenital vertical talus. The foot can be assessed by sections: hindfoot, midfoot, and forefoot, and deformities in each section can be assessed. The longitudinal arch of the foot should also be assessed. In infants, the arch is low or nonexistent. A high arch can indicate a neurologic abnormality. The number and appearance of toes should also be examined, noting extra toes, overlapping of toes, or syndactyly (**Fig. 4**).

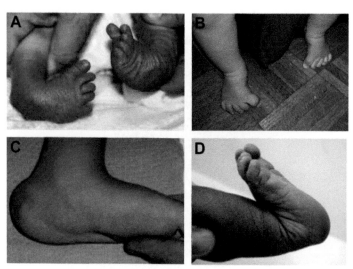

Fig. 4. Common foot deformities. (*A*) Clubfeet. (*B*) Metatarsus adductus. (*C*) Rocker bottom foot, congenital vertical talus. (*D*) Calcaneovalgus foot.

Once the assessment of the feet has been completed, the infant should be turned over onto its stomach to examine the back and spine.

Scapulae

Scapulae should be assessed, noting size, location, and symmetry. Any winging of the scapula or asymmetry should be noted.

Spine

Palpate the spine, noting abnormalities. If a hairy patch, dimples, deep pits that may lead to opening of spinal cord, or midline hemangioma are found on the lumbar region, this can indicate a spinal abnormality. Dimpling on the buttocks can also indicate a congenital anomaly of the femur.

Bending of the knee at a 90° angle allows for the measurement of the thigh foot angle (the angle between the axis of the thigh and axis of the foot), which measures the tibial torsion in the patient (**Fig. 5**).

Neurologic Examination

Several primitive reflexes are present in neonates and infants and are associated with normal development. Primitive reflexes are present at birth and disappear as the child matures. Other reflexes appear during infancy and young childhood, and some continue throughout life.[1]

Children and Adolescents

With the exception of the hip, most of the pediatric orthopedic examination of a child and adolescent is very similar. If evaluating a painful or injured site, one should start palpating with the noninjured or unaffected area far away from area of interest and watch facial expressions during examination; start with light pressure and then deeper pressure as tolerated. Note any edema, effusion, skin tension, adhesions, bony prominences/areas, temperature difference, pulses, and/or abnormal lumps/bumps.

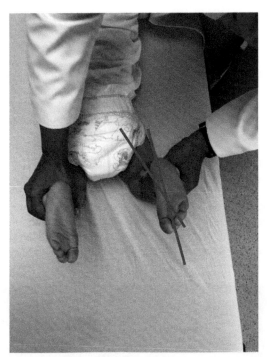

Fig. 5. Thigh-foot axis. In this patient, there is mild internal tibial torsion, which is common and physiologic in his age group (18 months).

♠ When examining the patient, *test the unaffected side first*, because this sets a baseline for the examination and gains patient trust and confidence. In addition, *perform painful movements last*, preventing pain from overcasting the next movement. Active ROM should first be assessed and then passive ROM, then follow with strength testing, flexion, extension, side bend, and rotation. If active ROM is full, give end range pressure for end feel of joint (soft means tissue is being compressed, if end feel seems hard, it is bony, implying bone hitting bone) and degree of motion. Repeated maneuvers are done if symptoms are complained of with multiple repetitions, in an attempt to elicit described symptomatology.

Although positive findings can strongly suggest a type of injury, condition, or disease, negative findings do not necessarily rule out an injury.

Last, perform neurologic assessments. To assess deep tendon reflexes (DTRs), the patient relaxes, with the tendon in a slight stretched position; if there is difficulty eliciting response, have the patient squeeze their hands together. Common DTRs include C5, C6, C7, L4, and S1. Generally, the authors perform initially only biceps, patellar, and Babinski reflexes and notice any asymmetries, hyperreflexia, or hyporeflexia, and if concerned, will then do a more expanded neurologic testing.

Head and Neck

Observe the posture of the head and neck. Is it in the midline/neutral position or is there head tilt or head rotation? When examining motion, evaluate flexion, extension, rotation, and lateral bend. Nodding occurs in the upper cervical spine; flexion occurs in the lower cervical spine. In side-bend, make sure the patient is not moving shoulder toward ear. Do resisted isometric movements in the cervical spine and shoulder/upper extremity (**Fig. 6**).

Shoulder

When examining the shoulder, it is important to have the patient remove enough clothing so that both shoulders can be viewed and compared. Evaluate both exposed shoulders and compare for asymmetry. If ecchymosis or swelling is present around the shoulder, this can indicate trauma with resultant fracture, subluxation of joint, or sprain.

Palpation of the shoulder should evaluate for areas of tenderness. Important areas to palpate include the sternoclavicular joint, clavicle, acromioclavicular joint, bicipital groove, glenohumeral joint line, subacromial space, and spine of the scapula.

Because the shoulder has the greatest ROM, both active and passive ROM should be assessed. When assessing range of elevation of the glenohumeral joint, stand behind the patient and immobilize the scapula by holding its inferior angle. To restrict the motion of the scapulothoracic joint, place a hand over the acromion of the upper

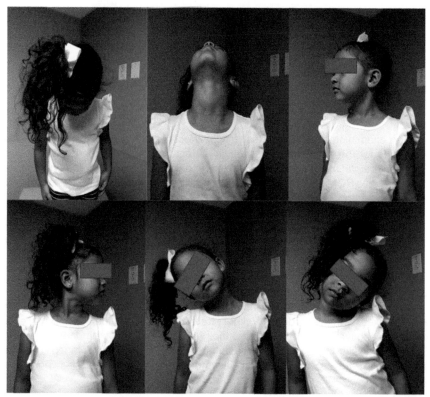

Fig. 6. A 4-year-old girl demonstrating cervical spine ROM with flexion, extension, lateral rotation, and lateral bending. Notice on right lateral rotation (*top right*) the shoulders are rotated, and this can be a compensatory maneuver to accommodate limitation of rotation. Make sure the shoulders are both facing forward. On the left lateral bending (*bottom right*), notice the patient brings the shoulder up to the ear. Again, this is a compensatory maneuver.

limb being tested. When the glenohumeral and scapulothoracic joints move together, the scapula rotates upward and anteriorly over the chest wall; the shoulder then elevates to 180° (see **Fig. 7** and **Table 5** for normal shoulder ROM values).

Again, do the muscle strength testing as going distal on the extremity while assessing ROM.

Elbow

The elbow is a hinge joint with 3 sites of movement: the ulnohumeral, radiohumeral, and radioulnar articulations, with an ROM from 0° to 150° of flexion and from 150° to 0° of extension.

When inspecting the elbow, look for swelling, redness, or warmth. Redness or warmth can suggest infection or trauma.

Palpation helps pinpoint the source of any potential elbow pain as anterior, posterior, lateral, or medial.

Strength testing is performed as restricted movements and should be evaluated with the following movements: supination and pronation of wrist, extension and flexion of wrist, resisted finger extension, elbow flexion, and extension.

The collateral ligaments of the elbow should be evaluated (the lateral and MCLs) for pain and/or laxity. Performed by having the shoulder in full external rotation and placing the elbow in 20° to 30° flexion. Place your palm over the lateral elbow and create a valgus stress to evaluate the MCL. A varus stress is done in the opposite direction to evaluate the LCL. Forearm rotation, which is combined motion of proximal and distal radioulnar joints and radiohumeral joints, is evaluated as pronation and supination. Normal pronation is 70° to 80°, and normal supination is 80° to 90° (**Fig. 8**). The authors find it useful to use pens to determine the angles. Functional ROM is 30°

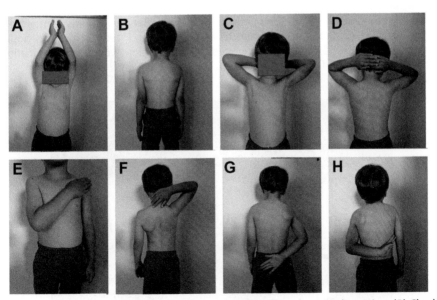

Fig. 7. (*A, B*) Shoulder elevation. (*C*) Horizontal abduction and external rotation. (*D*) Check levels of the scapular spine. (*E*) Adduction and internal rotation. (*F*) Elevation, internal rotation, and adduction. (*G*) Extension, adduction, and internal rotation. (*H*) Extension, internal rotation, and adduction.

Table 5
Shoulder range of motion

	Values (°)
Elevation	180
Internal rotation	50-60
External rotation	40-45
Extension	45-55
Internal rotation in 90 abduction	70
External in 90–90	100

to 130°. Certain forearm abnormalities can be associated with systemic disease as is the case of radial deficiency and hematologic issues.

Wrist and Hands

Inspect for deformities, asymmetries, radial or ulnar deviation of the wrist, and range of the wrist flexion and extension (**Fig. 9**). There are no true normalized values, and thus the evaluation is usually assessed from symmetry.

Examine the appearance of the hands as well as the number of fingers and thumbs. Note any syndactyly, webbing, or hypoplasia of any aspect of the hand, wrist, or forearm. Finally, check ROM of the wrist and fingers.

Check muscles strength after ROM going distally on the extremity with resisted ROM, and last, check for neurologic function. A quick motor test consists of making the "ok" sign (this checks for anterior interosseous nerve), "thumbs up" to check for posterior interosseous nerve, and crossing over the index and middle digits and then making the "peace sign." This is adduction and abduction of the digits. Check function of the interossei muscles innervated by the ulnar nerve. Sensation should be checked in all distributions. Last, assess pulses and perfusion. In an acute trauma situation or if there is any concern for perfusion, vascular examination should be performed first.

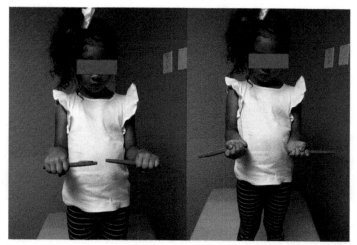

Fig. 8. Forearm pronation and supination. It is useful to have the child hold a pencil.

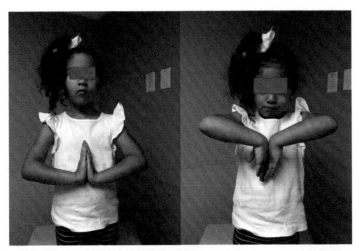

Fig. 9. Wrist flexion and extension; again look for symmetry more so than a particular range.

Hip

Inspect the hips from the front, back, and sides. Note any asymmetry or swelling. Observe gait up and down the hall for any signs of a limp. Note the resting position of the leg; assess weight-bearing amount on each leg, standing posture, any leg-length discrepancy, and the thigh folds.

Palpate the hip for tenderness in the anterior hip joint, anterior superior iliac spine, anterior inferior iliac spine, greater trochanter, iliotibial band, gluteus muscle, sciatic notch, ischial tuberosity, and proximal hamstring muscles.

Despite having a decreased ROM as compared with the shoulder, the hip's ROM varies with age. For example, newborns have greater external rotation and hip rotation, but decreased flexion and extension, because of the intrauterine position (**Fig. 10**, hip rotation). There are also small differences between male and female hips as described by Sankar and colleagues[7] (**Table 6**).

When evaluating the hips, observe the pelvis and make sure it is not tilting or rotating because it can mask a contracture and give an inaccurate ROM measurement.

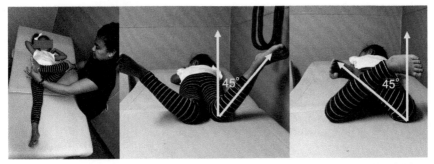

Fig. 10. Hip rotation supine, external rotation (*left*), prone internal rotation (*middle*), and prone external rotation (*right*). Notice the legs make an "X" for eXternal rotation.

Table 6
Normal hip range of motion in children at different ages in degrees[1,7]

Motion	Newborn	2–5 Male/ Female	6–10 Male/ Female	11–17 Male/ Female
Flexion	128	118/121	118/122	113/120
Extension	−30	21/21	19/21	15/22
Abduction	79	51/53	43/51	34/44
Adduction	17	17/18	15/18	14/17
Internal rotation in flexion	76	45/47	40/41	35/35
External rotation in flexion	92	51/49	44/48	40/46

Data from Sankar W, Laird C, Baldwin K. Hip range of motion in children: what is the norm? *J Pediatr Orthop.* 32(4):399-405.

Hip extension is evaluated with the Thompson test (completely flex both hips until the lumbar spine is flattened, then extend 1 hip while the opposite hip remains flexed until the pelvis rotates). The point where the hip can no longer be extended provides the angle between thigh and the examining table (degree of flexion deformity) (**Fig. 11**).

The presence and degree of abduction contracture of the hip are determined by the Ober test. With the patient lying on the side opposite the one being tested, the underneath hip and knee are maximally flexed to flatten the lumbar spine and stabilize the pelvis. The hip to be tested is then flexed to 90° (with the knee flexed to a right angle), fully abducted, and brought into full hyperextension and allowed to adduct maximally. During this maneuver, the knee of the tested extremity should always be kept at 90° of flexion. The angle of the thigh and a horizontal line parallel to the examination table represents the degree of abduction contracture. A normal limb will drop well below this horizontal line. If there is abduction contracture, the hip cannot be adducted to neutral position.

Check the thigh foot axis for tibial rotation assessment (see **Fig. 5**).

With the patient standing, assess for the *Trendelenberg sign*. Do not allow any assistance, such as holding onto table or wall. During a normal examination, the patient will elevate the unsupported pelvis by abducting the stance-leg hip, using the hip abductor musculature (primarily the gluteus medius) to bring the center of gravity over the stance leg. Normal examination indicates that the patient has adequate hip joint range and arc of motion, normal morphology, no inflammation in or around the joint, good to normal muscle strength, and normal central and peripheral neurologic functions. Video 3 shows a positive Trendelenberg test on a young adult patient

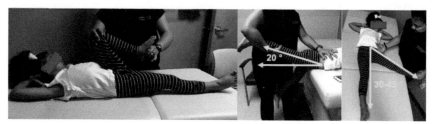

Fig. 11. Hip ROM. Hip extension 10°–20°, flexion 100°–120°, and abduction in extension 30°–45°.

with right-sided history of Legg-Calve-Perthes with resultant leg length inequality and abductor weakness. In the video, notice that the unsupported side drops when the patient attempts to stand on 1 leg, usually with exaggeration of lateral flexion of the lumbar spine in an attempt to place as much body mass as possible over the stance leg.

Knee

Observe lower-extremity alignment for genu valgum (intermalleolar distance) or genu varum (intercondylar distance) (**Fig. 12**).

Ensure the child is in shorts and note the resting position for the leg and the patient's standing posture and assess the weight-bearing amount on each leg. In addition, note any joint effusion, generalized swelling, scars, or rotational deformities.

Palpate the patella tibial tubercle, medial and lateral joint line, distal femoral condyle, medial collateral ligament (MCL), lateral collateral ligament (LCL), pes tendons, suprapatellar pouch, and hamstring tendons. Osteochondritis or inflammation at tendinous insertion is a common presentation in the growing child, particularly the tubercle, with Osgood-Schlatter and inferior pole, also known as Sinding-Larsen-Johannson.

When examining movement, evaluate flexion, extension, patellar mobility, patellar tilt, extensor lag, and flexion contracture (**Fig. 13**).

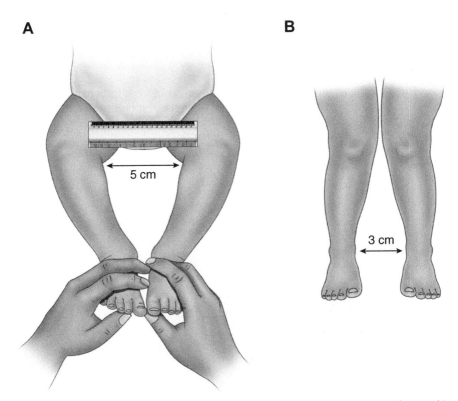

A

B

5 cm

3 cm

Fig. 12. Physiologic bowing. (*A*) Intercondylar distance to measure genu varum. Abnormal is greater than 6 cm. (*B*) Intermalleolar distance to measure genu valgum abnormality is greater than 8 cm.

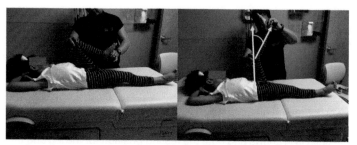

Fig. 13. Knee flexion and extension with popliteal angle measurement.

To test for collateral ligamental injuries, MCL and LCL stress tests can be performed. Similar to the collateral stress test performed on the elbow, a varus and valgus pressure is placed on the knee to differentiate between a potential MCL tear or an LCL tear. To identify a meniscal tear, perform the McMurray test. Finally, to identify an anterior cruciate ligament (ACL) tear, the anterior drawer test can be performed. Similarly, the posterior drawer test can identify a posterior cruciate ligament (PCL) tear (**Fig. 14**).

Ankle and Foot

Inspect the joints for redness, swelling, symmetry and alignment, muscle atrophy, deformities, nodules, and condition for overlying skin (ie, rashes) and assess contractures.

Palpate the ankle and foot for heat, instability, tenderness, crepitus, and/or nodules. The Silfverskiöld test can be used for differentiating between gastrocnemius and Achilles contractures (**Fig. 15**).

The ROM for the ankle and foot varies with age group; it is important to look for smooth, coordinated movements. Active ROM is most commonly used for this examination (**Fig. 16**). There are not true common ranges, but expected dorsiflexion, plantar flexion, inversion, and eversion should be symmetric.

One of the most common presenting chief complaints is flexible pes planovalgus deformities. On weight-bearing, the arch will collapse and usually can be re-created

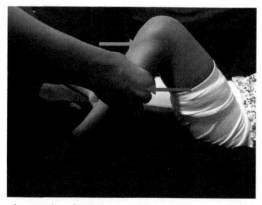

Fig. 14. Anterior and posterior drawer test to assess ACL and PCL stability, respectively. Green arrow shows direction of pressure applied for the stress test for PCL, and red arrow shows direction of pressure applied for the anterior drawer for ACL stability.

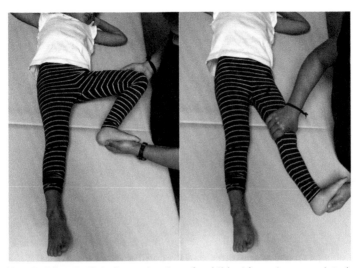

Fig. 15. Silfverskiöld test. Clinical examination of a child with equinus associated with cerebral palsy reveals an inability to fully dorsiflex the ankle. If the ankle can be passively dorsiflexed with the knee bent to 90° but cannot be dorsiflexed with the knee extended, it is thought that the gastrocnemius is tight, but the soleus is not contracted.

on a tiptoe stance or with dorsiflexion of the first metatarsophalangeal (MTP) joint (**Fig. 17**).

Another foot deformity is the cavus foot (**Fig. 18**), which is commonly seen in patients with Charcot-Marie-Tooth syndrome or a neuromuscular condition. It is important to recognize that this can be secondary to a tethered cord, and thus, a full neurologic evaluation and spinal MRI are warranted. If the condition is familial, genetic testing may be considered. To determine if the deformity is fixed or rigid, the hindfoot can be assessed with a Coleman block test, which is done by placing a block on the lateral aspect of the foot and thus allowing the first ray to plantarflex, because this removes one of the deforming forces driving the hindfoot varus.

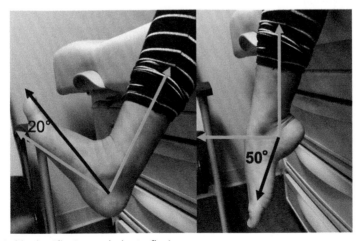

Fig. 16. Ankle dorsiflexion and plantarflexion.

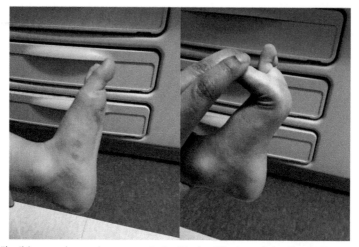

Fig. 17. Flexible pes planovalgus corrected with dorsiflexion of the first MTP.

Spine

Another common referral to the orthopedist is evaluation of spinal asymmetry or scoliosis. Part of the history should include any associated pain or whether there are any neurologic symptoms, such as radiating pain or loss of bowel or bladder control. Also ask if there is a family history of scoliosis or connective tissue disease, such as Marfan syndrome or neurofibromatosis, or neuromuscular disease, such as muscular dystrophy. Start by inspecting the skin over the spine for hairy patches, dimples, or hemangiomas. Look at the sagittal balance and assess thoracic kyphosis or if there is flat lower back with loss of lumbar lordosis. Such deformity may indicate the presence of spasms or spondylolisthesis. Notice the level of the shoulders, and iliac crests. Be sure to assess for leg length discrepancy here, driving pelvic obliquity. Ask the patient to bend forward and touch their toes with arms hanging freely. This position checks spinal flexibility and hamstring tightness and also checks for any evidence of rotational deformity secondary to scoliosis. Then run the fingers along the spine and note any defects of the vertebral bodies or spinous process and ask if there is pain with palpation.[1]

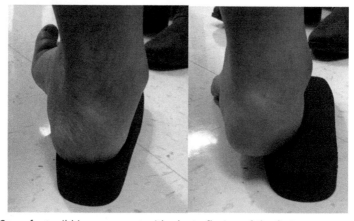

Fig. 18. Cavus foot mild improvement with plantarflexion of the first ray.

DISCLOSURE

No disclosures.

SUPPLEMENTARY DATA

Supplementary data related to this article can be found online at https://doi.org/10.1016/j.pcl.2019.09.004.

REFERENCES

1. Herring J. 5th edition. Tachdjian's pediatric orthopaedics: from the Texas Scottish rite hospital for children, vol. 1. Philadelphia: Elsevier; 2014.
2. Hanevold C. White coat hypertension in children and adolescents. Hypertension 2019;73(1):24–30.
3. Hornsby J, Mongan P, Taylor A, et al. "White coat" hypertension in children. J Fam Pract 1991;33(6):617–23.
4. Weinstein S, Flynn JM. Lovell and Winter's pediatric orthopaedics. 7th edition. Philadelphia: Lippincott Williams & Wilkins; 2014.
5. Ganel A, Dudkiewicz I, Grogan DP. Pediatric orthopedic physical examination of the infant: a 5-minute assessment. J Pediatr Health Care 2003;17(1):39–41.
6. Hauk L. Developmental dysplasia of the hip in infants: a clinical report from the AAP on evaluation and referral. Am Fam Physician 2017;96(3):196–7.
7. Sankar W, Laird C, Baldwin K. Hip range of motion in children: what is the norm? J Pediatr Orthop 2012;32(4):399–405.

Genetic and Metabolic Conditions

Lawrence M. Stankovits, MD[a],*, Alexander H. Lopyan, MD, MS[b,1]

KEYWORDS

- Skeletal dysplasia • Muscular dystrophy • Rickets • Down syndrome
- Ehlers-Danlos syndrome • Neurofibromatosis • Osteogenesis imperfecta

KEY POINTS

- Boys with Duchenne muscular dystrophy often develop scoliosis at a young age. Early referral for orthopedic intervention is necessary because the criteria to perform spinal fusion is lower than in other conditions.
- Many children with skeletal dysplasias develop basilar invagination or upper cervical spine instability; gait changes or changes in tone or reflexes should prompt an immediate investigation into a possible cervical spine condition.
- Individuals with Down syndrome have ligamentous laxity. Hip and patella instability is common.
- The diagnosis of rickets is made by radiographic irregularities, including bowing of the long bones and physeal changes.
- Osteogenesis imperfecta needs to be considered when evaluating a child for nonaccidental trauma. Blue sclera and dental changes, although characteristic, are often not present and not diagnostic.

DUCHENNE'S MUSCULAR DYSTROPHY
Introduction

This disorder, characterized by progressive muscle weakness, has a prevalence of 2 to 3 per 1000 and affects boys beginning between the ages of 2 and 6. Duchenne muscular dystrophy (DMD) is inherited in an X-linked recessive fashion, which is responsible for the male presentation, although it has been found to be caused by a spontaneous mutation in up to one-third of all cases. The gene responsible, Xp21.2,

Disclosure: None of the authors have a relationship with a commercial company that has a direct financial interest in the subject matter presented in this article or with a company making a competing product.
[a] Pediatric Orthopedic Surgery, Monmouth Medical Center, Long Branch, NJ, USA;
[b] Orthopedic Surgery, Monmouth Medical Center, Long Branch, NJ, USA
[1] Present address: 1 Melrose Terrace, Apartment 424, Long Branch, NJ 07740.
* Corresponding author. 1131 Broad Street, Suite 202, Shrewsbury, NJ 07702.
E-mail address: lstankovits@gmail.com

> **Key Points**
>
> - X-linked recessive mutation of dystrophin.
> - Presents in male children with proximal weakness, lordosis, calf hypertrophy.
> - Scoliosis should be monitored for early. Fusion is recommended for curves greater than 20° before deterioration of lung function.

encodes the protein dystrophin, and affected patients expectedly have absent dystrophin protein.[1,2]

Presentation

Male patients typically present between the ages of 2 and 6 years and may have a family history. These patients or their parents may describe progressive weakness affecting the proximal muscles (gluteal muscles first), which manifests with gait abnormalities, difficulty with stairs, and decreased motor skills.

Physical examination findings include calf pseudohypertrophy, which results from infiltration of normal muscle with connective tissue. In addition, the Gower sign is a classic finding, which involves the child being unable to stand up from a seated position independently without "walking" their hands up their legs. These patients, as opposed to those afflicted with spinal muscular atrophy, have intact deep tendon reflexes.

Diagnosis

In addition to the physical examination findings mentioned earlier, suspected abnormalities include the following to assist in formal diagnosis:

- Increased creatine phosphokinase (CPK) level, possibly 10 to 200 times normal
- Muscle biopsy with absent dystrophin
- DNA testing with absent dystrophin
- Electromyogram with myopathic pattern (decreased amplitude, short duration, polyphasic motor)

Orthopedic Manifestations

Beyond the muscle weakness previously identified, patients can be expected to be unable to ambulate independently by age 10 years, require a wheelchair by age 15 years, and succumb to cardiorespiratory complications by age 20 years.

Scoliosis is a serious concern in these patients because their curves progress rapidly (age 13–14 years) and should not be treated with bracing (**Fig. 1**). These patients require a spinal fusion procedure with curves exceeding 20°, those that are rapidly progressive, and those with rapidly deteriorating pulmonary function tests (functional vital capacity <35%) (**Fig. 2**).

Differential Diagnosis

Becker muscular dystrophy is a similar muscle wasting disorder that also presents with calf pseudohypertrophy, increased CPK level, and X-linked transmission. It carries a better prognosis with slower progression.

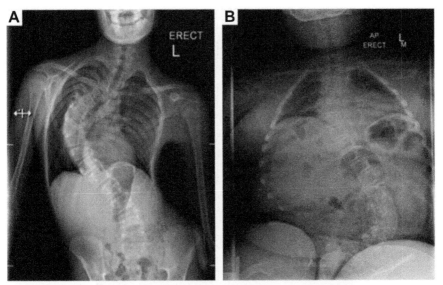

Fig. 1. The difference in curve pattern between that seen in adolescent idiopathic scoliosis and DMD scoliosis. (*A*) An anteroposterior radiograph of a patient with adolescent idiopathic scoliosis; (*B*) an anteroposterior radiograph of a patient with DMD with scoliosis showing the difference in curve pattern and location within the spine. (*From* Archer JE, Gardner AC, Roper HP, et al. Duchenne muscular dystrophy: the management of scoliosis. Journal of Spine Surgery [Online], 2.3 (2016): 185-194. Web. 2 Sep. 2019; with permission.)

MARFAN SYNDROME

Key Points

- Clinical suspicion is key to diagnosing Marfan syndrome.
- Manifestations are the result of defective elastin.
- Important to refer to orthopedics, cardiology, and ophthalmology.
- High prevalence of scoliosis and chest wall deformities.

Introduction

First described by French pediatrician Anton Marfan in 1896, the syndrome is characterized as a connective tissue disorder that can be associated with, among other things, tall stature. There is a prevalence of 1 in 5,000, with an equal distribution between gender and ethnicities. Inheritance of this syndrome is autosomal dominant, although there is an additional rate of spontaneous mutation identified as between 15% and 30%. Marfan is the result of a mutation of the *fibrillin-1* (*FBN1*) gene, located on chromosome 15 (locus CH 15q21), which is associated with elastin and is present in the aortic media, and suspensory ligaments of the lens, skin, tendon, cartilage, and periosteum.[3]

Presentation

Patients with Marfan have characteristic tall stature with lanky body type, although many patients have less florid manifestations, and thorough familiarity with the condition is necessary for appropriate diagnosis.

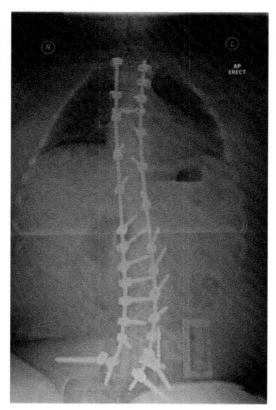

Fig. 2. A postoperative anteroposterior radiograph of the earlier patient with DMD after surgical instrumentation with fusion to the pelvis. The proximal extent of the instrumentation and fusion is T2; however, this patient had already lost the ability to self-feed. (*From* Archer JE, Gardner AC, Roper HP, et al. Duchenne muscular dystrophy: the management of scoliosis. Journal of Spine Surgery [Online], 2.3 (2016): 185-194. Web. 2 Sep. 2019; with permission.)

Physical examination findings include arm span greater than height (dolichostenomelia), long thin digits (arachnodactyly), chest wall deformity, myopia, and cardiac murmurs. These patients may show the thumb sign, in which, with the thumb clasped under the remaining digits in the palm, the thumb extends beyond the small digit. They may also present with the wrist sign, in which the distal phalanges of the thumb and small digits overlap when one hand is grabbing the opposite wrist (**Fig. 3**). Beyond the skeletal findings, these patients may also manifest with cardiac murmur related to dilatation of the ascending aorta or mitral valve insufficiency. In addition, the eyes must be closely evaluated for dislocated lens (ectopia lentis), which typically translates upward and laterally.[4]

Diagnosis

Despite identifying the defective gene in Marfan syndrome, the diagnosis of this condition is clinical, and many criteria systems have been refined for assistance in diagnosis. There are several major and minor criteria for Marfan syndrome. Patients with a definite family history or confirmed first-order relative with Marfan require 1 major

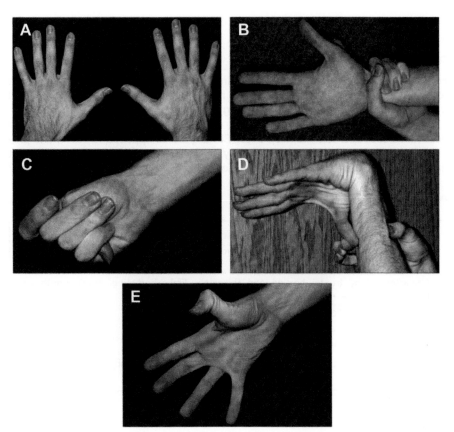

Fig. 3. Individuals with Marfan syndrome have characteristic arachnodactyly with joint hypermobility. (*A*) Long fingers. (*B*) Positive wrist sign (Walker sign). (*C*) Positive thumb sign (Steinberg sign). (*D, E*) Hypermobile joints. (*From* Adkinson, LR. Elsevier's Integrated Review Genetics, 2nd ed. Chapter 7; Philadelphia, PA: Elsevier; 2012; pp 114-132.)

criterion and involvement of a second organ system to complete diagnosis. For patients without a definite family history, major criteria in at least 2 different organ systems and involvement of a third are required to complete diagnosis.[4]

Orthopedic Manifestations

Scoliosis is often a presenting symptom of Marfan syndrome, and the incidence is 30% to 100%. For these patients, management is similar to idiopathic scoliosis, with bracing an option for curves between 25° and 45°. Importantly, before surgical intervention for scoliosis, MRI is advised to evaluate for the presence of dural ectasia, and these patients have an overall higher postoperative complication rate than those with idiopathic scoliosis.

Acetabular protrusion is another skeletal manifestation of Marfan syndrome, characterized by hip stiffness and pain clinically, as well as radiographic changes. Symptomatic patients may require surgical intervention with closure of the triradiate cartilage in patients from 8 to 10 years of age and should be referred appropriately.

Patients presenting with tall stature, flatfeet, joint instability, pectus excavatum, developmental dysplasia of the hip, or scoliosis should be carefully scrutinized for additional Marfan findings, and, if there is concern, consultation with cardiology and ophthalmology should be undergone.[3,4]

Differential Diagnosis

Homocystinuria is a metabolic disorder than can manifest clinically in a similar fashion to Marfan syndrome. These patients may have concomitant mental deficiency, and this diagnosis may be confirmed by testing the urine for excessive homocysteine.

Congenital contractual arachnodactyly, otherwise known as Beals syndrome, is associated with sporadic mutation of the FBN2 gene as opposed to FBN1, and presents with tall stature and arachnodactyly as well. These patients have joints that are stiff as opposed to lax, and problematic kyphoscoliosis as opposed to scoliosis.[3]

ACHONDROPLASIA

> **Key Points**
>
> - Autosomal dominant or spontaneous mutation of fibroblast growth factor receptor (FGFR) gene.
> - Characterized by frontal bossing and rhizomelic limb shortening. Trunk length and intelligence normal.
> - Genetic testing for FGFR gene mutation is diagnostic.
> - Sleep apnea, hypotonia, and hyperreflexia should alert the clinician to possible craniocervical stenosis.
> - Young achondroplastic children should be monitored for thoracolumbar kyphosis and spinal stenosis.

Introduction

The most common of conditions known as skeletal dysplasia, achondroplasia is a form of rhizomelic (proximal limb shortening) dwarfism. There is an incidence ranging between 1.3 per 100,000 to 1.5 per 10,000 live births. The inheritance is autosomal dominant and involves complete penetrance, although 90% of cases involve spontaneous mutation in the fibroblast growth factor receptor (*FGFR*) gene. Homozygous achondroplasia is typically fatal neonatally. The mutation involved is a glycine to arginine substitution encoding for FGFR-3 (chromosome 4p). This gain-of-function mutation increases inhibition of chondrocytes in the proliferative zone of the growth plate, resulting in deficient endochondral bone formation. As such, although the length of bones is shorter, bones that are formed through intramembranous ossification, such as the clavicles and skull, are normal, as is the width of the long bones.[5,6]

Presentation

The most striking finding in these patients is their short stature. As mentioned earlier, there is rhizomelic shortening of the extremities, such that the humerus is shorter than the forearm, and the femur shorter than the tibia. These patients retain a normal trunk length as well as normal intelligence.

Physical examination findings include frontal bossing, trident hands (**Fig. 4**) with fingers the same length and divergence of the ring and middle fingers, and possible excessive lordosis and thoracolumbar kyphosis, with an adult height of approximately 127 cm (50 inches).[6]

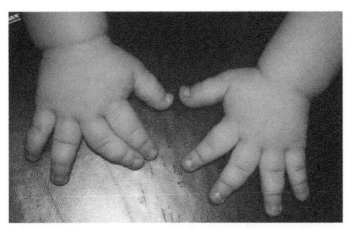

Fig. 4. Hands in achondroplasia, showing brachydactyly and (here, asymmetric) trident configuration: excess separation between the third and fourth fingers. (*From* Pauli, RM. Achondroplasia: a comprehensive clinical review. Orphanet J Rare Dis. 2019 Jan 3;14(1):1. https://doi.org/10.1186/s13023-018-0972-6; with permission.)

Diagnosis

There have been attempts at prenatal diagnosis of achondroplasia through the use of ultrasonography. When targeted at evaluation of femoral length for gestational age, sonographic diagnosis was accurate in 65% of fetuses, and, if the disorder is clinically more probable, confirmation of genetic testing for the FGFR gene can confirm the diagnosis.

Orthopedic Manifestations

Craniocervical stenosis is an important manifestation of achondroplasia, and is hypothesized to be one of the leading causes of mortality in up to 7.5% in the first year of life. Symptoms concerning for this condition include hypotonia and sleep apnea. Although decreased tone and developmental delay up to 6 months are common in achondroplasia, clonus and hyperreflexia are concerning findings that should prompt further work-up. Sleep apnea may be evaluated with sleep studies, and, if determined to be central sleep apnea caused by cervical compression, needs to be monitored closely at least. Patients with progressive symptoms require neurosurgical foramen magnum decompression. Radiographs, and MRI, are often necessary imaging modalities if there is concern.

Thoracolumbar kyphosis is typically seen in achondroplastic infants. This condition is theorized to stem from the larger head these children possess, as well as hypotonia. In greater than 90% of these patients, the kyphosis resolves as the child begins ambulation. In slightly older children, aged 3 to 5 years, with persistent thoracolumbar kyphosis there is a concern that the kyphosis may become progressive and, coupled with stenosis, may lead to neurologic complications. As such, in select patients in whom there is concern, bracing and potentially surgical intervention may be warranted.

Spinal stenosis is seen in nearly all achondroplastic patients secondary to anatomic changes in the bony architecture around the spinal cord. Not all patients are symptomatic, although presentation is typically around the third decade of life. Patients present with neurogenic claudication and, with persistent pain or progressive symptoms, may require advanced imaging and surgical intervention.[5,6]

MULTIPLE EPIPHYSEAL DYSPLASIA

Key Points

- Short-limbed skeletal dysplasia that may not be recognized at birth.
- Multiple inheritance patterns: autosomal dominant and autosomal recessive.
- May be mistaken on radiographs for Legg-Calvé-Perthes avascular necrosis. Key is symmetric involvement.
- Hip arthritis common in young adulthood.

Introduction

Multiple epiphyseal dysplasia (MED) is a form of dwarfism characterized by delayed appearance of the epiphysis, as well as symmetric irregular epiphyseal formation. There is a prevalence of 1 in 10,000 and it typically presents between the ages of 5 and 14 years. This condition is most commonly inherited in an autosomal dominant fashion when related to mutations in the cartilage oligomeric matrix protein (*COMP*) on chromosome 19 (the most common), mutations in type IX collagen (*COL9A1– 3*), and mutations in matrillin 3. However, this condition may also be inherited in autosomal recessive fashion with a mutation in the diastrophic dysplasia gene (*DTDST*).[6]

Presentation

These patients are difficult to recognize at birth. The diagnosis might not be made until early adolescence or when a delay in walking is perceived by the family. Symptoms at presentation may include joint stiffness or contractures, pain, or limp. These patients have normal intelligence, neurologic examination, and facies.

Physical examination findings include hip joint contractures, short and stubby fingers and toes, commonly with a normal spine and short limbs.[5]

Diagnosis

Typically made in early adolescence, this diagnosis is a combination of clinical and radiographic findings. Symmetric epiphyseal irregularity, primarily in the hips, is a common sign. Differential diagnosis includes Legg-Calvé-Perthes disease, which can mimic the hip pain and radiographic appearance of the femoral head. As previously stated, MED occurs symmetrically and synchronously in both hips, which sets it apart from the commonly unilateral and asynchronous symptoms in Legg-Calvé-Perthes. Hypothyroidism may cause similar radiographic findings, which can be distinguished with thyroid function tests. Spondyloepiphyseal dysplasia (SED) is distinguished from MED by involvement of the spine.

Orthopedic Manifestations

The primary symptom of MED is the bilateral hip deformity that is present in early childhood. Parents should be advised to work with the child on maintaining range of motion to prevent stiffness, as well to avoid weight gain as much as possible. Many of these patients develop osteoarthritis in their hips by 30 years of age and may require surgical intervention with progressive pain and disability.[5,6]

SPONDYLOEPIPHYSEAL DYSPLASIA

Key Points

- Involves both the epiphyses and spine.
- Characterized by short stature, short neck, waddling gait, short barreled chest, and protuberant abdomen.
- Monitor for atlantoaxial instability and basilar invagination.
- Frequently develop scoliosis and later arthritis in adulthood.

Introduction

There are 2 major forms of SED, a congenita type present at birth and a milder type that presents later in childhood. Both involve disproportionate dwarfism with involvement of the epiphyses, similar to MED, as well as involvement of the spine in contradistinction. The inheritance of this condition can be autosomal dominant, which is associated with SED congenita, and X-linked recessive (SED tarda). SED congenita is caused by a mutation in type II collagen gene (*COL2A1*), whereas the mutation in SED tarda is associated with the gene for the protein sedlin (*SEDL*).[5,6]

Presentation

These patients present with short stature associated with protuberant-appearing abdomen secondary to increased lumbar lordosis, and potentially waddling gait secondary to lower extremity contractures and deformity.

Physical examination findings include wide-set eyes, short neck, barrel-shaped chest, flattened facies, and decreased motion of the hips. Patients may also display cleft palate, myopia with retinal detachment, cataracts, and herniae, as well as, rarely, nephrotic syndrome.

Diagnosis

This condition, similar to MED, also involves a combination of clinical and radiographic findings. In addition to the clinical findings mentioned earlier, these patients may have delayed ossification of the femoral heads, the carpals, and tarsals radiographically. These patients require radiographs of the cervical spine to assess for atlantoaxial instability and other cervical anomalies. The appearance of the cervical spine can mimic that of Morquio and other mucopolysaccharidoses.

Orthopedic Manifestations

The spine, specifically the cervical spine, requires earliest treatment in these patients. Evidence of cervical instability includes hypotonia, sleep apnea, and respiratory problems, similar to achondroplastics. To prevent complications of this instability, flexion-extension radiographs of the cervical spine should be obtained before any anesthetic in patients with SED. These patients are likewise at risk for basilar invagination and malformation of the upper cervical vertebral bodies, which require surgical intervention. Additional spine involvement in these patients includes scoliosis and lumbar lordosis. Scoliosis is managed similar to idiopathic cases, whereas lumbar lordosis can be observed (**Fig. 5**).

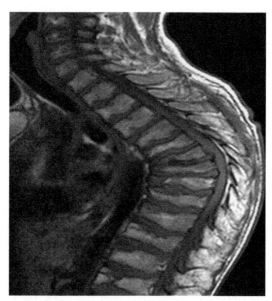

Fig. 5. Patient with spondyloepiphyseal dysplasia showing thoracic MRI of the patient with wedging, kyphosis, and disk herniations at T6YT9 causing spinal stenosis, cord compression, and myelomalacia. (*From* Yoleri O, Oz B, Olmez N, et al. Spondyloepiphyseal dysplasia tarda with progressive arthropathy complicated with paraplegia. Am J Phys Med Rehabil. 2011 Jun;90(6):490-4. https://doi.org/10.1097/PHM.0b013e3182063b01; with permission.)

Patients with SED may also have hip involvement, which manifests as deformity and pain. These symptoms should be monitored closely because they can progress to cause dislocation of the hip and may require surgical intervention. These patients may have activity-related joint pain and early-onset arthritis, similar to patients with MED.[5,6]

METAPHYSEAL CHONDRODYSPLASIAS
Introduction

This group of conditions is characterized by failure of normal bone mineralization. These patients therefore are short in stature and may have deformities of the limbs, although the epiphyses are unaffected, thus not predisposing these patients to arthritis. Jansen type is the most severe but rarest form, and is caused by a mutation of the parathyroid hormone (*PTH/PTHrP*) gene on chromosome 3. It is inherited in an autosomal dominant fashion. Schmid type is the most common form, and is also inherited in an autosomal dominant fashion via mutation of type X collagen (*COL10A1*). McKusick type is seen primarily in the Amish and Finnish, and results from an autosomal recessive mutation in the ribonuclease of mitochondrial RNA-processing (*RMRP*) gene on chromosome 9.[6]

Presentation

- Jansen-type metaphyseal chondrodysplasia is associated with mental deficiency, short-limbed dwarfism, wide-set eyes, and exophthalmos. These patients develop a monkeylike stance.
- Schmid type presents with short-limbed dwarfism, excessive lumbar lordosis, severe leg bowing, elbow contractures, and waddling gait.

- McKusick-type patients are shorter than Schmid type, and may develop ankle deformity; scoliosis; increased lumbar lordosis; and the distinguishing feature of fine, sparse, short, brittle hair.

Diagnosis

- Jansen type is typically diagnosed at birth clinically, with evaluation of the short stature, wide-set eyes, and exophthalmos. These patients also have severe hypercalcemia and hypophosphatemia despite normal or low levels of PTH, secondary to the mutation in the receptor.
- Schmid-type patients do not develop skeletal changes until weight bearing, at 3 to 5 years of age, when the lower extremity bowing becomes apparent. To formally diagnose Schmid-type dysplasia, nutritional and vitamin D–resistant rickets need to be ruled out with normal serum chemistry values.
- McKusick type can at times be mild at birth, causing a delay in diagnosis, and these patients require evaluation for immunologic deficiency and increased risk of malignancy.

Orthopedic Manifestations

- Jansen type primarily results in severe short stature and angular deformity of the limbs, which can primarily be managed conservatively except in severe progressive cases.
- Schmid type similarly manifests with lower extremity deformities of the knees and hips. Surgical intervention can more commonly be beneficial in these patients, with considerations for correcting the deformities through osteotomies versus growth modulation.
- McKusick-type management is directed at the ankle and the foot, with severe deformity necessitating surgical intervention to make a plantigrade foot.

MUCOPOLYSACCHARIDOSES
Introduction

This group of metabolic diseases is characterized by abnormal intracellular degradation of micromolecular compounds by lysosomal enzymes. Although there are 13 syndromes included in this category, the most common are discussed here. There is an incidence of 1 in 25,000 live births. Inheritance is typically in an autosomal recessive fashion, such as for Morquio, Hurler, and San Filippo syndromes. Hunter syndrome is the exception, with an X-linked inheritance.[6]

Presentation

- Morquio syndrome, which is associated with a mutation causing deficiency of either galactosamine-6-sulfate-sulphatase or beta-galactosidase, is characterized by normal intelligence, proportionate dwarfism, waddling gait, kyphosis, and corneal clouding (**Fig. 6**).
- Hurler syndrome is caused by deficiency of alpha-L-iduronidase, and although patients rarely live beyond the first decade of life, these patients may present with proportionate dwarfism, progressive mental deficiency, cloudy corneas (**Fig. 7**), and instability of the cervical spine.
- San Filippo syndrome is associated with multiple enzyme deficiencies, and patients accumulate heparan sulfate. These patients show mental deficiencies and proportionate dwarfism but, in contradistinction, have clear corneas.

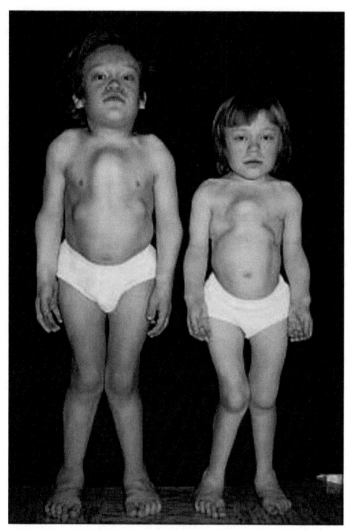

Fig. 6. Morquio disease in a brother and sister. Note the short trunk with pectus carinatum and knock-knees. (*From* Bukhari, MAS.. Mucopolysaccharidoses. In: Hochberg MC, Silman AJ, Smolen JS, et al. eds. Rheumatology (Sixth Edition), Philadelphia PA: Elsevier; 2015; with permission.)

- Hunter syndrome is caused by deficiency of sulphoiduronate sulfatase, leading to accumulation of dermatan and heparan sulfate. Similar to San Filippo syndrome, these patients are not expected to live beyond the second decade of life, have mental deficiencies, proportionate dwarfism, and clear corneas.

Diagnosis

For these lysosomal storage disorders, the diagnosis is suspected based on clinical and radiographic criteria. The definitive diagnosis is regularly delineated with urine studies, which show excess of keratan sulfate in Morquio, dermatan sulfate in Hurler and Hunter, and heparan sulfate in San Filippo or Hunter.

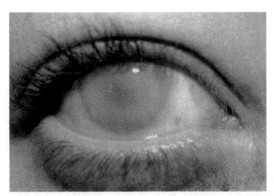

Fig. 7. Corneal clouding in a patient with Hurler syndrome. (*From* Ashworth JL, Biswas S, Wraith E, et al. Mucopolysaccharidoses and the eye. Surv Ophthalmol. 2006 Jan-Feb;51(1):1-17; with permission.)

Orthopedic Manifestations

All of the mucopolysaccharidoses have the potential to develop cervical instability, specifically atlantoaxial instability. This symptom is most pronounce in Morquio syndrome, with all patients affected. The first sign might not be evident until 4 to 6 years of age when patients complain of difficulty ambulating. Cervical radiographs aid in diagnosis, and progressive symptoms may require surgical intervention.

These patients commonly show kyphosis, as well as deformities of the lower extremity. Although bone marrow transplant has increased lifespan in patients with mucopolysaccharidosis, it has not been shown to affect the orthopedic complications.[5,6]

OSTEOGENESIS IMPERFECTA

Key Points

- Characterized by multiple fractures throughout childhood.
- Defect in type 1 collagen.
- May or may not present with characteristic blue sclera or dental problems.
- Should be considered when evaluating for nonaccidental trauma.
- Consider treatment with bisphosphonates.
- Monitor for basilar invagination.

Introduction

A condition characterized by brittle bones, osteogenesis imperfecta is a spectrum of disorders with varying degrees of disability. The prevalence ranges from 1 in 15,000 to 1 in 20,000 children, and it is typically caused by defects in collagen secretion and production. The inheritance can be either autosomal dominant or autosomal recessive for the most common types and is linked to the *COL1A1* and *COL1A2* genes. The milder forms, such as type I and IV, are autosomal dominant, with the more severe forms inherited in an autosomal recessive fashion (II and III). Type II is the most severe form, which is typically lethal in the perinatal period, and type III is the most severe survivable type.[7,8]

Presentation

These patients present with multiple fractures during childhood, even in mild cases, and in severe cases can have fractures at birth and even be fatal. The number and severity of fractures may be expected to decrease over time and after skeletal maturity.

Physical examination findings include bowing of the long bones, blue sclera, brownish teeth, and hearing loss. These patients may also develop mitral valve prolapse or aortic regurgitation. In the teenage years, patients may develop basilar invagination, which can present with apnea, altered consciousness, ataxia, or myelopathy.

It is important to include osteogenesis imperfecta in the differential diagnoses when a baby or child presents with multiple fractures in various stages of healing and nonaccidental trauma is under investigation (**Fig. 8**).

Diagnosis

Determined through family history and clinical and radiographic findings, this can be supplemented with evaluation of an increased alkaline phosphatase level, as well as skull radiographs to evaluate for wormian bones, fibroblast culturing, or biopsy.

Orthopedic Manifestations

The hallmark feature of patients with osteogenesis imperfecta is multiple fractures throughout childhood. These patients and their families should be counseled appropriately about lifestyle modifications to limit the risk for fracture. Patients should be started on bisphosphonates and early bracing to attempt to avoid limb deformities. With excessive deformity of the long bones, patients may require realignment procedures.

Scoliosis is also a frequent orthopedic complication in these patients. Bracing is typically ineffective and is not well tolerated because of the soft ribs and bones these patients have. In severe cases of osteogenesis imperfecta, scoliosis should be corrected at a lower degree of angulation.

Basilar invagination is a serious complication of osteogenesis imperfect and should be suspected with myelopathic findings on examination, as mentioned earlier. These patients require surgical intervention.[7,8]

DOWN SYNDROME

Key Points

- Orthopedic manifestations mostly result from ligamentous laxity.
- Atlantoaxial instability is common and should be considered when neurologic changes are present. Careful radiological screening is important when considering sports participation.
- Hip and patella instability are common.
- Scoliosis and slipped capital femoral epiphysis are more common than in the general population.

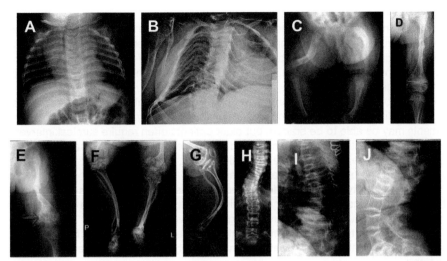

Fig. 8. Various skeletal manifestations of Osteogenesis Imperfecta. (*A*) Multiple rib fractures in various stages of healing. (*B*) Scoliosis. (*C*) Severe leg bowing from multiple fractures. (*D–G*) Thin tubular shafts of long bones with osteopenia. (*H–J*) Spinal deformity with 'codfish' vertebrae. (*From* Hrušková L, Mazura I, Marik I et al. COL1A2 gene analysis in a Czech osteogenesis imperfecta patient: a candidate novel mutation in a patient affected by osteogenesis imperfecta type 3. Advances in Genomics and Genetics. 2015. 275. 10.2147/AGG.S58766; with permission.)

Introduction

Down syndrome is the most common chromosomal abnormality in the United States, affecting 1 in 700 live births. Risk factors include advanced maternal age, with the incidence increasing to 1 in 250 births for women more than 35 years of age. It is caused by a maternal duplication of chromosome 21, which codes for type VI collagen (*COL6A1, COL6A2*).[3,4]

Presentation

These patients have involvement of several organ systems, causing manifestations such as mental delay, cardiac disease, endocrine disorders, duodenal atresia, Alzheimer disease, and premature aging.

Physical examination findings include flattened facies; epicanthal folds; single palmar crease, known as simian crease; ligamentous laxity, which can affect joints as well as cervical spine; scoliosis; and hearing loss.

Diagnosis

Prenatal screening is available for Downs syndrome, and can be evaluated by measuring the alpha-fetoprotein concentration during the second trimester, which are lower than in a pregnancy for an unaffected baby. In addition, the unconjugated estriol level is decreased, human chorionic gonadotropin level is increased, and serum inhibin A levels are increased. Ultrasonography can also be an important tool for noninvasive screening. Ultimately, amniocentesis and chromosome analysis are diagnostic in at-risk mothers.

Orthopedic Manifestations

These patients have generalized ligamentous laxity, and the most profound region affected is the cervical spine. Hypermobility of the cervical spine can cause significant complications, and, because these patients are hypermobile at baseline, they must be carefully scrutinized before any high-impact activity. At present, Special Olympics athletes are required to obtain flexion-extension radiographs of the cervical spine before participation in any at-risk event. With progressive symptoms and pain, patients may require surgical intervention.[3]

Hip instability is another common complication in patients with Down syndrome. This instability is secondary to the overall ligamentous laxity and hypotonia. Younger patients may be able to be braced, but older patients often require surgical intervention. These patients are also at increased risk of developing slipped capital femoral epiphysis because of endocrine abnormalities, and, if affected, should undergo prophylactic pinning of the contralateral hip as well.

Patellar instability commonly affects these patients, and, again, this is secondary to the generalized ligamentous laxity they display. Younger patients with symptomatic instability may require bracing versus surgical intervention.

Several different foot conditions may affect these patients, ranging from clubfoot to flatfoot, and should be treated conservatively with orthotics as symptoms demand.

NEUROFIBROMATOSIS

Key Points

- Scoliosis is common and requires MRI to evaluate for intraspinal abnormalities such as dural ectasia.
- Fibromas should be monitored and carry a risk of malignant transformation.

Introduction

There are 2 types of neurofibromatosis (NF), which is a hamartomatous disorder affecting multiple organ systems. Type 1 (von Recklinghausen disease) is caused by a mutation responsible for neurofibromin, a regulator of the Ras pathway (*NF1* gene on chromosome 17). It is also the most common genetic disorder caused by a new mutation of a single gene, occurring in 1 in 3000 births. NF2 (bilateral acoustic neurofibromatosis) is caused by a mutation on chromosome 22, and rarely causes orthopedic manifestations.[3,4]

Presentation

Often, the first presentation for patients with NF1 is associated with deformity of the tibia, commonly found to be bowing in an anterolateral direction. These patients may also present with bowing of the radius in similar fashion, although this is less commonly.

Physical examination findings include verrucous hyperplasia, hemihypertrophy, café-au-lait spots with a coast-of-California border, axillary freckling, scoliosis, and Lisch nodules of the iris.

Diagnosis

The National Institutes of Health (NIH) has developed guidelines for diagnosing patients with NF1:

Two or more of the following criteria are sufficient for diagnosis[3,4]:
- Six or more café-au-lait spots at least 15 mm diameter in adults, 5 mm in children

- Two or more neurofibromas or 1 plexiform neurofibroma
- Freckling in the axillary or inguinal region
- Optic glioma
- Two or more Lisch nodules (iris hamartomas)
- A distinctive osseous lesion such as sphenoid dysplasia or thinning of the cortex of a long bone, with or without pseudoarthrosis
- A first-degree relative (parent, sibling, or offspring) with NF1 by these criteria

Orthopedic Manifestations

The spine is the most common location of orthopedic involvement in patients with NF1. They typically develop scoliosis, which can affect the thoracic spine and can present as an abrupt curve over few vertebral segments. Because of the potential for intradural abnormalities in these patients, closer observation is required versus idiopathic patients, and advanced imaging is almost always a necessity.

As mentioned earlier, these patients develop deformity about the tibia, which begins as a bow in the anterolateral direction. This deformity may subsequently require bracing, and, if patients develop progressive bowing with nonhealing fracture, may require surgical intervention (**Fig. 9**).

Although rare, patients with NF1 may develop hemihypertrophy of 1 extremity, typically unilateral. This hemihypertrophy is theorized to stem from neurosegmental overgrowth, although it affects the soft tissues and bones. No surgical cure-all has been elucidated for this condition at this time, although attempts to diminish the growth of the larger limb via epiphysiodesis and debulking have been described.

The neurofibromas that are a hallmark of this condition have a risk of malignant transformation, especially as these patients age. Careful monitoring of the growth of the fibromas, as well as screening examinations, are important.

EHLERS-DANLOS SYNDROME

Key Points

- Spectrum of disorders with varying severity and inheritance patterns.
- Patients are at increased risk for chronic joint instability, especially in the shoulders and patellae.

Introduction

Characterized by hyperelastic skin, joint hypermobility, and ligamentous laxity, Ehlers-Danlos syndrome (EDS) describes a group of inherited disorders of connective tissue. Classic EDS involves a mutation in the gene for type V collagen (*COL5A1* and *COL5A2*) and is inherited in an autosomal dominant fashion. Variations of the classic-type EDS have been shown to be inherited in an autosomal recessive manner as well, and to affect similar collagen-forming genes. Furthermore, there are many children with joint hypermobility that do not meet specific criteria for the described forms of EDS who, nevertheless, have similar presentation.[3,4]

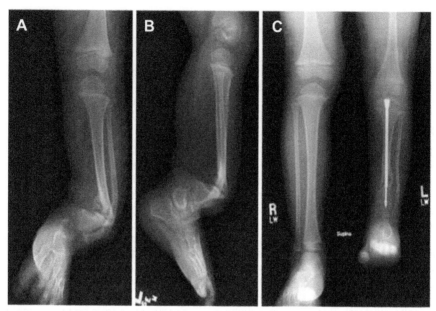

Fig. 9. Anterolateral tibia bowing with pseudoarthroses in a patient with neurofibromatosis. (*A*) Anteroposterior, (*B*) lateral, (*C*) postsurgical anteroposterior radiographs. (*From Wallace M.. Pseudarthrosis of the Tibia. In: Eltorai A, Eberson C, Daniels A. (eds) Orthopedic Surgery Clerkship. Springer International Publishing: Switzerland; 2017; with permission.*)

Presentation

Patients with EDS experience generalized laxity and joint hypermobility, stretchy and easily bruised skin, poor wound healing, and joint issues.

Diagnosis

The Beighton-Horan scale is a point-based system identifying joint hypermobility, with a score of 5 out of 9 defining joint hypermobility[3]:

- Passive hyperextension of each small finger greater than 90° (+1 point each)
- Passive abduction of each thumb to the surface of the forearm (+1 point each)
- Hyperextension of each knee greater than 10° (+1 point each)
- Hyperextension of each elbow greater than 10° (+1 point each)
- Forward flexion of trunk with palms on floor and knees fully extended (+1 point)

Orthopedic Manifestations

Most commonly in patients with EDS, as mentioned earlier, there is generalized ligamentous laxity and joint hypermobility, which causes hyperextensibility of all joints, sometimes to extreme positions and to dislocation. This mobility becomes associated with significant joint pain, and may lead to chronic joint dislocations in the shoulder and patella. These patients may also develop pseudotumors in sites of friction, such as the elbows and knees.

Skin complications are also seen in patients with EDS, with patients having easily bruised skin that might remain discolored and may develop wound healing issues with trauma or surgical intervention.

RICKETS

Key Points

- Rickets is characterized by long-bone bowing and characteristic physeal irregularity on radiographs.
- Serum and urine laboratory tests are required to characterize the specific defect.
- Orthopedic manifestations are often corrected by correcting the underlying metabolic disorder.

Introduction

Rickets is a condition defined by a defect in the mineralization of osteoid matrix, which leads to poor calcification of bones and overall calcium homoeostasis. There are multiple different forms of rickets, including nutritional (vitamin D deficient), familial hypophosphatemic (vitamin D resistant), vitamin D dependent (type I and II), hypophosphatasia, and renal osteodystrophy. Familial hypophosphatemia is inherited in an X-linked dominant fashion, the vitamin D–dependent type and hypophosphatasia are inherited in autosomal recessive fashion, and renal osteodystrophy is associated with kidney dysfunction.[7,8]

Presentation

These patients develop brittle bones that potentially show bowing, ligamentous laxity, flattening of the skull, enlargement of the costal cartilage (otherwise known as rachitic rosary), and kyphosis (known as cat back).

Diagnosis

Nutritional rickets, associated with poor nutrition and decreased intake of vitamin D, is still seen in premature infants, African American children older than 6 months who are still breastfed, patients with malabsorption, and immigrants, despite vitamin D being added to supplement milk. The absence of vitamin D leads to decreased calcium absorption, increased parathyroid hormone (PTH) level, and subsequent bone resorption. These patients have low to normal serum calcium, low serum phosphate, increased alkaline phosphatase, increased PTH, and low vitamin D levels.

Familial hypophosphatemic rickets, which is vitamin D resistant secondary to an impaired response to vitamin D_3, is X-linked dominant and can be associated with tibial bowing. It is caused by inability of renal tubules to absorb phosphate and as such has phosphate wasting. Laboratory findings include low serum phosphorus, increased alkaline phosphatase, and normal or low serum calcium levels.

Hereditary vitamin D–dependent rickets can be stratified into type I and type II, of which type II is more severe. Type I is caused by inability to convert vitamin D to its active form, and type II is caused by a defect in the intracellular receptor for activated vitamin D. Presentation for both conditions is similar to nutritional rickets, and laboratory values follow the same pattern. The distinguishing laboratory value in type II is a markedly increased activated vitamin D level.

Hypophosphatasia is caused by a mutation in alkaline phosphatase (*TNSALP*), and the laboratory values include increased calcium, increased phosphorus, and

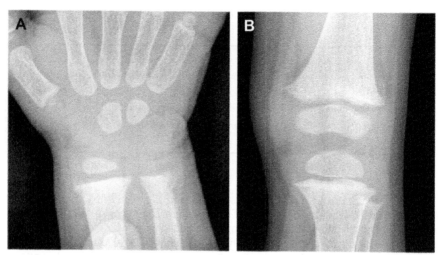

Fig. 10. Vitamin D deficiency rickets in a child ages 1 year 10 months. Rachitic findings include physeal widening and irregularity of the wrist (*A*) and knee (*B*). (*From* Shore RM, Chesney RW. Rickets: Part II. Pediatr Radiol. 2013 Jan;43(2):152-72. https://doi.org/10.1007/s00247-012-2536-6. Epub 2012 Nov 21; with permission.)

significantly decreased alkaline phosphatase levels. In addition, discovery of phosphoethanolamine in the urine is diagnostic for hypophosphatasia.[7,8]

Orthopedic Manifestations

Lower limb deformity, such as bowing, is a common finding in all patients with rickets (**Fig. 10**). This deformity is related to the lower quality of the bone, and as such can at times respond to appropriate medical management. Severe or progressive deformities may require surgical intervention.

Pathologic fractures are another typical complication from rickets. These fractures must be treated appropriately for the specific fracture type, and, again, investigation into the nature of the defect in bone health is essential for timely healing and prevention of future fractures.

REFERENCES

1. Mendell J, Shilling C, Leslie N, et al. Evidence-based path to newborn screening for duchenne muscular dystrophy. Ann Neurol 2012;71(3):304–13.

2. Shieh P. Muscular dystrophies and other genetic myopathies. Neurol Clin 2013; 31(4):1009–29.

3. Herring J. Orthopaedic-related syndromes. In: Tachdjians pediatric orthopedics. 4th edition. Philadelphia: Saunders; 2008. p. 1795–916.

4. Alman B, Goldberg M. Syndromes of orthopaedic importance. In: Flynn J, Weinstein S, editors. Lovell and Winter's pediatric orthopaedics. 7th edition. Philadelphia: Lippincott Williams & Wilkins; 2014. p. 218–77.

5. Sponseller P, Ain M. The skeletal dysplasias. In: Flynn J, Weinstein S, editors. Lovell and Winter's pediatric orthopedics. 7th edition. Philadelphia: Lippincott Williams & Wilkins; 2014. p. 177–217.

6. Herring J. Skeletal dysplasias. In: Tachdjian's pediatric orthopaedics. 4th edition. Philadelphia: Saunders; 2008. p. 1677–794.
7. Howard A, Alman B. Metabolic and endocrine abnormalities. In: Flynn J, Weinstein S, editors. Lovell and Winter's pediatric orthopaedics. 7th edition. Philadelphia: Lippincott Williams & Wilkins; 2014. p. 140–76.
8. Herring J. Metabolic and endocrine bone diseases. In: Tachdjians pediatric orthopedics. 4th edition. Philadelphia: Saunders; 2008. p. 1917–82.

Pediatric Neuromuscular Disorders

Christopher Michel, MD[a], Christopher Collins, MD[b],*

KEYWORDS

- Pediatric neuromuscular disorders • Cerebral palsy • Duchenne muscular dystrophy
- Meningocele • Myelomeningocele • Friedreich ataxia • Spinal muscular atrophy
- Marfan syndrome

KEY POINTS

- Neuromuscular disorders are pathologies that can severely affect the quality of life as well as longevity of patients.
- The most common disorders include cerebral palsy and myelodysplasia.
- The orthopedic manifestations of these disorders can be treated operatively or nonoperatively. Both focus on the prolongation of mobility and preservation of ambulatory capacity for patients.

INTRODUCTION

Neuromuscular disorders are diseases that affect the development and growth of the neuromuscular system in children. The pathology can present anywhere along the neuromuscular pathway, from the brain to the nerves to the muscle fibers. These diseases have a profound impact on the quality of life of not only the children but their families. Although there is a multitude of neuromuscular disorders recognized, this article highlights some common disorders with orthopedic manifestations.

CEREBRAL PALSY

Cerebral palsy (CP) is defined as a nonprogressive upper motor neuron disease due to injury of the immature brain. This is also known as a static encephalopathy. The affected portion of the musculoskeletal system, however, changes with growth. Upper motor neuron lesions, seen by periventricular leukomalacia on magnetic resonance imaging (MRI), result in weakness and spasticity. By definition, the onset must be before the first 2 years of life and it is the most common cause of chronic childhood disability.

[a] Monmouth Medical Center, 300 2nd Avenue, Long Branch, NJ 07740, USA; [b] Seaview Orthopaedic & Medical Associates, 1200 Eagle Avenue, Ocean, NJ 07712, USA
* Corresponding author.
E-mail address: collinch5765@gmail.com

Pediatr Clin N Am 67 (2020) 45–57
https://doi.org/10.1016/j.pcl.2019.09.002
0031-3955/20/© 2019 Elsevier Inc. All rights reserved.

CP leads to muscle imbalance in patients with a mixture of weakness and spasticity. Risk factors for CP include prematurity (<32 weeks' gestation) anoxic injuries, perinatal infections, meningitis, chorioamnionitis, placental bleeding, hypotension hypoxia, multiple pregnancies, and brain malformations.[1]

Orthopedic manifestations of CP include

- Abnormal tone
- Loss of motor control
- Spasticity
- Hypotonia
- Chore and athetosis

Secondary orthopedic manifestations related to growth and spasticity are

- Contractures
- Upper extremity deformities
- Hip subluxation and dislocation
- Foot deformities
- Gait disorders
- Fractures[2]

Classification of CP is done using the gross motor function classification scale (**Table 1**).

There are many different classification schemes for CP—some orthopedic generalizations regarding common classifications follow. Spastic CP is the most common and typical features include hyperreflexia, clonus, and velocity-dependent resistance to passive joint motion.[2] Hemiplegic CP manifests as upper and lower extremities on a single side affected. These children typically are able to ambulate. Diplegia CP typically has features of the lower extremities being affected more than the upper extremities. Most are able to ambulate. Quadriplegic CP patients have significant deficits and usually are unable to ambulate (**Fig. 1**).

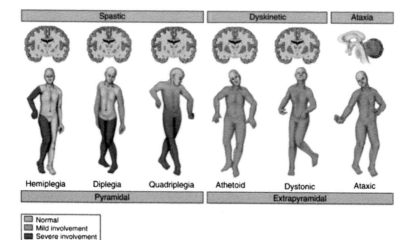

Fig. 1. Types of cerebral palsy with brain damage location. (*From* Pellegrino L. Cerebral palsy. In Batshaw ML, editor: Children with Disabilities, 4e. Baltimore, Maryland: Brookes Publishing; 1997; with permission.)

Table 1
Gross motor function classification scale

Level I	Near-normal gross motor function; independent ambulator
Level II	Walks independently but difficulty with uneven surfaces; minimal ability to jump
Level III	Walks with assistive devices
Level IV	Severely limited walking ability; primary mobility is wheelchair
Level V	Nonambulator with global involvement; dependent in all aspects of care

Data from Morris C. Definition and classification of cerebral palsy: a historical perspective. Dev Med Child Neurol Suppl. [Historical Article]. 2007 Feb;109:3-7.

Pertinent parts of the history include the mother's perinatal history and prior medical treatments as well as the patient's functional status and communication skills. Physical examination of patients with CP should include a general musculoskeletal examination to assess tone, range of motion, and gait, if possible. Carefully examine the patient's spine, checking for the presence and flexibility of scoliosis, spinal balance, shoulder height, pelvic obliquity, and resting head posture. Assess the patient's hips to check for contractures (typically flexion or adduction). It also is important to check leg length in sitting or supine position due to hip instability and dislocations being common in this patient population. Lastly, observe wear patterns of the foot and ankle and check for pressure points if the patient is immobile.[1]

Imaging of these patients should include anteroposterior (AP) and lateral radiographs of the hips as well as standing spine radiographs. In addition, brain MRI can be useful in diagnosis (**Fig. 2**).

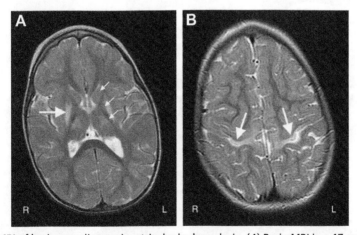

Fig. 2. MRI of brain revealing periventricular leukomalacia. (*A*) Brain MRI in a 17-month-old boy with history of hypoxic encephalopathy. Axial T2-weighted image demonstrates bilateral, symmetric signal abnormality and mild volume loss affecting the thalami (*arrows*). The basal ganglia are spared. (*B*) Brain MRI in a 3-year-old boy with right-sided seizures and right hemiplegia. Axial T2-weighted image demonstrates areas of cystic encephalomalacia in the left frontal and parieto-occipital regions due to parasagittal watershed infarcts (*arrows*) and ex vacuo ventricular dilatation, left thalamic gliosis, and volume loss (*arrow*). (*From* Reid SM, Dagia CD, Ditchfield MR. Grey matter injury patterns in cerebral palsy: associations between structural involvement on MRI and clinical outcomes. Dev Med Child Neurol. 2015 Dec;57(12):1159-67. https://doi.org/10.1111/dmcn.12800. Epub 2015 May 12; with permission.)

Associated conditions may include mental impairment, seizures, movement disorders, visual impairment, malnutrition, and hydrocephalus. If by 2 years of age there is the presence of 2 or more primitive reflexes or there is a lack of sitting balance, this predicts for a child to be a nonambulator.[1] Neuromuscular scoliosis is common in children with CP. The highest risk is recognized in children with spastic quadriplegia. One of the most significant and common disorders with CP is hip subluxation and dislocation.

Conservative treatment of patients with CP focuses on nonoperative management and is aimed at controlling spasticity. The treatment regimen typically includes physical therapy, bracing or orthotics, and medications to treat spasticity, including Botox or baclofen. Operative treatment may include soft tissue releases, such as tenotomies or tendon transfers (**Fig. 3**), selective dorsal rhizotomy to remove dorsal nerve rootlets that do not show a response to stimulation, and bone deformity correction to treat static contractures and progressive joint breakdown. The main goal of surgical intervention is to preserve painless function.[2]

MYELODYSPLASIA (MYELOMENINGOCELE AND SPINA BIFIDA)

Myelodysplasia is a group of congenital abnormalities secondary to the failure of fusion of neural folds during neurulation—the fetal spinal cord fails to completely close. Risk factors include folate deficiency in pregnancy as well as maternal diabetes,

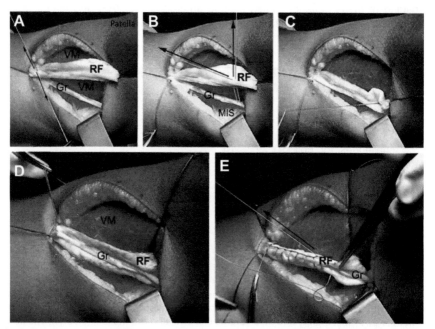

Fig. 3. Example of rectus femoris transfer for quadriceps out-of-phase firing. Transferring a portion of the rectus femurs (RF) to the Gracilis hamstring tendon (Gr) to improve knee function. (*A–E*) Anteromedial aspect of knee. MIS, medial intermuscular septum, VM, vastus medialis. (*From* Khouri N, Desailly E. Rectus femoris transfer in multilevel surgery: technical details and gait outcome assessment in cerebral palsy patients. Orthop Traumatol Surg Res. 2013 May;99(3):333-40. https://doi.org/10.1016/j.otsr.2012.10.017. Epub 2013 Mar 21; with permission.)

use of valproic acid during pregnancy, and maternal hyperthermia.[3] Forms of myelo-dysplasia include spina bifida occulta, which is a defect in the vertebral arch with a confined spinal cord and meninges; meningocele, where the sac protrudes without neural components; and myelomeningocele, where the sac protrudes with neural components. Diagnosis can be aided with evaluation of α-fetoprotein, which is elevated in up to 75% of patients with myelodysplasia in the second trimester.[4]

There are a multitude of orthopedic manifestations when considering a child with myelodysplasia. Spina bifida occulta typically has no symptoms or long-term effects. Other, more severe forms of myelodysplasia may have orthopedic manifestations, including pathologic fractures due to osteopenia, neuromuscular scoliosis, congenital kyphosis, hip dislocations and contractures, knee contractures, rotational deformities of the tibia, and club feet. Additionally, neurologic complications may have eventual orthopedic manifestations, including hydrocephalus, syrinx, Arnold-Chiari malformation, tethered spinal cord, and hydromyelia.[5]

Some basic orthopedic generalizations when treating children with myelodysplasia are well understood and have implications later in life. For instance, when categorizing myelodysplasia, the lowest functional level is of importance. This can be used to guide treatment in the future—L4 level allows for functioning quadriceps, which portends the ability for independent ambulation. All patients with myelodysplasia should treated as if they have latex allergy, which is IgE mediated and particularly common. There is also a higher postoperative infection rate recognized in children with myelo-dysplasia—noted to be as high as 25% of postoperative children with myelodyspla-sia (**Table 2**).[4]

It has been recognized early in the orthopedic evaluation for children with myelodys-plasia that ambulation can be predicted by the age of 2 years. If a child is not commu-nity ambulatory by the age of 6 years, it is often unlikely the child will reach that goal.[4]

Some areas requiring close monitoring by an orthopedic surgeon for patients with myelodysplasia include the hip and spine. There are many potential issues beyond the scope of this article; however, hip and spine potential deformities should be mentioned. Conservative measures, including brace wear, physical therapy, and, at times, medication, are all conservative treatments that are typically exhausted before surgical intervention is contemplated.

Hip challenges for children with spina bifida often are dictated by the level affected. Hip flexion contractures are common, in particular, for patients with thoracic and high lumbar levels affected. This is secondary to unopposed hip flexors and adductors. Hip flexion contractures may lead to hip flexion and adduc-tion deformities. When conservative measures fail, tenotomies or tendon lengthen-ings are used. The goal is to maintain a concentric, painless hip. This preserves and maintains the ability to sit comfortably and preserves the ability to ambulate. Indeed, 50% of children show hip subluxation or frank dislocation in the first 10 years of life. If ambulation is achieved, preservation of hip congruency is partic-ularly important. Hip and pelvic osteotomies (reshaping the proximal femur and pelvis) may be required in addition to soft tissue procedures, such as tendon lengthenings.[5]

Spinal deformity is also common with patients with myelodysplasia. This deformity can be severe and progressive and also depend heavily on the myelodysplasia level. Indeed, 90% of children with an L1 level or higher develop scoliosis. Tethered cord and hydrocephalus are features of myelodysplasia that show rapid progression. Any child with myelodysplasia that has been diagnosed with scoliosis with a Cobb angle greater than 25° is typically fitted for an orthosis in an attempt to limit progression. In cases in which scoliosis is progressive, surgical fixation that typically extends

Table 2
Expected functional levels depending on most distal functional motor level with corresponding mobility predictions

Functional Motor Level	Expected Muscle Function	Functional Mobility	Equipment Use	Orthotic Use
Thoracic	Abdominals, paraspinals, quadratus lumborum	Nonfunctional ambulation/standing during therapy, school or at home, wheelchair for mobility	Standing frame, wheelchair, parapodium	Trunk–hip–knee–ankle–foot orthosis
High lumbar L1-L3	Hip flexion, hip adduction	Limited household ambulation, wheelchair for mobility	Wheelchair, walker, forearm crutches	Reciprocating gait orthosis, hip-knee–ankle–foot orthosis
Midlumbar L3-L4	Knee extension	Household, limited community ambulation	Wheelchair, walker, forearm crutches	Knee–ankle–foot orthosis
Low lumbar L4-L5	Hip abduction, knee flexion, ankle dorsiflexion, ankle inversion, toe extension	Household, community ambulation, wheelchair for long distances	Wheelchair, forearm crutches	Ankle-foot orthosis
Sacral S1S2	Hip extension, ankle plantar flexion, ankle eversion, toe flexion	Community ambulation	—	Supramalleolar-foot orthosis, foot orthotic

(*From* Apkon SD, Grady R, Hart S. Advances in the care of children with spina bifida. Adv Pediatr. 2014 Aug;61(1):33-74. https://doi.org/10.1016/j.yapd.2014.03.007; with permission.)

down to the pelvis is required. With current surgical techniques, this can be achieved with posterior spinal fusion and instrumentation. There are higher rates of postoperative infection and pseudoarthrosis for patients with myelodysplasia.[6]

SACRAL AGENESIS

Sacral agenesis is characterized by partial or complete absence of the sacrum and/or the lower lumbar spine. This condition is highly associated with maternal diabetes. One of the differing features of sacral genesis and myelodysplasia is the preservation of sensation distal to the affected levels.

The classic physical examination findings are buttock dimpling, postural abnormalities, and multiple joint contractures. There often are a multitude of associated conditions, including imperforate anus, advanced kyphosis, and genitourinary and cardiovascular abnormalities.

Children may improve with physical therapy. A majority of patients respond well to conservative measures and typically become community ambulators. Ambulation is aided by addressing lower extremity deformities and may improve significantly with amputations of nonfunctional extremities and fitting for prostheses. Similar to myelodysplasia, patients with sacral agencies often require spinal stabilization procedures for progressive scoliosis.[5]

FRIEDREICH ATAXIA

Friedreich ataxia is the most common form of spinocerebellar degenerative diseases and is characterized by lesions in the dorsal root ganglia, corticospinal tracts, the cerebellum, and the peripheral sensory nerves. It is autosomal recessive secondary to an unstable trinucleotide repeat. This results in a defect in frataxin. Associated orthopedic conditions include gait abnormalities, a pes cavovarus foot, and scoliosis. Symptoms are staggering wide-based gait with the classic triad being ataxia, areflexia, and positive plantar response (Babinski reflex).[3]

Often recognized is an unstable gait (from imbalance not weakness), dysarthria, and cardiomyopathy. First to be affected are hip extensors and abductors that result in the common waddling gait. Cavovarus foot can be treated operatively and typically is treated only nonoperatively in a patient who is not ambulatory. Scoliosis is recognized in nearly all patients and is treated with posterior spinal fusion with instrumentation if the Cobb angle is greater than 40°.[3] Death may be common in the fourth or fifth decade of life and usually is associated with cardiomyopathy, pneumonia, or pulmonary compromise secondary to aspiration.

SPINAL MUSCULAR ATROPHY

Spinal muscular atrophy (SMA) is a disease of progressive motor weakness secondary to progressive loss of motor neurons in the anterior horn of the spinal cord. It has been associated with a defect in the survival motor neuron gene.

Type I SMA, Werdnig-Hoffmann, is the most severe. Patients affected typically never sit without support. Type II SMA is intermediate. Patients typically survive until the fourth to fifth decades. It is associated with proximal muscular weakness, tongue fasciculations, and hip subluxation/dislocations. Patients are able to sit unassisted but rarely have the ability to ambulate. Scoliosis is extremely common and early surgical stabilization is recommended to maintain forced vital capacity on pulmonary function testing.[7] Type III SMA, Kugelberg-Welander, is milder and patients have normal life expectancies. Waddling gaits are common secondary to proximal muscle weakness. Scoliosis typically is less severe and managed conservatively with physical therapy and brace wear.[8]

Symptoms include symmetric progressive weakness that is typically more pronounced in the lower extremity and proximally than upper extremity and distally. Patients with SMA often have absent deep tendon reflexes.[9]

ARTHROGRYPOSIS

Arthrogryposis is a nonprogressive congenital disorder involving multiple rigid joints (usually symmetric), leading to severe limitation in motion. Contractures are due to immobilization in utero and are 90% neurogenic, with 10% being myopathic. Joint contractors are due to limitation of intrauterine movement and may improve with age; 25% of children with arthrogryposis may sustain birth fractures.[10] On birth, a lack of normal joint skin creases is evident (**Fig. 4**). Patients with arthrogryposis have normal intelligence.

Arthrogryposis may be myopathic, neuropathic, or mixed. Common types of arthrogryposis include arthrogryposis multiplex congenita, distal arthrogryposis syndrome (autosomal dominant), Larsen syndrome, and multiple pterygium syndrome (autosomal recessive).

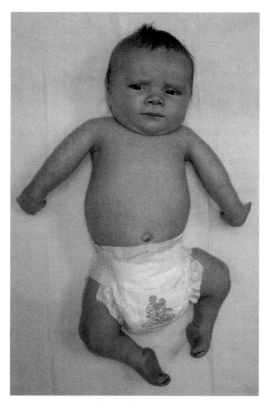

Fig. 4. Child with arthrogryposis. Note lack of flexion creases. (*From* Bamshad M, Van Heest AE, Pleasure D.Arthrogryposis: a review and update. J Bone Joint Surg Am. 2009 Jul;91 Suppl 4:40-6. https://doi.org/10.2106/JBJS.I.00281; with permission.)

Associated orthopedic conditions include upper extremity deformities, hip subluxation and dislocation, knee contractures, scoliosis, and club feet. Indeed, 90% of children with arthrogryposis are diagnosed with club foot,[10] a majority of which require surgical intervention to achieve a plantigrade foot to include a posteromedial release with or without talectomy. Patients with arthrogryposis typically have a teratologic hip dislocation. Treatment with a Pavlik harness is contraindicated in such patients. Surgical intervention with soft tissue releases, open reduction, and possible osteotomies typically are required to address such hip dislocations.

On physical examination, patients with arthrogryposis have their shoulders adducted and internally rotated with elbows extended, wrists flexed and ulnarly deviated, and with their thumb adducted. In addition, their hips are flexed, abducted, and externally rotated. Treatment of the upper extremity deformity is passive manipulation with serial casting or soft tissue releases, tendon transfers, and osteotomies.

MARFAN SYNDROME

Marfan syndrome is a connective tissue disorder in which patients have long limbs, cardiac abnormalities including aortic root dilatation and mitral valve prolapse, and ocular abnormalities with superior lens dislocations and potential for spontaneous pneumothorax in addition to orthopedic manifestations. These manifestations include arachnodactyly, scoliosis (50%), ligamentous laxity, protrusion acetabuli, meningocele, recurrent dislocations, pectus excavatum, and carinum.[5]

Marfan syndrome is autosomal dominant with multiple genetic mutations identified. The primary genetic aberration is of the fibrillin-1 gene located on chromosome 15. There is no gender or ethnic predilection appreciated and an incidence of 1:10,000 births. Patients may present with a history of multiple ankle sprains, patella dislocations, and scoliosis. It is typical to identify particular features on physical examination to include a positive thumb sign, arachnodactyly (long slender fingers and toes), dolichostenomelia (patient arm span is greater than height), significant per planovalgus (flat feet), and scoliosis (**Fig. 5**).[11]

As in most conditions and as a standalone diagnosis, scoliosis can be treated nonoperatively with bracing or operatively with spinal fusion. The joint laxity seen in these patients can be treated with observation and orthotics. Importantly, recognition of the nonorthopedic manifestations is paramount when treating patients with Marfan syndrome. Appropriate clearances should be obtained from pediatricians, cardiologists, and geneticists prior to any surgical procedure.

DUCHENNE MUSCULAR DYSTROPHY

Duchenne muscular dystrophy is a disorder of worsening neurologic dysfunction characterized by progressive muscle weakness due to absent dystrophin protein in skeletal muscle. It only affects young boys due to its X-linked recessive inheritance pattern. The defect is usually a spontaneous mutation of the gene coding for dystrophin—synthesis of an unstable dystrophin protein is rapidly degraded. Muscle biopsy is required for diagnosis, which reveals connective tissue infiltration.

Associated orthopedic manifestations include scoliosis, equinovarus foot deformity, and joint contractures. On physical examination, these patients have progressive weakness affecting proximal muscles, beginning with gluteal muscles and hip extensors. This leads to delayed walking and toe walking. Patients have calf pseudohypertrophy and deep tendon reflexes are present. Gowers sign, where patients rise by walking hands up legs to compensate for gluteus maximus and quadriceps weakness, is common in these patients. The clinical features are apparent by ages 3 years to

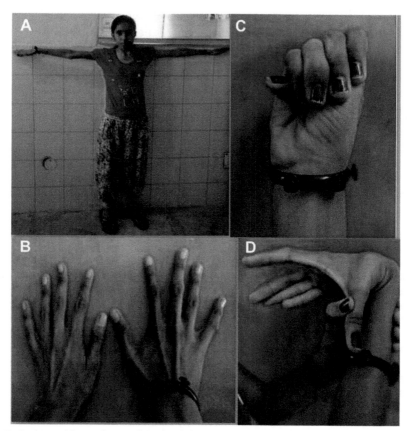

Fig. 5. Patient with Marfan syndrome exhibiting (*A*) dolichostenomelia, (*B*) arachnodactyly, (*C*) thumb in palm test, and (*D*) ligamentous laxity testing. (*From* Jain E, Pandey RK, Marfan syndrome BMJ Case Rep. 2013 Dec 11;2013. pii: bcr2013201632. https://doi.org/10.1136/bcr-2013-201632; with permission.)

6 years. Children afflicted typically have loss of independent ambulation by age 10 years to 12 years and are often wheelchair bound by the age of 15 years.[9]

Nonoperative treatment is aimed at maintaining ambulatory capacity as long as possible with steroid therapy and bracing. These acutely improve strength and slow progressive weakening. Patients also benefit from physical therapy to increase their range of motion. Operative treatment includes soft tissue releases to prolong ambulation. Scoliosis is a common feature and significant. Rapid, relentless progression of scoliosis is the rule and is exacerbated once relegated to a wheelchair. As opposed to most other types of scoliosis, which are not treated surgically until a Cobb angle is greater than 40°, patients with Duchenne muscular dystrophy are treated surgically once the curve approaches 20° to 30°. Scoliosis corrective surgery improves quality of life and sitting balance; however, it has no effect on pulmonary function and its age-related decline or patient longevity. Patients typically expire from cardiopulmonary complications by the age of 20.[9]

BECKER MUSCULAR DYSTROPHY

As opposed to Duchenne muscular dystrophy, Becker muscular dystrophy is much less severe. It is also X-linked recessive. Levels of dystrophin, however, are present but abnormal. This is from a truncated but stable protein. Boys affected also are color blind. Onset is later in life, with slower disease progression and a longer life expectancy. Patients typically live well beyond their third decade without respiratory support. The only way to differentiate between Duchenne muscular dystrophy and Becker muscular dystrophy is via muscle biopsy. Orthopedic manifestations and treatments of Becker muscular dystrophy are similar to those of Duchenne muscular dystrophy.[9]

NEUROFIBROMATOSIS

Neurofibromatosis is an autosomal dominant disorder of neurologic origin—neural crest origin. The incidence is 1:3000 and is the most common disorder caused by a single mutation in a single gene. The defect is a mutation in the *NF-1* gene on chromosome 17, which encodes for the neurofibrillin protein. This protein is important for the Ras-dependent MAPK (mitogen-activated protein kinase) activity, which is important for appropriate osteoclast function, hence, the reason for the number of orthopedic manifestations in neurofibromatosis. The abnormal Ras signaling also can lead to osteoclast death and certain neoplasias. The classification of Neurofibromatosis includes neurofibromatosis type 1 (von Recklinghausen disease), neurofibromatosis type 2, and segmental neurofibromatosis. Neurofibromatosis type 1 is the most common.[5]

Associated conditions include higher incidence of malignancies, hypertension due to renal artery stenosis, scoliosis, dural ectasias, long bone pseudoarthrosis, anterolateral bowing of the tibia, and hemihypertrophy. Associated malignancies include Wilms tumor, rhabdomyosarcoma, and neurofibrosarcoma. Diagnostic criteria are well established and include café au lait spots (6 or more with diameter >5 mm before puberty and >15 mm after puberty), neurofibromas, axillary freckling, optic glioma, Lisch nodules, iris hamartomas, a distinctive osseous abnormality, and having a first-degree relative with neurofibromatosis (**Box 1**).[5]

The 2 most important orthopedic manifestations of neurofibromatosis are scoliosis and tibial bowing with potential pseudoarthrosis. Scoliosis associated with

---

Box 1
Clinical criteria for neurofibromatosis type 1

1.Greater than or equal to 6 café au lait macules greater than 5 mm in greatest diameter in prepubertal individuals and greater than 15 mm in greatest diameter in postpubertal individuals

2.Greater than or equal to 2 neurofibromas of any type or greater than 1 plexiform neurofibroma

3.Freckling in the axillary or inguinal regions

4.Optic glioma

5.Greater than or equal to 2 Lisch nodules (iris hamartomas)

6.A distinctive osseous lesion, such as sphenoid dysplasia or thinning of the long bone cortex, with or without pseudoarthrosis

7.A first-degree relative (parent, sibling, or offspring) with neurofibromatosis type 1 according to the above criteria

From Wang Z, Liu Y. Research update and recent developments in the management of scoliosis in neurofibromatosis type 1. Orthopedics. 2010 May;33(5):335-41. https://doi.org/10.3928/01477447-20100329-20.

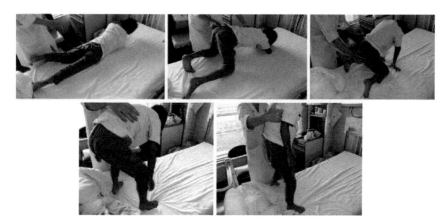

Fig. 6. Pictorial of Gowers sign evident in Duchenne muscular dystrophy. (*From* Koike Y, Aoki N, Zhu Y. Gowers' sign as an indication of recovery from Guillain-Barré syndrome. From J Pediatr. 2012 Jul;161(1):163-4. https://doi.org/10.1016/j.jpeds.2012.01.038. Epub 2012 Feb 28; with permission.)

neurofibromatosis is treated like idiopathic scoliosis, which includes bracing for curves greater than 20° and operative intervention for curves greater than 40°. Importantly, because of the association of neurofibromatosis and interspinal abnormalities, such as dural ectasias and intraspinal neurofibromas, an MRI of the cervical, thoracic, and lumbar spines is crucial in the preoperative work-up. Typical radiographic features of scoliosis in neurofibromatosis include vertebral scalloping, enlarged foramina, rib penciling, short segmented sharp curves, and kyphoscoliosis.[5]

Anterolateral bowing of the tibia is also a common feature of neurofibromatosis. If left unaddressed, it may lead to pseudoarthrosis of the tibia, which is a difficult problem to correct. Pseudoarthrosis may lead to a nonfunctional limb. A pseudoarthrosis may be seen in the radius, ulna, clavicle, and femur. Treatment of anterolateral bowing of the tibia (most common) is bracing, if mild. If a pseudoarthrosis is established, surgical intervention with intramedullary rod fixation (**Fig. 6**), vascularized bone grafts, and possible distraction osteogenesis is required. In cases of failed surgical intervention to address tibia pseudoarthrosis, below-the-knee amputation is typically required because the gait pattern is markedly improved opposed to attempts at limb salvage.

REFERENCES

1. Panda NK, Kaiser S. "Cerebral palsy." Orthopaedic knowledge update: pediatrics 5. Rosemont (IL): American Academy of Orthopaedic Surgeons; 2016. p. 123–36.

2. Koman LA, Smith BP, Shilt JS. Cerebral palsy. Lancet 2004;363(9421):1619–31.

3. Chan BW, Chan K-S, Koide T, et al. Maternal diabetes increases the risk of caudal regression caused by retinoic acid. Diabetes 2002;51(9):2811–6.

4. Drennan JC. Orthotic management of the myelomeningocele Spine. Dev Med Child Neurol 2008;18:97–103.

5. Weinstein SL. 7th edition. Lovell and Winter's pediatric orthopaedics, vol. 1. Philadelphia: Wolter Kluwer, Lippincot Willams et Wilkins; 2014.

6. Swaroop V. "Myelomeningocele." Orthopaedic knowledge update: pediatrics 5. Rosemont (IL): American Academy of Orthopaedic Surgeons; 2016. p. 137–52.

7. Aprin H, Bowen JR, Macewen GD, et al. Spine fusion in patients with spinal muscular atrophy. J Bone Joint Surg Am 1982;64(8):1179–87.

8. Pandolfo M. Friedreich ataxia: the clinical picture. J Neurol 2009;256(S1):3–8.

9. Shieh PB. Muscular dystrophies and other genetic myopathies. Neurol Clin 2013; 31(4):1009–29.

10. Doughty K, Cho R, Stutz C. "Arthrogrypotic syndromes." orthopaedic knowledge update: pediatrics 5. Rosemont (IL): American Academy of Orthopaedic Surgeons; 2016. p. 153–64.

11. Shirley LED, Sponseller PD. Marfan syndrome. J Am Acad Orthop Surg 2009; 17(9):572–81.

Pediatric Musculoskeletal Infections

Kristen DePaola, MS[a], Justin Fernicola, MD[b], Christopher Collins, MD[c],*

KEYWORDS

- Bone • Infection • Joint • Osteomyelitis • Soft tissue

KEY POINTS

- Pediatric musculoskeletal infections vary in presentation.
- Any soft tissue, joint, or bone is vulnerable to infection.
- Implanted hardware may increase the possibility of infection and provide challenges to treatment.
- A multidisciplinary approach with open communication allows for improved outcomes and patient experiences.
- Early care may decrease potential complications.

INTRODUCTION

Pediatric populations are prone to infections and most can be managed appropriately in a primary care setting. There are, however, some infectious processes that require intervention or management from an orthopedic surgeon. The most serious infectious processes in the pediatric population from an orthopedic standpoint are osteomyelitis and septic arthritis. Early recognition of these conditions and prompt referral of serious infections, as well as the ability to differentiate which infections should be referred for specialist evaluation is critical.

In general, pediatric musculoskeletal infections range in presentation. The multitude of presentations can make diagnosis and treatment challenging. Equally as challenging is obtaining information from patients who often are unable to provide details. Many symptoms can remain subacute and onset may be insidious. Musculoskeletal injections may also vary, of course, location. Any extremity—skin, muscle, tendon, joint, spine—may be involved. Pediatric musculoskeletal infections may be isolated or involved with a systemic issue such as disseminated infections. Location of

[a] Medical Student, Rowan University School of Osteopathic Medicine, 1 Medical Center Drive, Stratford, NJ 08084, USA; [b] Orthopedic Resident, Monmouth Medical Center, 300 2nd Avenue, Long Branch, NJ 07740, USA; [c] Pediatric Orthopedics, Seaview Orthopedics and Medical Associates, 1200 Eagle Avenue, Ocean, NJ 07712, USA
* Corresponding author.
E-mail address: collinch5765@gmail.com

Pediatr Clin N Am 67 (2020) 59–69
https://doi.org/10.1016/j.pcl.2019.09.001
0031-3955/20/© 2019 Elsevier Inc. All rights reserved.

infection may also dictate how it presents and is treated. The presence of any orthopedic hardware (plates, screws, wires, anchors) from surgical intervention may increase the risk of infection. Retained orthopedic hardware may also complicate medical treatment. This highlights the need for a complete history and physical examination for any pediatric patient with a potential musculoskeletal infection.

One of the most important features of treating pediatric musculoskeletal infections is the requirement of a multidisciplinary approach. Communication among all practitioners and levels is paramount to appropriate treatment: pediatrician, orthopedists, pediatric infectious disease, radiologist, emergency room physicians, and nurses among others. The multidisciplinary approach improves outcomes and allows for standardized treatment protocols, appropriate resource utilization, and reduction of costs and decrease complication rates. Treatment complications may also be reduced by allowing for earlier transition of oral antibiotics treatment and potentially shorter hospital stays.

OSTEOMYELITIS

Osteomyelitis is defined as the seeding of bacteria into bone. In the pediatric population, osteomyelitis usually develops via hematogenous spread, often with a history of recent minor trauma. Osteomyelitis, if progresses, may lead to contiguous infections that may spread to other structures. Septic arthritis, tenosynovitis, and other soft tissue infections may result.

Staphylococcus aureus is by far the most common organism in all age groups; however, certain circumstances are associated with different organisms that the primary care provider should be aware of. Group B streptococcus species are the most common organism in the neonatal population, whereas pseudomonal infections have been linked to puncture wounds of the foot.[1]

Evaluation

Physical examination

The most often symptom of a child presenting with osteomyelitis is pain. Tenderness to palpation overlying the suspected area of osteomyelitis is the most common theme on physical examination. Because osteomyelitis may increase pressure away from the area in question, it is often helpful to palpate in concentric areas from the primary site. To differentiate from septic arthritis, which presents as exquisite pain with any active or passive range of motion of a joint, osteomyelitis presents with diffuse pain compartmentally and away from joints.

Other common physical findings include fever, unwillingness to use the affected extremity, edema, warmth, and an overall toxic appearance. Children may also present differently depending on the offending bacterial species. MSSA osteomyelitis may present more subtly and methicillin-resistant *Staphylococcus aureus* (MRSA) osteomyelitis may present as a significantly more ill patient. Interestingly, patients with cellulitis, other soft tissue infections, and septic arthritis have lower rates of bacteremia and hospital stay. Acute osteomyelitis may lead to significant adverse outcomes such as growth plate sequelae (limb length discrepancy due to physeal arrest) and avascular necrosis. Patients with acute osteomyelitis also typically require much longer schedules of antibiotic treatment and have higher rates of recurrence.

Diagnostic imaging and testing

For any potential musculoskeletal infection, one of the first steps is to obtain plain radiographs. Plain radiographs may quickly aid in excluding or decreasing the differential diagnosis from other potential disease processes such as injury and neoplasms for example. Plain radiographs may also reveal chronicity of disease. Other findings on plain radiographs such as soft tissue swelling of joint effusions are equally as important. Of note, the effects of osteomyelitis on bone is typically delayed when evaluating with plain radiographs, as nearly a 33% loss of the bone mineral density is required to be visualized.[1] CT scan may be performed and offer additional information not provided by plain radiographs (**Fig. 1**).

One of the most useful imaging modalities is MRI. MRI allows for the potential differentiation of infection versus neoplasm. It may allow for complete visualization of periosteal abscesses, sequestrum, cortical erosion, and the general extent of the disease. Often, obtaining an MRI in a younger child may be challenging — often, MRI with sedation is required. Timeliness of a sedation MRI may be challenging in many hospital scenarios. Certain protocols such as sedation MRI with continuation of sedation evolving into surgical intervention have shown many benefits. This may decrease hospital stays by increasing efficiency of appropriate treatment again highlighting the benefits of a multidisciplinary approach and maximizing communication among practitioners.

When evaluating for osteomyelitis, an MRI with and without contrast should be obtained. Efficient interpretation by radiologists aids in the overall efficiency of treatment. The goal of most centers is to obtain an MRI with and without contrast within the first 24 hours after admission.

Blood cultures should be obtained, but the provider must be aware that they are only positive in 30% to 50% of patients.[1] In addition, erythrocyte sedimentation rate (ESR), C-reactive protein (CRP), and a complete blood count (CBC) are evaluated during the initial evaluation. These laboratory tests are typically trended to evaluate for efficacy of treatment. Studies have shown CRP levels to be the most reliable predictor of response to treatment. Of course, other laboratory testing may be required.

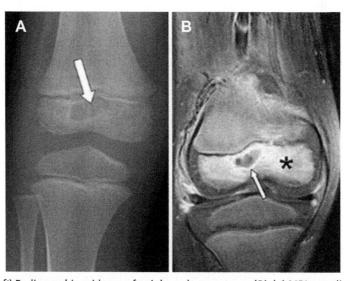

Fig. 1. (*Left*) Radiographic evidence of epiphyseal sequestrum. (*Right*) MRI revealing sequestrum with surrounding edema consistent with osteomyelitis. (*From* Desimpel J, Posadzy M, Vanhoenacker F. The Many Faces of Osteomyelitis: A Pictorial Review. J Belg Soc Radiol. 2017 May 11;101(1):24. https://doi.org/10.5334/jbr-btr.1300.)

Management

Antibiotics

Again emphasized is the multidisciplinary approach. For instance, stable patients would benefit from withholding antibiotics until appropriate cultures can be obtained. Cultures may be obtained via aspiration, interventional radiology, or surgically. Of course, any patient showing signs of sepsis require immediate empirical antibiotic administration. Early interdisciplinary communication is imperative. Results of blood cultures and other appropriate cultures may guide narrowing the antibiotic coverage.

In all patients, blood cultures and laboratory tests (including CBC with differential, ESR, and CRP) should be performed. Infectious disease practitioners may assist in antibiotic selection by their understanding of local and national trends. For instance, Group B streptococcal osteomyelitis is common in infants but rare in older children. Kingella kingae is most common in children younger than 4 years. The most common organism causing osteomyelitis is methicillin-susceptible S aureus. Understanding and noting other chronic disease, mode of infection, potential pathogen common to patient age and general epidemiology, and likely pathogen susceptibility greatly aids in antibiotic selection.[2]

Community-acquired MRSA is now responsible for a considerable amount of osteomyelitis and other soft tissue musculoskeletal infections. As such, increasing amounts of vancomycin, clindamycin, and bactrim are used. Vancomycin use requires cautious monitoring of vancomycin trough and serum creatinine levels to assess for renal complications. Infectious disease practitioners provide important guidance secondary to their knowledge of local epidemiology and antibiotic resistance patterns, both local and national.

As peripherally inserted central catheters have become more commonplace, antibiotic protocols have been subject to changes. The increased safety and ease of parenteral antibiotic administration in the outpatient environment has led to a short course of intravenous antibiotics as an inpatient followed by extended parental treatment as an outpatient. Oral antibiotic administration following an appropriate parenteral course is common as well. Oral therapy may extend 3 to 6 weeks depending of many factors.

Cessation of antibiotic therapy is dictated by many factors. Primarily, antibiotic schedule is changed or ceased by normalized inflammatory markers (CRP, ESR, white blood cells [WBC]) and normal physical findings. Typical hospital discharge criteria include a painless, afebrile patient who is able to achieve physical therapy clearance. If complete resolution of symptoms is not achieved, antibiotic therapy may be continued. Reassessing physical examination and inflammatory markers is continued weekly until resolution. If resolution is not achieved in a standard antibiotic regimen schedule, additional evaluation is required. Treatment failure may require additional imaging to be obtained such as a repeat MRI. This may reveal a sequestrum, area of necrotic bone, often intramedullary that may require surgical intervention, as this would be sine qua non of chronic osteomyelitis. Consideration for additional cultures should be entertained to further guide treatment.

Surgery

Barring recognition of an abscess or sequestrum, osteomyelitis is a medical diagnosis and treated medically. Surgery is generally indicated when the aforementioned is identified; culture is required to guide treatment, failure of medical treatment, or if a patient is unstable demonstrating hemodynamic instability. If a collection is identified that would not likely respond to medical treatment alone, incision, irrigation, drainage, and debridement may be indicated. Indeed, in certain patients, multiple surgical interventions may be required—multiple studies show the need for repeat surgical interventions is dictated by the severity at initial presentation. Of note, it seems there is recognized higher rate of surgical intervention with increasingly commonplace of MRSA osteomyelitis.

Surgical technique depends on the severity of disease. Surgical intervention for osteomyelitis may include abscess drainage, corticotomy (creating a bone window), debridement of infected bone or necrotic material, and irrigation. The orthopedic colloquialism "the solution to pollution is dilution" quips at the need to debulk necrotic bone and reduce the bacterial load with irrigation to improve surgical results. Unfortunately, although decompressing an abscess, debriding necrotic bone, and decreasing bacterial load improve symptoms and aid in the treatment of osteomyelitis, it also may reduce perfusion and hence antibiotic delivery. Increased complication rates may occur depending on the proximity of the abscess or osteomyelitis to the physis. Damage to the physis or the perichondrial ring that provides physeal blood supply may result in physeal injury resulting in growth plate sequelae.[1] Adjuvant therapies may also be beneficial such as local delivery of antibiotics—antibiotic impregnated absorbable beads for instance.

If laboratory or clinical findings do not improve within 72 to 96 hours following surgical debridement, repeat irrigation and debridement should be considered. Additional imaging is of little use unless there is suspicion for another focus of infection or if inadequate decompression is suspected. The virulence of the bacterial species may also influence the need to additional or repeat surgical debridements. It should be noted that postoperative MRI scans should be viewed with some clinical skepticism, as they may mislead, as they often seem to show a worsening condition as the infection progresses through its normal course.[1]

Key points

- Physical examination is often significant for bone tenderness over the area of interest.
- Clinical findings may include fever, pain, tenderness, refusal to bear weight or decreased limb use, warmth, and edema.
- Deep soft-tissue swelling is the most important plain radiographic finding.
- MRI provides better understanding of the area of interest and should be obtained within 24 hours.
- Continuing anesthesia for immediate surgery following MRI improves patient outcomes.
- ESR, CRP, CBC, and blood cultures are typically performed on admission. Antibiotics can be withheld until cultures are returned in stable patients. Early empirical antibiotics should be considered in unstable patients.
- Group B streptococcal osteomyelitis is common in infants but rare in older children. *K kingae* is most common in children younger than 4 years.
- Community-acquired MRSA is responsible for many bone, joint, and soft-tissue infections.
- Normal protocol includes in-hospital antibiotic therapy followed by parenteral or oral antibiotics therapy at home.
- Lack of clinical findings and normalized inflammatory markers indicate conclusion of antibiotic therapy.
- Treatment of osteomyelitis is started with empirical antibiotics and in most cases is sufficient to treat the condition. Patients who improve within 48 hours do not usually require surgery. Surgical debridement is reserved for cases with deep periosteal abscesses or those that do not respond to antibiotic therapy.

- Surgery tends to be indicated for unstable patients and is helpful in certain patients with collections or abscesses requiring decompression.

CHRONIC RECURRENT MULTIFOCAL OSTEOMYELITIS
Evaluation

Chronic recurrent multifocal osteomyelitis (CRMO) or chronic nonbacterial osteomyelitis is a poorly understood disease that varies in course and location. However, it is thought that genetic predisposition may play a role or be a contributing factor in some patients. CRMO is described as a self-limiting disorder. CRMO has some distinguishing characteristics when compared with acute osteomyelitis. It is not typically associated with any type of trauma. It is uncommon to occur in the very young and primarily occurs in late childhood and adolescence. There is a gender preponderance toward women with a female to male ratio of 4:1.[2]

The usual presentation is a female patient with ill-defined complaints insidious in nature. There are usually no systemic symptoms such as fever. Physical complaints may be mild to severe, and CRMO can be associated with other inflammatory diseases. Although it is common to recognize elevated ESR, a lack of leukocytosis and a normal CRP are the norm. Opposed to acute osteomyelitis, it is common to have patients complain of multiple sites of pain and present with multiple sites of edema and tenderness to palpation.

Plain radiographs may show soft tissue swelling; however, advanced imaging such as MRI shows patchy areas of bony edema often in multiple locations. Blood cultures and areas of interest aspiration or cultures are sterile. CRMO is typically a diagnosis of exclusion after consideration of acute osteomyelitis and other disorders are ruled out (**Fig. 2**).

Management

Management of CRMO is challenging, as it is a diagnosis of exclusion. Patients are typically worked up for a diagnosis of acute osteomyelitis. This usually includes antibiotic treatment and at times, surgical debridement and/or biopsy. Interestingly, one of the distinguishing features of CRMO is that pain typically responds to nonsteroidal antiinflammatory drugs (NSAIDs) and other conservative measures, opposed to acute osteomyelitis.

Key points

- CRMO primarily occurs in late childhood and adolescence.
- CRMO is more common in women than men.
- Presentation shows gradual onset without evidence of systemic infection.
- Imaging often shows multiple bone lesions.
- Biopsy typically shows inflammatory changes with sterile cultures. CRMO is a diagnosis of exclusion and is often mistaken for acute osteomyelitis.
- CRMO can be well managed with NSAIDs, activity modification, and immobilization.

SEPTIC ARTHRITIS

Septic arthritis is defined as an intraarticular infection. Septic arthritis is an orthopedic surgical emergency. Bacterial colonization and bacterial byproducts are caustic to cartilage. Urgent surgical intervention reduces the risk of complications of delayed treatment. Complications of septic arthritis include early, significant degenerative disease, deformity, limb length discrepancy, pain, sepsis, and osteomyelitis. Incidence

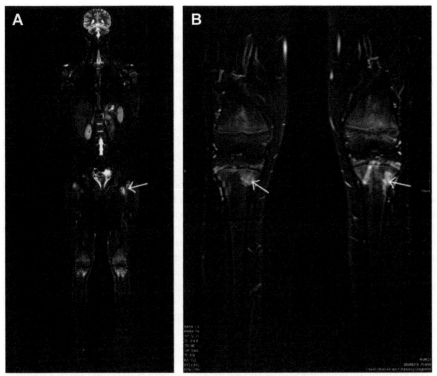

Fig. 2. MRI of revealing chronic recurrent multifocal osteomyelitis. Arrow in (*A*) signifying proximal femoral osteomyelitis. Arrows in (*B*) showing left and right proximal tibial metaphyseal osteomyelitis. (*From* Hofmann SR, Roesen-Wolff A, Hahn G, Hedrich CM. Update: Cytokine Dysregulation in Chronic Nonbacterial Osteomyelitis (CNO). Int J Rheumatol. 2012;2012:310206. https://doi.org/10.1155/2012/310206. Epub 2012 May 21; with permission.)

peaks in first few years of life. This condition usually occurs from trauma or hematogenous seeding and can often develop from direct spread of previous osteomyelitis. Septic arthritis typically involves large joints such as knee, hip, shoulder, and elbow. Smaller joints such as ankle and wrist may also be involved less commonly.

Evaluation

A typical patient will present with pain, limp or refusal to bear weight, and fever as well as other systemic complaints. Complaints of pain can be quite significant. Mostly with regard to the diagnosis of a septic hip, the Kocher criteria have been developed to aid in expedient diagnosis:

- Serum WBC greater than 12,000
- Inability to bear weight
- Fever greater than 101.3
- ESR greater than 40

Four out of four Kocher criteria predicts nearly 100% the diagnosis of septic arthritis in the appropriate patient and setting. Physical examination reveals exquisite pain with any type of micromotion, active or passive, about the joint.[3]

In general, neonates have an increased risk of bone, joint, and soft tissue infections. In infants, a common isolate of septic arthritis, osteomyelitis, and pyomyositis is *Streptococcus agalactiae*. Neonates are also at risk for developing septic arthritis from hospital-acquired species, including MRSA, candida species, and mulitdrug-resistant gram-negative organisms because of their hospital presence and the need for vascular access, catheters, and other medical devices. In general, the most common cause of septic arthritis, and indeed all musculoskeletal infections, other than the aforementioned is *S aureus*. Immunocompromised children, whether it be from a lack of immunizations or systemic illness or syndrome, are at risk of developing septic arthritis secondary to *Streptococcus pneumoniae*. Presentation usually occurs during admission in neonates; however, indolent forms may present weeks to months later in their home settings.

Diagnosing neonates for musculoskeletal infections, particularly septic arthritis, can be extremely challenging. Because they are unable to communicate and explain location of pain, onset, and duration, this requires a higher level of suspicion in the practitioners caring for them. One would expect classic symptoms of pain, fever, and to show leukocytosis and elevated inflammatory markers. This is often not so for neonates; they can present with none of the aforementioned. If fever of unknown origin, it is appropriate to search for any source, as up to 40% of neonates with a musculoskeletal infections have multifocal disease.[3] Neonates have multiple joints with intracapsular metaphases, such as the hip and knee, which increases the likelihood of septic arthritis associated with osteomyelitis. As typical with suspicion for osteomyelitis or other musculoskeletal infections, advanced imaging is supported except for one particular case. If a septic hip arthritis is suspected, ultrasound is used, as it is typically quick and may be used to aspirate joint fluid.

The authors' protocol for suspected septic hip arthritis is to obtain serial inflammatory markers to include CBC, CRP, and ESR. Afterward, a hip ultrasound is performed with aspiration for cell count and culture obtained. If ultrasound is unavailable, the child is taken to operating room for aspiration for cell count and culture. In the appropriate setting and with supporting supplemental laboratory tests such as leukocytosis greater than 12,000 cells/mL, serum CRP greater than 2 mg/dL, admission ESR greater than 40 mm/h, and a cell count greater than 40,000 nucleated cells/mL with greater than 75% neutrophils, a diagnosis of septic arthritis is made.[3] If the cell count is consistent with septic arthritis, a formal incision, irrigation, drainage, and debridement is performed. Patients are followed closely during the postoperative period.

Management

Antibiotics

Antibiotic therapy is typically initiated with antistaphylococcal parenteral antibiotics. Closely following patients after the initiation of antibiotics is required. A typical protocol includes attempts to transition patients to oral antibiotics once efficacy is proved by an improvement in symptoms and a decrease in inflammatory markers. Thus, of course, assuming culture sensitivities proves an oral antibiotic may be effective. At times, long-term parenteral antibiotics are required. Typically, antibiotic treatment times are 2 to 3 weeks for septic arthritis and 4 to 8 weeks when associated with osteomyelitis.[3]

Surgery

When surgical intervention is deemed necessary, multiple techniques may be used. The gold standard, an open incision, irrigation, drainage, and debridement (I and D), is performed. In many cases, an arthroscopic I and D is appropriate. Many joints including ankle, knee, hip, shoulder, elbow, and wrist are candidates for this type of I and D. Many sources have shown that arthroscopic I and D efficacy is comparable to open I and D (**Fig. 3**). In addition, arthroscopic I and D may reduce adjacent soft tissue disruption, decrease postoperative pain, and decrease hospital stays. If clinical improvement is not appreciated 48 to 72 hours after I and D, consideration for repeat I and D or advanced imaging techniques such as MRI should be considered.[2]

Key points

- *S agalactiae* is a common cause of septic arthritis in neonates. *S aureus* is the most common cause of musculoskeletal infection past early infancy. *K kingae* is a common cause of septic arthritis in children aged 6 months to 4 years. *S pneumoniae* can occur in immunocompromised children. Neonates are at high risk of hospital-acquired pathogens.
- Clinical presentation may often include lack of fever, less than expected pain, and normal inflammatory markers.
- Up to 40% of neonates have multifocal infections.
- Joints with intracapsular metaphyses are most susceptible to adjacent osteomyelitis, and advanced imaging should be considered except in the case of septic hip arthritis.
- Ultrasound should be used to examine capsular distention in suspected septic hip arthritis.
- Peripheral WBC, ESR, and CRP results aid in diagnosis. Antistaphylococcal parenteral antibiotics are typically used to initiate antibiotic therapy.
- Arthroscopic drainage is a safe and effective surgical option.

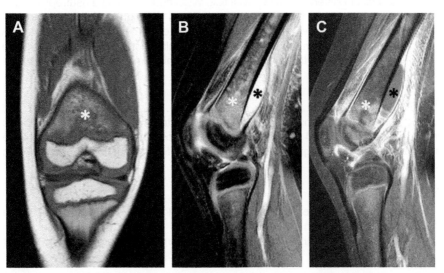

Fig. 3. (*A*) Coronal MRI showing metaphyseal osteomyelitis. (*B*) Sagittal MRI showing periosteal abscess and (*C*) effusion consistent with septic arthritis. White asterisk is showing metaphyseal osteomyeltiis and Black asterisk is showing subperiosteal abscess. (*From* Schallert EK, Kan JH, Monsalve J, et al. Metaphyseal osteomyelitis in children: how often does MRI-documented joint effusion or epiphyseal extension of edema indicate coexisting septic arthritis? Pediatr Radiol. 2015 Jul;45(8):1174-81. https://doi.org/10.1007/s00247-015-3293-0. Epub 2015 Feb 20.)

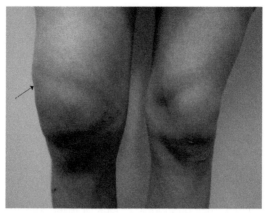

Fig. 4. Knee effusion (*arrow*). (*From* Wikimedia. Available at: https://upload.wikimedia.org/wikipedia/commons/e/eb/Kneeffusion.JPG.)

- If no improvements are seen within 48 to 72 hours postoperatively, repeat I and D and/or advanced imaging should be considered.

SPECIAL CIRCUMSTANCE: LYME ARTHRITIS
Evaluation

Lyme septic arthritis is challenging to differentiate from bacterial septic arthritis in children. In cases of confirmed lyme septic arthritis, it has been shown that there is no statistically significant difference in synovial fluid WBC count, absolute neutrophil count, and percentage of segmented neutrophils. Increased levels of suspicion for lyme septic arthritis is required in geographic areas shown where lyme exposure is endemic. A very common presentation is a child with monoarticular joint effusion (such as a knee) for an extended period of time. In addition, the patient will not exhibit systemic symptoms (**Fig. 4**).[2]

Management

Lyme arthritis is well managed with oral antibiotic treatment. Duration of antibiotic treatment is typically for 4 weeks. It is uncommon for lyme septic arthritis to require surgical intervention. Prognosis is improved with efficient initiation of oral antibiotic treatment.

Key points

- Where Lyme is endemic, an acutely swollen knee is more likely to be Lyme arthritis versus septic arthritis.
- Children with Lyme arthritis have excellent prognosis after oral antibiotic therapy for 4 weeks.

SUMMARY

Careful evaluation, vigilant follow-up, and increased levels of clinical suspicion are required when treating children with suspected and confirmed musculoskeletal infections. Bone, joint, and muscle infections are common but may be mimicked by other conditions (eg, neoplasms, inflammatory disorders, and trauma). Evidence-based clinical algorithms, improved communication between the interdisciplinary team, and coordination of care have all been shown to improve patient outcomes.

REFERENCES

1. Castellazzi L, Mantero M, Esposito S. Update on the management of pediatric acute osteomyelitis and septic arthritis. Int J Mol Sci 2016;17(6):855.
2. Lovejoy JF, Lawson CAB. "Musculoskeletal infection." Orthopaedic knowledge update: pediatrics 5. Rosemont (IL): American Academy of Orthopaedic Surgeons; 2016. p. 35–43.
3. Pääkkönen M. Septic arthritis in children: diagnosis and treatment. Pediatric Health Med Ther 2017;8:65–8.

Pediatric Anesthesia Concerns and Management for Orthopedic Procedures

Jeffrey P. Wu, MD

KEYWORDS

- Pediatric anesthesia • Local anesthetic • Caudal • Peripheral nerve block
- Pediatric fracture • SCFE • Club foot • Scoliosis

KEY POINTS

- Pain management for pediatric orthopedic patient includes a multimodal pharmacologic approach and regional anesthesia.
- Regional anesthesia performed on pediatric patient under general anesthesia has been shown to be safe.
- Anesthetic concerns during scoliosis surgery include optimizing neuromonitoring signals, blood loss management, positioning-related injuries, and postoperative visual loss.

INTRODUCTION

Anesthesiologists are presented with unique challenges when caring for pediatric patients undergoing orthopedic surgeries. The anesthetic approach must consider a child's psychological development and frequent predilection to respiratory infections. Surgeries can range from simple ambulatory procedures to complex and extensive operations. A large part of the anesthetic care includes pain management, management of concomitant disease, and risk reduction for adverse events. This article reviews select anesthetic perioperative concerns, discusses various methods of pain control used for orthopedic surgeries, and reviews anesthetic considerations for select pediatric orthopedic surgeries.

SELECT PEDIATRIC PERIOPERATIVE CONCERNS
Anxiety in the Pediatric Patient

Pediatric patients presenting for orthopedic surgery can express variable levels of anxiety and distress. Preoperative stressors can include new surroundings,

Disclosure Statement: The author has no relationship with a commercial company that has a direct financial interest in subject matter or materials discussed in article or with a company making a competing product.
Department of Anesthesiology, Jersey Shore University Medical Center, 1945 Route 33, Neptune, NJ 07753, USA
E-mail address: Jeffrey.Wu@hackensackmeridian.org

procedures, hunger, anticipation of pain, and parental separation. Some risk factors for preoperative anxiety include the age group of 1 year olds to 5 year olds, shy temperament, poor prior medical experiences, high cognitive levels, and high parental anxiety.[1,2]

The degree of preoperative anxiety can have an impact on postoperative outcomes. Unrelieved anxiety can be associated with postoperative behavioral changes, including generalized anxiety, separation anxiety, aggression toward authorities, and nighttime crying.[3] These behaviors can persist up to 1 year after surgery.[4] Other postoperative outcomes can include higher pain scores and higher requirements of pain medications after surgery for at least 3 days postoperatively.[5]

Several strategies can be used to mitigate preoperative anxiety in children. Presurgical preparation programs can include site visits, videos, books, and child-life interventions. Parental presence during induction of anesthesia can allay separation anxiety. Pharmacologic intervention, such as oral midazolam, improves compliance and shows some reduction in negative behavior changes in the near term postoperatively.[6,7]

Upper Respiratory Tract Infections

The pediatric patient presenting for orthopedic surgery with a current or recent upper respiratory tract infection (URI) is a complicated dilemma for anesthesiologists and surgeons. Young children frequently are infected with a URI, presenting with runny nose, cough, and fever. Common implicating viruses include rhinoviruses, adenoviruses, and coronaviruses. Although the viral infection may reside in the nasopharynx, the lower respiratory tract can have increased sensitivity for up to 6 weeks after the URI symptoms have resolved.[8,9] Patients are at increased risk for perioperative laryngospasm, bronchospasm, and oxygen desaturation during this time with perhaps the greatest risk within the first 2 weeks after the URI has resolved.[8] Delaying surgery for 6 weeks after resolution of the URI is impractical because the child most likely will contract another URI.

For elective surgery, delaying surgery is prudent for severe symptoms, such as fever (>100.4°F), purulent nasal drainage, behavioral changes such as lethargy or poor feeding, and lower respiratory tract involvement such as wheezing.[10] In contrast, an uncomplicated URI limited to clear nasal discharge in an otherwise healthy patient usually can proceed with elective surgery. In-between these spectrums post a more difficult clinical decision-making challenge. Various factors are incorporated into determining postponing surgery, including age of patient, comorbidities, prior cancellations, complexity of surgery, and urgency of surgery. If elective surgery is delayed, most clinicians would postpone 2 weeks to 4 weeks after resolution of URI symptoms.[8,11]

For urgent surgeries, the risk of postponement should outweigh the increased respiratory risk of a sick child.

Induction of Anesthesia

Inhalational induction of anesthesia via a mask is a common approach to pediatric patients because it avoids the fear of IV placement. Sevoflurane is the primary volatile anesthetic used for inhalational induction. It is the least pungent of the modern inhaled anesthetics and the least irritating to the airway. The odor of sevoflurane, however, can still upset children. Nitrous oxide often is first administered because it is odorless and provides rapid anxiolysis and sedation. These effects can increase acceptance of increasing levels of sevoflurane.[12]

The progression of an inhalational induction to general anesthesia is a critical time. After the child becomes unconscious, the brain goes through a hyperreflexic, excitable phase of anesthesia before relaxation. Eyes may show nystagmus or may roll up. Respiratory patterns can change to rapid and shallow. Snoring may begin, signifying decreased muscle tone and ensuing partial upper airway obstruction. Sudden movements of the arms and legs can occur from the excited state.[12] External stimulation during this phase of anesthesia should be avoided. This includes tourniquet/IV placement, dressing changes, cast removal, or physical examinations. Such stimulation during the excitement phase may lead to laryngospasm.[13] IV placement and airway management are performed after the excitement phase has passed.

Contraindications to inhalational induction can include history of malignant hyperthermia, full stomach, difficult airway, and cardiac conditions. An IV placed prior to induction may be necessary.

STRATEGIES FOR PAIN MANAGEMENT

A multimodal strategy for perioperative pain management is often used for children undergoing orthopedic surgery. Pharmacologic adjuncts to narcotics act synergistically for enhanced analgesia, thus minimizing overall opioid use. Often these adjuncts are continued postoperatively as well. Regional anesthesia is invaluable to treat acute postoperative pain.[14] Blockage of pain conduction from the surgical site decreases the need for systemic pain medications. Decreased opioid use can minimize side effects and complications, such as nausea, vomiting, constipation, sedation, and apnea.

Acetaminophen

Acetaminophen is a widely used analgesic. Its mechanism of action is unclear and likely involves several pain pathways both peripherally and centrally. These include blocking prostaglandin synthesis by inhibiting a variant cyclooxygenase (COX) enzyme, enhancing the cannabinoid pathway, activating serotonergic pathways, and inhibiting the L-arginine/nitric oxide pathway.[15]

Overdosing of acetaminophen resulting in hepatic failure is always of concern. Acetaminophen can be administered orally, rectally, and IV. Oral narcotics often are formulated with an acetaminophen component so all previous forms of acetaminophen given must be confirmed prior to additional administration.

Nonsteroidal Anti-inflammatory Drugs

Nonsteroidal anti-inflammatory drugs (NSAIDs) are commonly used adjuncts, although as a class, their use is debatable for certain orthopedic surgeries. NSAIDs provide analgesia by reducing prostaglandin synthesis via inhibiting the COX pathway. Peripherally, at tissue injury sites, there is decreased inflammation.[14] There may be centrally mediated actions blocking hyperalgesic responses and activation of serotonin pathways.[16]

Ketorolac is a commonly used NSAID. It is usually administered IV and provides pain relief similar to opioids. Usage is limited to less than 5 days due to its reduction in renal blood flow.[14] Ibuprofen is one of the oldest used oral NSAIDs and is available IV as well.

NSAIDs use is not without risk. As a class, their use is debatable for certain orthopedic surgeries. They affect platelet adhesion and aggregation. Measured bleeding times are increased, although usually within normal range and clinically insignificant.[16] They should still be used with caution for surgeries with high risk for perioperative bleeding.

NSAIDs have the potential to affect bone formation via their action on prostaglandin. Thus, controversy exists using NSAIDs during orthopedic surgeries such as spinal fusion. Animal studies suggest altered bone healing after fractures and surgeries. NSAIDs have been used, however, after various orthopedic surgeries without adverse effects. In a subset of healthy children undergoing idiopathic scoliosis surgery, no adverse effects, such as curve progression, hardware failure, and reoperation, were found with ketorolac use.[17]

Opioids

Opioids often are required if postoperative pain is expected to be moderate to severe. Commonly used opioids include short-acting narcotics, like fentanyl, or longer-acting narcotics, like morphine or hydromorphone. IV dosing allows for close titration in the recovery room. Delivery postoperatively can be in the form of as-needed basis, nurse-controlled analgesia pump, or patient-controlled analgesia pump, depending on patient age and cognitive ability.[18]

Oral opioids usually are prescribed once the child tolerates oral intake. Commonly prescribed oral opioids, however, should be used with caution. Many oral opioids undergo metabolism through the hepatic cytochrome P450 2D6 (CYP2D6). Codeine, a prodrug, is metabolized into morphine through this pathway. Tramadol is converted to its active form O-desmethyltramadol. Polymorphisms of CPY2D6 can lead to poor metabolizers of codeine, leading to lack of efficacy. Ultrarapid metabolizers of codeine, however, result in higher than intended morphine formation and possible toxicity and respiratory depression.[19]

In 2013, the US Food and Drug Administration issued a boxed warning contraindication of using codeine for postoperative pain in a subset of children.[20] The Food and Drug Administration further restricted the use of codeine in 2017 and included tramadol. Codeine and tramadol are contraindicated in all children under 12 years old and recommended against their use for children 12 years old to 18 years old with obesity, sleep apnea, or severe lung disease.[21] Still in question are the safety profiles of hydrocodone and oxycodone in children. Currently, there is not enough evidence to conclude that ultrarapid metabolizing phenotypes of CYP2D6 are at increased risk with use of these 2 opioids.[19]

Regional Anesthesia

Regional anesthesia involves using local anesthetic agents, such as lidocaine, bupivacaine, and ropivacaine, to temporarily block nerve conduction from a specific part of the body. Sensory input is blunted, and motor blockade can be achieved as well. Immobility and muscle relaxation from an extremity can aid in providing optimal conditions for the orthopedic surgeon. Systemic anesthesia medications usually can be decreased. Duration of analgesia from a regional anesthetic depends on many factors, including type of local anesthetic, concentration used, volume used, and use of other pharmacologic additives. For multiday pain management, local anesthetics can be infused continuously via a catheter.

Caudal and lumbar epidural anesthesia

Neuraxial anesthesia is a form of regional anesthesia targeting nerves of the central nervous system (CNS). Such techniques include spinal, epidural, and caudal blocks. Contraindications include spina bifida, increased intracranial pressure, coagulopathy, or infection at the insertion site.

Caudal blocks are the most widely used regional technique in pediatric anesthesia and have been proved very safe.[22,23] It is appropriate for surgeries below the umbilicus, such as the hip, leg, knee, and foot. There is no laterality in this block; thus, both lower extremities are affected. A caudal block is performed by inserting a needle through the sacral hiatus and into the epidural space. The sacral hiatus is an opening at the caudad end of the sacrum and is due to a nonunion of the fifth sacral vertebral arch. Bordering the sacral hiatus laterally are the sacral cornu, which are bony prominences representing remnants of the inferior articular processes of the fifth sacral vertebra.[24] The sacral cornu are easily palpated in infants and younger children. Once a needle enters the epidural space, local anesthetic can be given as a single injection or a catheter can be threaded up to a desired epidural level to provide continuous analgesia.

Lumbar epidural catheters can also be placed if there is difficulty placing a catheter at the caudal level. The procedure in children is like that of adults. A Tuohy needle typically is used with a midline approach between the spinous processes of the targeted level. The needle with a syringe attached is advanced until a loss of resistance is felt from the syringe. This signifies that the tip of the Tuohy needle has entered the epidural space after passing the ligamentum flavum. An epidural catheter is then passed, or a single injection of local anesthetic is administered.[25]

Peripheral nerve blocks

Peripheral nerve blocks are techniques used to deliver local anesthetics to nerve bundles. Nerves can be localized with either nerve stimulation or ultrasound techniques. Nerve stimulation localizes nerve bundles using knowledge of anatomic landmarks along with an insulated needle with exposed metal at its tip to deliver electrical impulses. As the metal tip approaches the targeted nerve, the electrical impulse depolarizes the nerve and stimulates a muscle contraction. Once the expected muscle group is stimulated, local anesthetic is injected through the needle to surround the nerve bundle. A catheter can be placed as well.

The use of ultrasound is gaining popularity in pediatric regional anesthesia. It allows for visualization of the needle position in relation to the nerve bundle and of the distribution of local anesthetic. Compared with nerve stimulation techniques, the use of ultrasound has been shown to decrease the volume of medication needed for a successful block, thus decreasing risk of toxicity. Evidence has suggested increased rate of success, decreased procedure time, and decreased needle passes when using ultrasound guidance.[26,27]

Table 1 summarizes common peripheral nerve blocks, the location of surgery they can be used for and associated complications.[28,29]

Safety when performing regional techniques under general anesthesia

Approach to regional anesthesia is different between pediatric and adult patients. Regional anesthesia for adults is usually performed in an awake or mildly sedated state. This allows for feedback from the patient regarding paresthesia and pain during needling or local anesthetic injection. This may signify potential nerve injury. In contrast, pediatric patients may not have the cognitive ability to accurately report paresthesia. Poor patient cooperation, needle-phobia, and inability to lie still make regional anesthesia difficult to perform in awake or sedated children. Unexpected movements may cause inadvertent injuries or complications.[30] Thus, most regional anesthetics for pediatric patients have been performed after children are under general anesthesia.

Investigations have been done evaluating issues of safety and nerve injury while performing regional anesthesia in an unconscious pediatric patient. In 2014, the first

Table 1
Peripheral nerve blocks, usage, and complications

Nerve Block	Location of Surgery	Complications
Upper extremity		
Interscalene	Shoulder, upper arm	Spinal cord injury, intrathecal injection, pneumothorax, vertebral artery puncture, phrenic nerve blockade, Horner syndrome
Supraclavicular	Arm below shoulder, elbow, forearm, wrist, hand	Pneumothorax, phrenic nerve blockade, intravascular injection
Infraclavicular	Elbow, forearm, hand	Intravascular injection, pneumothorax
Axillary	Elbow, forearm, hand	intravascular injection
Lower extremity		
Lumbar plexus block	Hip, fractures femoral head/shaft, knee	Hematoma in muscle sheath, retroperitoneal space, or kidney; epidural spread
Fascia iliaca block	Hip surgery, femur	Intravascular injection
Femoral nerve block	Thigh, femur, knee	Intravascular injection; persistent strength deficits
Saphenous nerve block	Sensory medial lower leg, knee	Motor weakness with large volume; intravascular injection
Sciatic nerve block	Knee, leg, ankle, foot	Intravascular injection

Data from Flack S, Lang RS. Regional anesthesia. In: Davis PJ, Cladis FP, editors. Smith's anesthesia for infants and children, 9th edition. St. Louis: Elsevier; 2017. p. 487-506; and Gray AF, Collins AB, Eilers H. Peripheral nerve blocks. In: Stoelting RK, Miller RD, editors. Basics of anesthesia, 5th edition. Philadelphia: Churchill Livingstone; 2007. p. 276-86.

prospective study investigating this issue used data from 50,000 regional pediatric blocks from the Pediatric Regional Anesthesia Network database.[31] The study showed pediatric complication rates consistent with adult data. A follow-up study published in 2018 used data from 100,000 pediatric blocks.[22] More than 93% of patients were under general anesthesia during regional blockade. No permanent neurologic deficits were found. Transient neurologic deficits occurred in 2.4 of 10,000 patients. They were sensory in nature and resolved over weeks to months. Severe local anesthetic toxicity occurred in 0.76 of 10,000 patients, which is lower than reported adult data. Risk of neurologic and toxicity events were higher in the awake/sedated pediatric patient compared to that under general anesthesia. This study confirms safety of performing regional techniques in children under general anesthesia.[22]

Local anesthetic systemic toxicity

Local anesthetic systemic toxicity (LAST) produces serious reactions to the CNS and cardiovascular system. In general, lower plasma levels of local anesthetic produce CNS effects compared with higher plasma levels needed for cardiovascular effects. Thus, early signs of toxicity may include CNS signs, such as circumoral numbness, lightheadedness, dizziness, tinnitus, restlessness, and slurred speech. Increasing levels produce tonic-clonic seizures and eventual coma. As plasma levels further increase, cardiovascular signs develop. Short-acting local anesthetics like lidocaine tend to cause bradycardia and hypotension from vasodilation and myocardial depression. Cardiac arrest later ensues. Long-acting local anesthetics like bupivacaine and ropivacaine, however, may lead to ventricular arrythmias, peaked T waves, or complete cardiovascular collapse. Bupivacaine has a small threshold for cardiac toxicity and thus CNS and cardiovascular signs may occur simultaneously or, occasionally, cardiovascular signs may precede CNS signs.[32,33]

Because regional anesthesia for pediatric patients usually is performed under general anesthesia, seizure or cardiovascular signs like tachyarrhythmias or complete collapse is the first symptom of toxicity.[34] As discussed previously, severe local anesthetic toxicity is a rare event.[22] Adults can report early signs of CNS toxicity and have a tachycardic response when a local anesthetic and epinephrine test dose is initially injected. In the anesthetized pediatric patient, early signs of intravascular injection from a test dose can be EKG changes, such as peaked T waves or increased blood pressure.[35] Sensitivity and specificity of test dosing in pediatric patients under anesthesia, however, have not been conclusive and do not provide early warning signs of rapid local anesthetic intravascular absorption.[34] Pediatric patients at highest risk for severe LAST seem to be infants less than 6 month old, with all incidences associated with bolus dosing.[22] Some investigators advocate a 30% reduction in local anesthetic dosing in this population.[33]

Compartment syndrome

Compartment syndrome is a serious orthopedic emergency which, if unrecognized, can result in muscle ischemia or limb loss. Regional anesthesia often has been avoided in orthopedic patients with fractures due to the possibility of masking early signs of ensuing compartment syndrome. Classic signs include pain, pallor, paresthesia, paralysis, and pulselessness. The sensitivity and positive predictive value of these signs in children, however, are low. Some suggest signs of increased agitation, anxiety, and analgesia requirements are more useful in children.[36]

Currently, there is no evidence suggesting that regional anesthesia would delay the diagnosis of compartment syndrome in children. Increasing breakthrough pain from a working regional anesthetic, however, may be pathognomonic for acute compartment syndrome. Strategies to minimize complications include identifying high-risk patients, such as those undergoing tibial compartment surgery; using dilute solutions of local anesthetics and cautious use of additives to decrease the density of the block; appropriate monitoring of symptoms; and measurement of compartment pressure if compartment syndrome is suspected.[37,38]

SPECIAL CONSIDERATIONS FOR SELECT PEDIATRIC ORTHOPEDIC SURGERIES
Fractures and Trauma

An orthopedic fracture is one of the most common reasons for a pediatric emergency department visit. In one epidemiology study, the most common fracture in the pediatric population involves the forearm accounting for 17.8%, followed by the finger and the wrist. Few of these patients require anesthetic care, because only 1 of 18 fractures required hospitalization.[39] In contrast, of the pediatric traumas requiring inpatient care, femur fractures were the most common orthopedic injury, accounting for 21.7% of fractures, followed by tibia/fibula fractures (21.5%), humerus fractures (17%), and radius/ulna fractures (14.7%). These trauma patients have on average 3 concomitant injuries. Patients with pelvis or vertebral fractures have on average 5 concomitant injuries.[40] For infants presenting with a fracture, nonaccidental trauma should be considered because it accounts for approximately 25% of fractures under 1 year of age.[41]

Anesthetic care for pediatric orthopedic traumas should begin with a review of concomitant injuries. Potential intracranial, cervical, chest, or abdominal injuries should be evaluated. Bleeding and hypovolemia need to be assessed. Urgency of the orthopedic surgery must be determined and may take precedence over appropriate presurgical fasting times, thus placing patients at risk for aspiration during induction of anesthesia. Therefore, airway management with a rapid-sequence intubation may be needed. Pain management with a regional anesthetic should be discussed because it may interfere with postoperative evaluation of nerve injury and motor function.

Slipped Capital Femoral Epiphysis

Slipped capital femoral epiphysis (SCFE) is a common hip disorder of adolescence. There is a gradual or acute displacement of the femoral head from the femoral neck through the physis. Patients present with a limp and pain in the groin, anterior thigh, or knee. The average age of diagnosis is 12 years to 13 years, corresponding to a growth spurt.[42] Typical patients are obese, with approximately half of patients above the 95th percentile in weight.[43,44] SCFE is classified as stable or unstable based on the ability to bear weight. Surgical management usually involves in situ screw fixation to prevent further slippage.[42]

Anesthetic management may require a rapid-sequence intubation if a patient presents emergently. Underlying obstructive sleep apnea associated with obesity may make postoperative opioids problematic. A multimodal approach to pain management can reduce opioid requirements. Central or peripheral regional techniques have been used for pain management as well.

Club foot

Congenital club foot is a common deformity that is usually treated with the Ponseti method, which involves a series of foot manipulation and casting, an Achilles tenotomy, and bracing.[45] A percutaneous Achilles tenotomy is needed 80% to 90% of the time. It is performed at a mean age of 9.5 weeks, with a range of 4 weeks to 12 weeks of age.[45]

The Achilles tenotomy can be performed in an office on an awake infant with local anesthetics or in the operating room under anesthesia. Various methods of anesthesia have been used, including sedation, general anesthesia, and spinal anesthesia.[45–48] Caution for postoperative apnea regardless of anesthetic type should be taken for patients born full term but less than 30 days old or born preterm and less than 60 weeks postconceptual age.[49] Extended hospital stay or overnight stay should be planned in this subset of patients.

For club foot requiring more extensive surgery, postoperative pain is of concern. Anesthesia care usually involves general anesthesia combined with a neuraxial or sciatic block.

Scoliosis—Posterior Spinal Fusion

The anesthetic management of a patient undergoing posterior spinal fusion for scoliosis surgery is complex and extensive. Some issues are discussed, although this section is not meant to be comprehensive.

Neuromonitoring

Paralysis or sensory loss is one of the most devastating complications associated with scoliosis surgery. There are various causes for neural injury, including direct cord or nerve injury from instrumentation and pedicle screws, stretch injury from deformity correction, and spinal cord ischemia from poor perfusion.[50] Spinal cord and nerve root injuries have been reported to be between 0.26% and 1.75% for idiopathic scoliosis.[50] Intraoperative neuromonitoring allows for early detection of possible nerve injury, giving the surgeon and anesthesiologist a chance to reverse the cause of injury.

Neuromonitoring usually combines somatosensory evoked potentials (SSEPs), motor evoked potentials (MEPs), and electromyography. SSEPs involve peripheral nerve stimulation and measuring responses via scalp electrodes. MEPs involve transcranial stimulation of the motor cortex and tracking responses peripherally. Electromyography can monitor nerve roots during manipulation and instrumentation. Most anesthetic agents depress neuromonitoring signals, with inhalational anesthetics doing so to a greater extent. IV anesthetics are often used to minimize use of inhalational anesthetics.[51]

The wake-up test is the gold standard and still has a role intraoperatively. The wake-up test assesses gross motor function and may be used to confirm persistent SSEP and MEP changes.[51] The depth of anesthesia is reduced to allow patients to follow commands to move upper and lower extremities. Risks of extubation, intraoperative recall, and air embolism exist.

Blood management strategies

The anesthesiologist must be prepared for large blood loss and hemodynamic instability during scoliosis correction surgery. There are large areas of bone bleeding and constant venous oozing at osteotomy sites and around screws.[52] Identification of high-risk patients is crucial. Blood loss is estimated to be approximately 750 mL to 1500 mL for posterior spinal fusion for idiopathic scoliosis or 65 mL to 150 mL per vertebral level. Patients with cerebral palsy have slightly elevated blood loss of 1300 mL to 2200 mL or 100 mL to 190 mL per vertebral level. Duchenne muscular dystrophy patients have the highest blood loss of 2500 mL to 4000 mL or 200 mL to 280 mL per vertebral level.[53] Other factors associated with increased blood loss include male gender, degree of kyphosis, operative time, lower body mass index, number of levels fused, and Cobb angle greater than 50°.[54–56] Rate of blood loss was shown to be greatest during the reduction and deformity correction stage at 9.08 mL/min for idiopathic scoliosis versus 3.43 mL/min during exposure, 5.05 mL/min during screw placement, and 3.28 mL/min during closure.[52]

Several strategies are used to decrease blood loss and transfusion of allogenic blood products, including preoperative iron or erythropoietin, preoperative autologous blood donation, and intraoperative blood salvage. Strategies used by the anesthesiologist include controlled hypotension, normovolemic hemodilution, and use of antifibrinolytic agents. Controlled hypotension has been shown to decrease blood loss, although increases the risk of poor end-organ perfusion, including the spinal cord. Hemodilution techniques involve removing and storing patient's blood and replacing it with crystalloid/colloid prior to start of surgery. Fewer red cells are lost during surgical blood loss, and patient's own blood can be transfused intraoperatively when needed. Antifibrinolytic agents, such as epsilon-aminocaproic acid and tranexamic acid inhibit the degradation of fibrin. Their use have been shown to decrease intraoperative blood loss as well. Of these techniques, intraoperative blood salvage and antifibrinolytic agents are the most widely used.[57,58]

Positioning related injuries

Careful positioning of patients is paramount to reducing adverse events. Padding on pressure points from bony prominences is needed to minimize skin breakdown. Peripheral neuropathies, such as brachial plexopathy and ulnar nerve injury, usually are due to stretch or compression injury due to positioning.[59,60] Care must be taken to reevaluate the arms as positioning may change during surgery.

Visual loss

Visual loss is a rare and devastating complication. There are various causes of post-operative visual loss. Ischemic optic neuropathy, posterior greater than anterior, is the most common cause during spine surgery in the adult population.[61] It is thought to be due to decreased perfusion pressure of the optic nerve.[62] Retinal artery occlusion can be caused by direct pressure on the globe.[63] Lastly, cortical blindness is due to injury of the visual cortex, which may be prone to insult from hypoperfusion and ischemic injury to due to its watershed blood supply.[63]

Incidence of visual loss for pediatric spine surgery was estimated to be 0.29%.[62] A more recent study looking at more than 42,000 pediatric scoliosis patients found post-operative visual loss to be 0.16%.[63] Their findings showed cortical blindness as the predominant cause in the pediatric population. This contrasts with a study of predom-inantly adults where ischemic optic neuropathy accounted for 89% of visual losses in spine surgeries.[61] Risk factors for the pediatric patient included younger age, male gender, fusion of 8+ levels, and preexisting iron deficiency anemia.[63] Although there are no data supporting specific prevention strategies, it is suggested to avoid hypo-tension, anemia, increased crystalloid administration, long surgical time, and head down position.[63] Frequent checks on the eyes are needed to prevent inadvertent pres-sure on the globe.

SUMMARY

Anesthetic care for the pediatric orthopedic patients is uniquely challenging. Preoper-ative concerns include children's psychological development, heightened anxiety, and frequent predilection to respiratory infections. Pain management is an essential part of perioperative care and often involves a multimodal approach. The goal of mini-mizing opioid use is especially important given the concerns of unexpected meta-bolism of oral opioids. Regional anesthetic in the form of neuraxial or peripheral nerve blocks are valuable to combat perioperative pain. The safety in performing these blocks in the anesthetized pediatric patient has been confirmed in recent studies. Certain pediatric orthopedic surgeries can have unique anesthetic concerns. Under-standing these concerns is necessary for optimal anesthetic care and outcomes.

REFERENCES

1. Kain ZN, Mayes LC, Weisman SJ, et al. Social adaptability, cognitive abilities, and other predictors for children's reactions to surgery. J Clin Anesth 2000;12(7): 549–54.

2. Davidson AJ, Shrivastava PP, Jamsen K, et al. Risk factors for anxiety at induction of anesthesia in children: a prospective cohort study. Paediatr Anaesth 2006; 16(9):919–27.

3. Kain ZN, Wang SM, Mayes LC, et al. Distress during the induction of anesthesia and postoperative behavioral outcomes. Anesth Analg 1999;88(5):1042–7.

4. Kain ZN, Mayes LC, O'Connor TZ, et al. Preoperative anxiety in children: predic-tors and outcomes. Arch Pediatr Adolesc Med 1996;150(12):1238–45.

5. Kain ZN, Mayes LC, Caldwell-Andrews AA, et al. Preoperative anxiety, postoper-ative pain, and behavioral recovery in young children undergoing surgery. Pedi-atrics 2006;118(2):651–8.

6. Kain ZN, Mayes LC, Wang SM, et al. Postoperative behavioral outcomes in chil-dren: effects of sedative premedication. Anesthesiology 1999;90(3):758–65.

7. Gulur P, Kain ZN, Fortier MA. Psychological aspects of pediatric anesthesia. In: Davis PJ, Cladis FP, editors. Smith's anesthesia for infants and children. 9th edition. St Louis (MO): Elsevier; 2017. p. 275–7.
8. Becke K. Anesthesia in children with a cold. Curr Opin Anaesthesiol 2012;25(3): 333–9.
9. Regli A, Becke K, von Ungern-Sternberg BS. An update on the perioperative management of children with upper respiratory tract infections. Curr Opin Anaesthesiol 2017;30(3):362–7.
10. Tait AR, Malviya S, Voepel-Lewis T, et al. Risk factors for perioperative adverse respiratory events in children with upper respiratory tract infections. Anesthesiology 2001;95(2):299–306.
11. Tait AR, Malviya S. Anesthesia for the child with an upper respiratory tract infection: still a dilemma? Anesth Analg 2005;100(1):59–65.
12. Deutsch N, Ohliger S, Motoyama EK, et al. Induction, maintenance, and recovery. In: Davis PJ, Cladis FP, editors. Smith's anesthesia for infants and children. 9th edition. St Louis (MO): Elsevier; 2017. p. 375–6.
13. Schwartz D, Connelly NR, Gutta S, et al. Early intravenous cannulation in children during sevoflurane induction. Paediatr Anaesth 2004;14(10):820–4.
14. Kraemer FW, Rose JB. Pharmacologic management of acute pediatric pain. Anesthesiol Clin 2009;27:241–68.
15. Jozwiak-Bebenista M, Nowak JZ. Paracetamol: mechanism of action, applications and safety concern. Acta Pol Pharm 2014;71(1):11–23.
16. Kokki H. Nonsteroidal anti-Inflammatory drugs for postoperative pain. a focus on children. Paediatr Drugs 2003;5(2):103–23.
17. Vitale MG, Choe JC, Hwang MW, et al. Use of ketorolac tromethamine in children undergoing scoliosis surgery. an analysis of complications. Spine J 2003;3(1): 55–62.
18. Monitto CL, yaster M, Kost-Byerly S. Pain management. In: Davis PJ, Cladis FP, editors. Smith's anesthesia for infants and children. 9th edition. St Louis (MO): Elsevier; 2017. p. 437–8.
19. Crews KR, Gaedigk A, Dunnenberger HM, et al. Clinical pharmacogenetics implementation consortium guidelines for cytochrome P450 2D6 genotype and codeine therapy: 2014 update. Clin Pharmacol Ther 2014;95(4):376–82.
20. US Food and Drug Administration. Safety review update of codeine use in children; new Boxed Warning and Contraindication on use after tonsillectomy and/or adenoidectomy. In: FDA Drug Safety Communications. 2013. Available at: https://www.fda.gov/downloads/Drugs/DrugSafety/UCM339116.pdf. Accessed February 14, 2019.
21. US Food and Drug Administration. FDA restricts use of prescription codeine pain and cough medicines and tramadol pain medicines in children; recommends against use in breastfeeding women. In: FDA Drug Safety Communication. 2017. Available at: https://www.fda.gov/Drugs/DrugSafety/ucm549679.htm. Accessed February 14, 2019.
22. Walker BJ, Long JB, Sathyamoorthy M, et al. Complications in pediatric regional anesthesia: an analysis of more than 100,000 blocks from the Pediatric Regional Anesthesia Network. Anesthesiology 2018;129(4):721–32.
23. Suresh S, Long J, Birmingham PK, et al. Are caudal blocks for pain control safe in children? An analysis of 18,650 caudal blocks from the Pediatric Regional Anesthesia Network (PRAN) database. Anesth Analg 2015;120(1):151–6.
24. Kao SC, Lin CS. Caudal epidural block: an updated review of anatomy and techniques. Biomed Res Int 2017;2017:9217145.

25. Bernards CM. Epidural and spinal anesthesia. In: Barash PG, Cullen BF, Stoelting RK, et al, editors. Clinical anesthesia. 6th edition. Philadelphia: Lippincott Williams & Wilkins; 2009. p. 934–6.

26. Lam DK, Corry GN, Tsui BC. Evidence for the use of ultrasound imaging in pediatric regional anesthesia: a systematic review. Reg Anesth Pain Med 2016;41(2): 229–41.

27. Guay J, Suresh S, Kopp S. The use of ultrasound guidance for perioperative neuraxial and peripheral nerve blocks in children: a cochrane review. Anesth Analg 2017;124(3):948–58.

28. Flack S, Lang RS. Regional anesthesia. In: Davis PJ, Cladis FP, editors. Smith's anesthesia for infants and children. 9th edition. St Louis (MO): Elsevier; 2017. p. 487–506.

29. Gray AF, Collins AB, Eilers H. Peripheral nerve blocks. In: Stoelting RK, Miller RD, editors. Basics of anesthesia. 5th edition. Philadelphia: Churchill Livingstone; 2007. p. 276–86.

30. Neal JM, Bernards CM, Hadzic A, et al. ASRA practice advisory on neurologic complications in regional anesthesia and pain medicine. Reg Anesth Pain Med 2008;33(5):404–15.

31. Taenzer AH, Walker BJ, Bosenberg AT, et al. Asleep versus awake: does it matter?: pediatric regional block complications by patient state: a report from the Pediatric Regional Anesthesia Network. Reg Anesth Pain Med 2014;39(4): 279–83.

32. Liu SS, Lin Y. Local anesthetics. In: Barash PG, Cullen BF, Stoelting RK, et al, editors. Clinical anesthesia. 6th edition. Philadelphia: Lippincott Williams & Wilkins; 2009. p. 542–4.

33. Suresh S, Polaner DM, Cote CJ. Regional anesthesia. In: Cote CJ, Lerman J, Anderson BJ, editors. A practice of anesthesia for infants and children. 6th edition. Philadelphia: Elsevier; 2019. p. 943–5.

34. Lönnqvist PA. Toxicity of local anesthetic drugs: a pediatric perspective. Paediatr Anaesth 2012;22(1):39–43.

35. Polaner DM, Zuk J, Luong K, et al. Positive intravascular test dose criteria in children during total intravenous anesthesia with propofol and remifentanil are different than during inhaled anesthesia. Anesth Analg 2010;110(1):41–5.

36. Lin JS, Balch Samora J. Pediatric acute compartment syndrome: a systematic review and meta-analysis. J Pediatr Orthop B 2019. Available at: https://journals.lww.com/jpo-b/Abstract/publishahead/Pediatric_acute_compartment_syndrome__a_systematic.98946.aspx. Accessed February 14, 2019.

37. Gadsden J, Warlick A. Regional anesthesia for the trauma patient: improving patient outcomes. Local Reg Anesth 2015;8:45–55.

38. Lönnqvist PA, Ecoffey C, Bosenberg A, et al. The European society of regional anesthesia and pain therapy and the American society of regional anesthesia and pain medicine joint committee practice advisory on controversial topics in pediatric regional anesthesia I and II: what do they tell us? Curr Opin Anaesthesiol 2017;5:613–20.

39. Naranje SM, Erali RA, Warner WC Jr, et al. Epidemiology of pediatric fractures presenting to emergency departments in the United States. J Pediatr Orthop 2016;36(4):e45–8.

40. Galano GJ, Vitale MA, Kessler MW, et al. The most frequent traumatic orthopaedic injuries from a national pediatric inpatient population. J Pediatr Orthop 2005; 25(1):39–44.

41. Flaherty EG, Perez-Rossello JM, Levine MA, et al. Evaluating children with fractures for child physical abuse. Pediatrics 2014;133(2):e477–89.
42. Purcell D, Varthi A, Lee MC. Slipped capital femoral epiphysis: current concepts review. Curr Orthop Pract 2011;22(1):81–9.
43. Aronsson DD, Loder RT, Breur GJ, et al. Slipped capital femoral epiphysis: current concepts. J Am Acad Orthop Surg 2006;14(12):666–79.
44. Aversano MW, Moazzaz P, Scaduto AA, et al. Association between body mass index-for-age and slipped capital femoral epiphysis: the long-term risk for subsequent slip in patients followed until physeal closure. J Child Orthop 2016;10(3): 209–13.
45. Radler C. The Ponseti method for the treatment of congenital club foot: review of the current literature and treatment recommendations. Int Orthop 2013;37(9): 1747–53.
46. Parada SA, Baird GO, Auffant RA, et al. Safety of percutaneous tendoachilles tenotomy performed under general anesthesia on infants with idiopathic clubfoot. J Pediatr Orthop 2009;29(8):916–9.
47. Tobias JD, Mencio GA. Regional anesthesia for clubfoot surgery in children. Am J Ther 1998;5(4):273–7.
48. AlSuhebani M, Martin DP, Relland LM, et al. Spinal anesthesia instead of general anesthesia for infants undergoing tendon Achilles lengthening. Local Reg Anesth 2018;3(11):25–9.
49. Ghazal EA, Vadi MG, Mason LJ, et al. Preoperative evaluation, premedication, and induction of anesthesia. In: Cote CJ, Lerman J, Anderson BJ, editors. A practice of anesthesia for infants and children. 6th edition. Philadelphia: Elsevier; 2019. p. 64–6.
50. Murphy RF, Mooney JF III. Complications following spine fusion for adolescent idiopathic scoliosis. Curr Rev Musculoskelet Med 2016;9(4):462–9.
51. Strike SA, Hassanzadeh H, Jain A, et al. Intraoperative neuromonitoring in pediatric and adult spine deformity surgery. Clin Spine Surg 2017;30(9):E1174–81.
52. Wahlquist S, Wongworawat M, Nelson S. When does intraoperative blood loss occur during pediatric scoliosis correction? Spine Deform 2017;5(6):387–91.
53. Shapiro F, Sethna N. Blood loss in pediatric spine surgery. Eur Spine J 2004; 13(Suppl 1):S6–17.
54. Ialenti MN, Lonner BS, Verma K, et al. Predicting operative blood loss during spinal fusion for adolescent idiopathic scoliosis. J Pediatr Orthop 2013;33(4): 372–6.
55. Yu X, Xiao H, Wang R, et al. Prediction of massive blood loss in scoliosis surgery from preoperative variables. Spine 2013;38(4):350–5.
56. Kim HJ, Park HS, Jang MJ, et al. Predicting massive transfusion in adolescent idiopathic scoliosis patients undergoing corrective surgery: association of preoperative radiographic findings. Medicine 2018;97(22):e10972.
57. Oetgen ME, Litrenta J. Perioperative blood management in pediatric spine surgery. J Am Acad Orthop Surg 2017;25(7):480–8.
58. Wilton NC, Anderson BJ. Orthopedic and spine surgery. In: Cote CJ, Lerman J, Anderson BJ, editors. A practice of anesthesia for infants and children. 6th edition. Philadelphia: Elsevier; 2019. p. 741–3.
59. Schwartz DM, Drummond DS, Hahn M, et al. Prevention of positional brachial plexopathy during surgical correction of scoliosis. J Spinal Disord 2000;13(2): 178–82.
60. Kamel I, Barnette R. Positioning patients for spine surgery: avoiding uncommon position-related complications. World J Orthop 2014;5(4):425–43.

61. Lee LA, Roth S, Posner KL, et al. The American Society of Anesthesiologists Post-operative Visual Loss Registry: analysis of 93 spine surgery cases with postoperative visual loss. Anesthesiology 2006;105(4):652–9.
62. Patil CG, Lad EM, Lad SP, et al. Visual loss after spine surgery: a population-based study. Spine 2008;33(13):1491–6.
63. De la Garza-Ramos R, Samdani AF, Sponseller PD, et al. Visual loss after corrective surgery for pediatric scoliosis: incidence and risk factors from a nationwide database. Spine J 2016;16(4):516–22.

Congenital Deformities of the Hands

Alice Chu, MD*, Jason Chan, MD, Omkar Baxi, MD

KEYWORDS

- Pediatric hand • Congenital deformity • Upper extremity • Syndactyly
- Thumb duplication

KEY POINTS

- Evaluation of the pediatric musculoskeletal system may be difficult because of differences between children and adults.
- As children mature, their physical structure approaches that of an adult.
- Varying stages of ossification and developmental timelines may confuse the average clinician.

BRACHIAL PLEXUS INJURIES

Obstetric brachial plexus palsy can have differing presentations and natural history depending on the extent of injury. In general, most birth palsies result in a traction neuropraxia that is expected to resolve spontaneously over time. However, injuries resulting in avulsion of the brachial plexus nerve roots have minimal expected recovery and may benefit from surgical intervention to improve upper extremity function.[1] The overall incidence of brachial plexus birth injury is reported at 0.38 to 1.56 per 1000 live births with risk factors including macrosomia, maternal diabetes, prolonged labor, breech delivery, shoulder dystocia, and difficult delivery requiring assistive devices.[2,3]

Plexus injury is described in several ways, with anatomic descriptions indicating the level of nerve roots involved or the location of expected injury within the plexus branching pattern. The pathophysiology and expected recovery of the injury are described with the Sunderland classification. This includes neurapraxia, axonotmesis, neurotmesis, and avulsion. Although neurapraxia and axonotmesis injuries are expected to recover spontaneously, neurotmesis and avulsion injuries are expected to require surgical intervention. Narakas and Slooff have classified plexus injuries into 4 categories: type 1 describes the mildest injury pattern with C5-6 injury and the classic presentation of Erb palsy with the arm held adducted, internally

Department of Orthopedics, Doctor's Office Center, 90 Bergen Street, Newark, NJ 07101-1709, USA
* Corresponding author.
E-mail address: a_chuparrott@yahoo.com

Pediatr Clin N Am 67 (2020) 85–99
https://doi.org/10.1016/j.pcl.2019.09.011
0031-3955/20/© 2019 Elsevier Inc. All rights reserved.

rotated, and extended at the elbow; type 2 describes the extended Erb palsy with C5-7 involvement indicated by the loss of wrist and finger extension; type 3 describes a flail extremity; and type 4 includes infants with an associated Horner syndrome.[1,4]

Radiographs of the affected extremity provide useful information because clavicular fractures may occur with brachial plexus injury, whereas a humeral fracture may mimic a plexus injury. The diagnosis of brachial plexus injury remains primarily based on serial physical examinations documenting the extent of injury and recovery potential. Return of biceps function by 6 months of age is an indicator of prognosis, as well as a means of determining need for microsurgical treatment. Near-complete recovery can be expected in patients who have return of antigravity biceps function at well younger than 6 months of age. On the other hand, patients with upper trunk palsy, without any biceps function at or approaching 6 months, may benefit from surgical intervention.[5] Patients with partial biceps recovery represent a more complicated cohort because functional limitations are expected, but the best treatment strategy remains controversial. The identification of global palsy, Horner syndrome, an elevated hemidiaphragm, or a winged scapula are predictors of a preganglionic avulsion injury that will not resolve. These may be reasons to intervene with earlier microsurgery by 3 months of age.

Although the specific surgical interventions are beyond the scope of this work, preganglionic or avulsion injuries cannot be treated with nerve repair. One surgical technique is the use of nerve transfers, most commonly taking the intercostal nerves or spinal accessory nerve as donors for needed recipient nerves. Postganglionic injuries requiring surgical intervention can be treated with either nerve transfers or primary nerve repair and grafting, depending on surgeon preference and extent of injury[1] (**Fig. 1**). Nerve transfers are gaining popularity, as they allow targeting of specific muscles, a shorter recovery time, and the ability to delay surgical timing.[6–9] Antigravity motor function may return as quickly as 3 to 6 months postoperatively. If unsuccessful, further intervention with tendon transfers may be indicated. The outcomes of specific surgical interventions for birth-related brachial plexus palsy are poorly described because of the wide variety in pathology and surgical technique. However, for patients with absence of antigravity biceps at

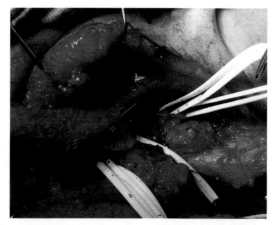

Fig. 1. Brachial plexus dissection. On the left, the clavicle is retracted with a Raytec sponge; on the upper right, the C5 and C6 nerve roots have been isolated.

6 months, microsurgical intervention seems to result in better recovery than natural progression alone.

CONGENITAL RADIAL HEAD DISLOCATION

Congenital radial head dislocation is an atraumatic dislocation of the radiocapitellar joint that is often bilateral. It occurs due to dysmorphic changes in the capitellum and radial head[10] and is the most common congenital anomaly of the elbow.[11] The genetic etiology is unclear, but it has been postulated that congenital radial head dislocation can be related to 2 major pathways: structural weakness in the annular ligaments (eg, collagen abnormalities) versus abnormal contact pressures about the radiocapitellar joint causing malformation of radial head and/or capitellum.[12] In approximately one-third of cases, congenital radial head dislocation is associated with other skeletal dysplasias, such as radioulnar synostosis, ulnar dysplasia, and syndromes such as Klinefelter, Cornelia de Lange, Ehlers-Danlos, and nail patella syndrome.[12]

At presentation, patients may have loss of elbow extension but will certainly have minimal forearm rotation. Presentation for evaluation is often delayed until a child is noticed having difficulty with activities of daily living. Findings on physical examination depend on direction of dislocation. Anterior dislocation will have a palpable radial head in the cubital fossa. If dislocated posteriorly, the radial head is palpated lateral to the capitellum.[11] It is important to distinguish between congenital and traumatic etiologies. Traumatic dislocation is almost always associated with known trauma, has normally formed osseous structures, and is rarely bilateral. Congenital dislocation is often bilateral and has associated shortened ulna as well as dysplastic-appearing radial head. On radiographic examination of the elbow, radiocapitellar dislocation can be identified through a line drawn along the axis of the radius that does not intersect with the capitellum.[13] In congenital cases, the radial head is dome shaped, the ulna is bowed and short, there is dysplasia of the capitellum, and there may be ulnar-positive variance of the wrist. In unclear cases, MRI may be obtained. Congenital dislocation will typically have an intact joint capsule, whereas traumatic dislocation will typically have a torn joint capsule.[10] Classification is based on direction of dislocation (Bado).

Treatment includes observation, reduction plus or minus annular ligament repair, or radial head excision. Observation is preferred, as children tend to have minimal functional limitations.[14] Reduction with annular ligament repair, although an option, has had poor outcomes.[15] In adulthood, patients may develop pain and require radial head excision. This has demonstrated significant improvement in pain; however, up to 25% of patients require reoperations because of development of wrist pain.[16]

CONGENITAL TRIGGER THUMB

Pediatric trigger thumb is an acquired triggering of the thumb caused by a mismatch in size of the flexor pollicis longus and the A1 pulley of the thumb.[17] It is a stenosing tenosynovitis of the flexor pollicis longus (FPL) tendon. The term congenital is a misnomer, as many studies have shown that trigger thumb is absent at birth and thus is developmental in nature.[18,19] Pediatric trigger thumb should not be confused with adult trigger thumb, which has a different anatomic cause.[20,21]

Patients typically present at approximately 2 years of age. There may not be a history of triggering, but patients often hold their thumb in a fixed, flexed position at the interphalangeal joint. Physical examination may elicit clicking or popping at the joint or simply a thumb held in flexion with difficulty in extension. There may be a palpable mass on the volar side of at the level of the metacarpophalangeal joint, known as a Notta nodule. A quarter of patients have bilateral triggering. Radiographs do not need to be obtained, as this is a clinical diagnosis. In addition, this diagnosis should not be confused with congenital clasped thumb, which is flexed at the metacarpophalangeal joint.

Conservative, nonsurgical management includes splinting and passive extension exercises. However, although improvement in range of motion was reported in multiple studies, results are inconclusive.[22,23] Patients may be observed until up to 3 years old, if the parents desire. If spontaneous resolution does not occur, then surgical release of the A1 pulley of the thumb has shown good results with low rates of recurrence.[24]

MADELUNG DEFORMITY

Madelung deformity of the wrist is characterized by a radius that is shortened and curved ulnarly and volarly. The ulna is typically subluxated dorsally and is very prominent, accentuated by a volar sag of the hand and wrist.[25] It is most often found in adolescent girls more than boys from approximately 6 years to 13 years, going unnoticed prior, but becoming more prominent as the patient grows.[26]

Madelung deformity is usually congenital, but can be acquired. It is caused by an abnormal growth arrest on the ulnar and volar aspect of the distal radial physis causing these areas to become relatively shortened as the patient grows.[26] In congenital cases, an abnormal ligament (Vickers ligament) that runs on the palmar side of the wrist, tethering the lunate to the volar-ulnar aspect of the distal radius is thought to contribute to the deformity.[27] Acquired deformity can be caused by prior trauma, repetitive loading or infection, and lesions such as osteochondroma or multiple hereditary exostosis causing the distal radial growth arrest. These causes are not associated with a Vickers ligament. There is an association with Leri-Weill dyschondrosis.[26]

At presentation, most common chief complaints are either diffuse pain or concern about the cosmetic appearance of the distal ulna prominence, and may be bilateral. Physical examination demonstrates dorsally prominent distal ulna, dorsal concavity laterally of the distal radius, and a proportionately short forearm.[26] Range of motion may be decreased in extension and ulnar deviation. However, there is not typically a significant loss of function. Radiographic analysis will show that the distal radius is deviated ulnar and volar with a dorsally subluxed distal ulna.[28] MRI may be obtained to evaluate for the presence of Vickers ligament.

Treatment is not necessarily required in painless deformity, but one may consider Vickers ligament excision and physiolysis in skeletally immature patients who are asymptomatic to prevent progression of deformity. In cases of painful deformity, the conservative treatment includes activity modification, nonsteroidal anti-inflammatory medication, and splinting. If conservative management fails and the patient continues to have pain, treatment is dictated by skeletal maturity.[29] In the skeletally immature, as in asymptomatic cases, surgical management may be physiolysis with release of Vickers ligament, combined with distal ulna epiphysiodesis. Vickers and Nielsen[27] reported that all skeletally immature patients who underwent physiolysis had improvement of pain symptoms as well as improved range of motion and subjective appearance of deformity. Symptomatic patients who are skeletally mature can be treated with a corrective radial osteotomy and may need an additional corrective ulnar osteotomy. In a series reported by Harley and colleagues,[30] all patients had improved radiographic parameters, increased range of motion, and improvement of pain.

PHALANGEAL NECK FRACTURES

Phalangeal neck fractures happen mostly in the pediatric population. They account for approximately 1% to 14% of all hand fractures in children.[31] In younger children (1–3 years), injuries are attributed to crush-type mechanism. In older children, phalangeal neck fractures are more often attributed to events occurring during sports.[32,33] Phalangeal neck fractures typically occur at border digits.[32] They are unique compared with other phalanx fractures because of the lower remodeling potential due to the distance of the fracture in relationship to the physis.[34] They often heal with unsatisfactory alignment if treated nonoperatively[31] (**Fig. 2**).

The patient often reports a history of trauma to the finger. The timing of injury should be elicited, as subacute presentation may mean healing has occurred. In the acute setting, there is tenderness to palpation and swelling about the injured site. Lack of tenderness to palpation may suggest that fracture healing has already occurred and an open procedure would be needed to reset the bone. Inspection of the hand will reveal decreased range of motion of the joint with inability to make a full fist.

Radiographs, including anteroposterior, oblique, and lateral, of the hand should be obtained. Fluoroscopy may be helpful if unable to visualize the injured digit well. Advanced imaging such as computed tomography is usually not required. Al-Qattan[32] classified these fractures in the following manner: type 1, nondisplaced; type 2, displaced but with maintained bone-to-bone contact with proximal segment; and type 3, loss of bone-to-bone contact and 3a, 90° rotation of fragment, 3b, 180° rotation of fragment, 3c, complete dorsal displacement of fragment, and 3d, complete volar displacement of fragment.

In acute fractures, nondisplaced fractures without coronal or rotational deformities are treated conservatively with splinting or cast immobilization for 3 to 4 weeks.[33,35] Displaced fractures require closed reduction and percutaneous pinning.[36] If the closed reduction is unsuccessful, then reduction using percutaneous osteoclasis followed by percutaneous pinning should be attempted. If this is unsuccessful, surgery should progress with open reduction and percutaneous pinning.

In healed fractures with mild extension deformity, if remodeling criteria are met, no coronal or rotation malalignment, congruent adjacent interphalangeal joint, bony union

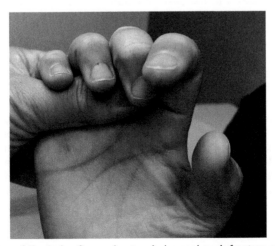

Fig. 2. Malrotation of the index finger due to phalangeal neck fracture malunion.

achieved, significant remaining growth potential, patient tolerates decrease in adjacent joint movement, and patient/family amenable to follow-up, the patient may be allowed a chance to remodel the fracture.[37] If these criteria are not met, then percutaneous osteoclasis may be performed to aid in reduction. If this is unsuccessful, then an open procedure with osteotomy may be required to attain adequate reduction.[33]

RADIAL DEFICIENCY

One of the most common forms of forearm malformation is radial longitudinal deficiency with a reported incidence of 1 in 30,000 to 100,000 live births.[38] The limb bud develops concurrently with the renal and cardiac systems, resulting in associated conditions involving multiple organs.[39] VACTERL syndrome describes a constellation of developmental deformities occurring at a similar time during embryonic development, including vertebral anomaly, anal atresia, cardiac anomaly, tracheal and esophageal anomaly, renal abnormality, and limb deficiency.[38] Holt-Oram syndrome describes cardiac defects with upper extremity malformations, whereas TAR syndrome describes thrombocytopenia, anemia, and an absent radius. TAR is unique with its upper extremity presentation, as the thumb is preserved despite the radial deficiency. Timely diagnosis of radial deficiency is critical to evaluate for these diseases and allow early treatment. In particular, Fanconi anemia results in bone marrow failure and a fatal aplastic anemia. Early diagnosis can allow more time to find a bone marrow donor and prevent mortality. All patients with radial deficiency should be screened with renal ultrasounds, echocardiograms, laboratory analysis, chromosomal analysis, and consultation with a geneticist.[38,39]

Classification of radial deficiency was originally based on the length of residual radius within the Bayne and Klug classification. With the James modification of the Bayne and Klug classification, the thumb, carpus, and proximal radius are also evaluated, but the distinguishing factor remains the variability of the distal radius.[40] Type 0 radial deficiency describes a normal radius with hypoplasia of the carpus or thumb. Type 1 arms have a distal radius slightly shorter than the distal ulna, whereas type 2 arms have a hypoplastic distal and proximal radius. Type 3 radial deficiency describes an absent physis of the distal radius, whereas type 4 deficiency has a completely absent radius.[40] In addition to the skeletal deformity, the radial soft tissues are also involved with absence of the radial wrist extensors, extrinsic thumb muscles, and frequently the radial nerve and radial artery.

Treatment of mild radial deficiency in type 1 or mild type 2 may simply involve soft tissue stretching of the radial forearm or tendon transfers and soft tissue releases if the radial deviation is severe.[41] In cases of more severe deficiency, including severe type 2 and type 3 arms, centralization of the carpus on the ulna is preferred.[42] However, careful evaluation of the elbow must be performed, as centralization is contraindicated in patients with elbow contracture because the radially deviated position of the wrist allows hand to mouth motion in these children. Centralization is performed by incising over the wrist capsule, freeing the radial carpus from any soft tissue contractures, and reducing and pinning the third metacarpal and carpus onto the distal ulna.[43] In cases in which the carpus cannot be easily reduced onto the ulna, some surgeons prefer soft tissue release and best possible centralization, whereas others will advocate for partial carpectomy and limited shaving of the ulnar epiphysis to ease the reduction.[39] Regardless of the technical procedure, treatment of radial deficiency remains difficult, with recurrence of the radial deviation almost universally, if wrist motion is not sacrificed.[44]

SEYMOUR FRACTURE

Phalangeal fractures in the pediatric population are common and account for a large number of emergency room visits in the United States with a historical incidence of 185 fractures per 100,000 patients aged 5 to 14 years.[45] Crush injuries to the pediatric hand are likely to result in tuft fractures, which can be managed with alumifoam splints or casting if minimally displaced. Although the vast majority of these fractures can be treated conservatively, practitioners need to be vigilant for the Seymour fracture, which represents an open injury to the phalangeal physis.[46] The epiphysis of the distal phalanx ossifies at approximately 16 to 30 months of age, after the appearance of the proximal and middle phalanx epiphyses; however, physeal closure proceeds from distal to proximal beginning at 14 years of age.[47] Presence of subungual hematoma should raise the possibility of a Seymour fracture and should be investigated with nail-plate removal and examination for nailbed injury. In addition, radiographs should be carefully assessed to compare the physeal width between the injured and non-injured distal phalanges; a widened physis and apex dorsal angulation is evident in the Seymour fracture and represents possible interposition of the nailbed into the physeal fracture.

Once recognized, the Seymour fracture should be treated as an open fracture with administration of prophylactic antibiotics and thorough debridement of fracture edges, removal of the interposed nailbed tissue, and fracture reduction with Kirschner wire immobilization as necessary.[47] To fully visualize the fracture, the nailplate should be removed and small longitudinal incisions are created at both corners of the nailfold to retract the dorsal nailfold. Care is taken to preserve the insertion of the terminal extensor tendon onto the distal phalanx epiphysis. Once the interposed tissue is removed, the distal phalanx is reduced and pinned to provide a stable base for nailbed repair with fine suture. Classically, the nailplate is replaced to stent the nailfold and prevent synechiae formation, although this traditional teaching is being questioned with ongoing randomized controlled trials.[48]

Failure to recognize the Seymour fracture can lead to infection and damage to the distal phalanx physis.[49] Reyes and Ho[50] found that 31% of Seymour fractures referred to their center had delayed treatment defined as more than 24 hours to treatment and had an infection rate of 45% compared with zero in those patients receiving acute and complete treatment. Krusche-Mandl and colleagues[51] retrospectively reviewed their cohort of 24 Seymour fractures and found no infections at a follow-up of 10 years, but did note radiographic growth disturbance in 20% of their patients.

SYNDACTYLY

Syndactyly is a congenital malformation of the hands in which adjacent fingers fail to separate during development. A syndactyly is considered "simple" when fingers are connected only by skin.[52] A syndactyly is considered complex when adjacent fingers are connected via bony or cartilaginous connections.[53] Syndactyly is relatively common, occurring in 1 or 2 of 3000 births.[52] The male to female ratio is 2:1 and is bilateral in half of affected patients. Associated risk factors are maternal smoking, poor nutrition in utero, lower socioeconomic status, and increased consumption of meat and eggs during pregnancy.[54] Simple syndactyly is caused by a failure in apoptosis, whereas complex syndactyly is most likely caused by the apical ectodermal ridge persisting in inappropriate locations.[55,56]

Evaluation of syndactyly should include an examination of the entirety of the affected limb up to the chest wall to assess for additional differences. Simple syndactyly is most common between long and ring fingers (50%), second most common between ring and small fingers, and least common in the first web space.[56] Complex syndactyly is also most common between the ring and long fingers.[53] In addition, radiographs should be obtained to assess for osseous involvement in cases of complex syndactyly, an MRI or ultrasound may be obtained to assess other soft tissue involvement. The evaluation of complex syndactyly also should include screening for associated syndromes, such as Poland or Apert syndrome.[57]

Syndactyly is broadly categorized into 4 groups: simple incomplete, only soft tissue involvement without involvement of the nailfold; simple complete, only soft tissue involvement including the nailfold; complex, osseous or cartilaginous connections between digits; and complicated, anything that is more than side-to-side fusions (accessory phalanges, abnormal tendons/nerves/muscles).[52]

Syndactyly is typically treated surgically with a release at approximately 12 months of age, although timing should be on the earlier side for border digits, and later for digits of similar length (Fig. 3). The goal is to create as many functional and independent digits as possible. If multiple digits are fused, it may be prudent to perform a staged procedure to prevent vascular compromise.[54] Complications include neurovascular injury, web creep, joint contractures, nail deformities, and graft/flap failure.[55]

Apert syndrome is a brachial arch syndrome that is caused by a defect in the FGF-2 gene that is usually a sporadic occurrence, but can be inherited in an autosomal dominant fashion.[57,58] The orthopedic manifestations are characterized by acrosyndactyly, symphalangism, and thumb radial clinodactyly.[58] More broadly, the syndrome includes craniosynostosis, hyperhidrosis, decreased eyesight/hearing, strabismus, and impaired development of language/motor skills. Apert hand is categorized into 3 types (Table 1).[57] The treatment for hand deformities is often surgical, with goals to achieve adequate separation of digits, and obtain thumb function and small finger mobilization.[59]

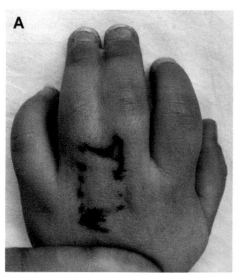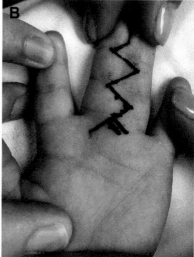

Fig. 3. (A) Simple syndactyly of the third webspace, with dorsal markings for the commissure flap. (B) Palmar appearance with reciprocal flaps outlined.

Table 1
Classification of Apert hand

Type	Description
I: spade hand	Radially deviated and small thumb. Swallow first webspace. Index/long/ring fingers with complete or complex syndactyly. Small finger with simple syndactyly
II: mitten/spoon hand	Radially deviated thumb with syndactyly with index. Index/long/ring fingers fused at tips causing curved palm
III: rosebud hand	Thumb/index/long/ring fingers distally fused with cartilaginous or bony attachments. May also be proximal fusions of fourth to fifth metacarpal and carpal fusions

THUMB DUPLICATION

Pre-axial polydactyly or thumb duplication is a congenital deformity of the hand that occurs on the radial side of the hand. It is more common in White and Asian populations, and tends to be unilateral and typically a sporadic occurrence without other associated conditions.[60] Thumb duplication occurs at a rate of 0.8 to 1.4 of 1000 births.[61] It is caused by a defect in the radial-ulnar axis that is governed by the sonic hedgehog protein that is expressed at the zone of polarizing activity.[60]

The Wassel-Flatt classification (**Table 2**) is based on the morphology of the thumb duplication. This consists of 7 types of duplicated thumbs, ranging from bifid distal phalanx to the triphalangeal thumb.[62] However, this classification does not include all possible variations of thumb duplications. In 2008, Zuidam[63] proposed the Rotterdam classification system that was found to be able to classify 100% of thumb duplication as opposed to 60% in the Wassel-Flatt system.[64] For the time being, the Wassel-Flatt classification is still the most prevalent, with type 4 being most prevalent and type 2 being second most prevalent (**Fig. 4**).

During evaluation of thumb duplication, the practitioner must closely observe the morphology as well as function. In particular, the passive motion, active motion, presence of thenar musculature, and stability of the joints to varus/valgus stress should be noted. In addition, one must observe the functionality of the digit, specifically which thumb is being used for pinch. Finally, radiographs of the hand will identify bone or joint abnormalities. The role of surgical treatment includes improvement of thumb function as well as improvement of cosmetic appearance.[61]

Table 2
Wassel-Flatt classification of thumb duplication

Classification	Description
Type 1	Bifid distal phalanx
Type 2	Duplicated distal phalanx
Type 3	Bifid proximal phalanx
Type 4	Duplicated proximal phalanx
Type 5	Bifid metacarpal
Type 6	Duplicated metacarpal
Type 7	Triphalangeal component

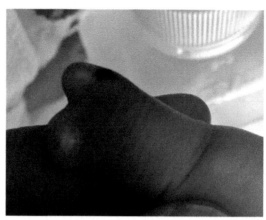

Fig. 4. Example of Wassel-Flatt type 2 thumb duplication.

Subtle type 1 and type 2 duplicated thumbs may not require surgery if they have a common nail and are properly aligned. However, most thumb duplications require operative interventions. Asymmetric thumbs can be treated by ablation of the smaller thumb (usually radial) and transfer of the radial collateral ligament and centralization of the extensor tendon to maintain adequate thumb axis.[65] Care should be exercised to identify and treat connections between the flexor and extensor tendons, as in a pollex abductus. The Bilhaut- Cloquet procedure of fusing 2 thumbs has largely fallen out of favor because of poor outcomes and cosmesis.[65] In type 3 and type 4 duplicated thumbs, exact surgical technique depends on what is found intraoperatively, but typically involves ablation of the lesser counterpart and using its soft tissues and attachments to augment the retained thumb to make it functional and aligned.[61] If the duplication is symmetric, typically the radial thumb is ablated to retain the ulnar collateral ligament (UCL) for pinch activities.[61] It is also important to take into consideration the functionality of interphalangeal joints, as this may determine which digit to keep. In higher Wassel types, operative goals remain the same, except with the added complexity of needing to reconstruct interosseous muscle attachments.

Outcomes are related to preoperative function and complexity of thumb duplication. Type 1, 2, and 4 duplications often have more satisfactory results than Type 3, 5, 6, and 7.[66] The Bilhaut-Cloquet procedure often produces a wide, stiff thumb, and is a technique that is now used only for very distal duplications.[67]

THUMB HYPOPLASIA

Thumb hypoplasia without radial deficiency can still be part of a syndromic presentation and should initiate workup for related anomalies, as discussed in the radial deficiency section.[68] The diagnosis of thumb hypoplasia can be straightforward when presenting with radial deficiency or a significantly shortened thumb. However, mild hypoplasia may present as the child grows older and begins to use his or her hand for more complex activities, such as writing and sports.[69] Knowledge of normal thumb anatomy is important for both diagnosis and as goals for thumb reconstruction: the thumb should reach just short of the index finger proximal interphalangeal joint clinically or to 70% of the index finger proximal phalanx on radiographs, whereas thumb girth should be approximately 133% of the index finger.[70]

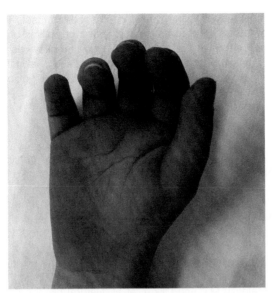

Fig. 5. Example of subtle, Blauth 2 thumb hypoplasia. Note hypoplasia of the thenar mound and diminished first webspace. The patient also had UCL laxity.

The Blauth classification of thumb hypoplasia is widely used because it helps guide diagnosis and management. Blauth class 1 thumbs have minor findings of hypoplasia and treatment is largely unnecessary. In class 2, the thumb is characterized by absence of the thenar muscles, incompetency of the UCL, and a narrow web space (**Fig. 5**). These thumbs can be reconstructed with an opposition transfer, web space deepening, and UCL reconstruction. Type 3 thumbs have further deficiencies with lack of extrinsic thumb musculature and skeletal deficiency. The critical diagnostic decision is the stability of the thumb carpometacarpal joint, as a type 3A thumb with a stable carpometacarpal (CMC) can be reconstructed satisfactorily, whereas a type 3B with an unstable CMC is best treated with ablation and pollicization.[71] Diagnosis of an unstable CMC is best accomplished by repeated clinical examination; children with unstable thumbs will frequently avoid use of the thumb and compensate with index and long finger scissor pinch. Radiographs may show a tapered thumb metacarpal but are frequently not helpful, as the trapezium will not ossify until age 6. In cases in which diagnosis is difficult, MRI or ultrasound can add further information of the presence and stability of the CMC joint.[68] Type 4 thumbs are described as "floating thumbs," with a small skin bridge connecting the hand to the remnant thumb. Type 5 hypoplasia describes a complete absence of the thumb.[71]

Pollicization of the index finger offers the best functional treatment for type 3B and higher thumb hypoplasia. Although there are variations in surgical technique, the basic scheme of pollicization converts the shortened index finger metacarpal into the new trapezium, and the index proximal phalanx into the thumb metacarpal with the middle and distal phalanges serving as the phalanges of the new thumb.[72] The extrinsic flexor and extensor tendons to the index finger serve as surrogates of the FPL and extensor pollicis longus, respectively, and do not need to be shortened as they adapt over time.[68] The index palmar interosseous muscle needs to be transferred into the ulnar lateral band of the proximal interphalangeal joint to function as the adductor pollicis. Similarly, the dorsal interosseous muscle insertion is transferred to the radial lateral band to act as the abductor pollicis brevis.[72] Outcomes of pollicization are dependent on the index finger mobility, as a mobile reconstructed thumb can allow near normal function. In cases of a stiff digit, the reconstructed thumb will act as a stable post for pinch.[72,73] The pollicization outcomes as a child generally persist into adulthood, with long-term studies showing integration of the thumb into daily life.[72,74]

REFERENCES

1. Cornwall R, Waters PM. Pediatric brachial plexus palsy. In: Wolfe SW, Hotchkiss RN, Pederson WC, et al, editors. Green's operative hand surgery. 7th edition. Amsterdam: Elsevier; 2017. p. 1391–425.
2. Foad S, Mehlman C, Ying J. The epidemiology of neonatal brachial plexus palsy in the United States. J Bone Joint Surg Am 2008;90:1258–64.
3. Hudic I, Fatusić Z, Sinanovic O, et al. Etiological risk factors for brachial plexus palsy. J Matern Fetal Neonatal Med 2006;19:655–61.
4. Al-Qattan MM, El-Sayed AA, Al-Zahrani AY, et al. Narakas classification of obstetric brachial plexus palsy revisited. J Hand Surg Eur 2009;34:788–91.
5. Pondaag W, Malessy MJ, van Dijk J, et al. Natural history of obstetric brachial plexus palsy: a systematic review. Dev Med Child Neurol 2004;46:138–44.
6. Blauuw G, Slooff AC. Transfer of pectoral nerves to musculocutaneous nerve in obstetric upper brachial plexus palsy. Neurosurgery 2003;53:338–42.
7. Little K, Zlotolow DA, Soldado F, et al. Early functional recovery of elbow flexion and supination following median and/or ulnar nerve fascicle transfer in upper neonatal brachial plexus palsy. J Bone Joint Surg Am 2014;96:215–21.
8. Vekris M, Lykissas MG, Beris A, et al. Management of obstetrical brachial plexus palsy with early plexus microreconstruction and late muscle transfers. Microsurgery 2008;28:252–61.
9. Waters PM. Comparison of the natural history, the outcome of microsurgical repair, and the outcome of operative reconstruction in brachial plexus birth palsy. J Bone Joint Surg Am 1999;81:649–59.
10. Kelly DW. Congenital dislocation of the radial head: spectrum and natural history. J Pediatr Orthop 1981;1:295–8.
11. Mardam-Bey T, Ger E. Congenital radial head dislocation. J Hand Surg Am 1979; 4:316–20.
12. Al-Qattan MM, Abou Al-Shaar H, Alkattan WM. The pathogenesis of congenital radial head dislocation/subluxation. Gene 2016;586:69–76.
13. Reichenbach H, Hormann D, Theile H. Hereditary congenital posterior dislocation of radial heads. Am J Med Genet 1995;55:101–4.
14. Kaas L, Struijs PA. Congenital radial head dislocation with a progressive cubitus valgus: a case report. Strategies Trauma Limb Reconstr 2012;7:39–44.
15. Miura T. Congenital dislocation of the radial head. J Hand Surg Br 1990;15: 477–81.
16. Bengard MJ, Calfee RP, Steffen JA, et al. Intermediate-term to long-term outcome of surgically and nonsurgically treated congenital, isolated radial head dislocation. J Hand Surg Am 2012;37:2495–501.
17. Rodgers WB, Waters PM. Incidence of trigger digits in newborns. J Hand Surg Am 1994;19:364–8.
18. Dinham JM, Meggitt BF. Trigger thumbs in children. A review of the natural history and indications for treatment in 105 patients. J Bone Joint Surg Br 1974;56:153–5.

19. Shreve M, Chu A. Pediatric thumb flexion deformities. Bull Hosp Jt Dis 2016; 74(1):97–108.
20. Shah AS, Bae DS. Management of pediatric trigger thumb and trigger finger. J Am Acad Orthop Surg 2012;20:206–13.
21. Cardon LJ, Ezaki M, Carter PR. Trigger finger in children. J Hand Surg Am 1999; 24:1156–61.
22. Baek GH, Lee HJ. The natural history of pediatric trigger thumb: a study with a minimum of five years follow-up. Clin Orthop Surg 2011;3:157–9.
23. Nemoto K, Nemoto T, Terada N, et al. Splint therapy for trigger thumb and finger in children. J Hand Surg Br 1996;21:416–8.
24. Slakey JB, Hennrikus WL. Acquired thumb flexion contracture in children: congenital trigger thumb. J Bone Joint Surg Br 1996;78:481–3.
25. Arora AS, Chung KC, Otto W. Madelung and the recognition of Madelung's deformity. J Hand Surg Am 2006;31:177–82.
26. Zebala LP, Manske PR, Goldfarb CA. Madelung's deformity: a spectrum of presentation. J Hand Surg Am 2007;32:1393–401.
27. Vickers D, Nielsen G. Madelung deformity: surgical prophylaxis (physiolysis) during the late growth period by resection of the dyschondrosteosis lesion. J Hand Surg Br 1992;17:401–7.
28. McCarroll HR Jr, James MA, Newmeyer WL 3rd, et al. Madelung's deformity: quantitative assessment of x-ray deformity. J Hand Surg Am 2005;30:1211–20.
29. Knutsen EJ, Goldfarb CA. Madelung's deformity. Hand (N Y) 2014;9:289–91.
30. Harley BJ, Brown C, Cummings K, et al. Volar ligament release and distal radius dome osteotomy for correction of Madelung's deformity. J Hand Surg Am 2006; 31:1499–506.
31. Barton NJ. Fractures of the phalanges of the hand in children. Hand 1979;11: 134–43.
32. Al-Qattan MM. Phalangeal neck fractures in children: classification and outcome in 66 cases. J Hand Surg Br 2001;26:112–21.
33. Matzon JL, Cornwall R. A stepwise algorithm for surgical treatment of type II displaced pediatric phalangeal neck fractures. J Hand Surg Am 2014;39:467–73.
34. Mintzer CM, Waters PM, Brown DJ. Remodelling of a displaced phalangeal neck fracture. J Hand Surg Br 1994;19:594–6.
35. Al-Qattan MM, Al-Qattan AM. A review of phalangeal neck fractures in children. Injury 2015;46:935–44.
36. Karl JW, White NJ, Strauch RJ. Percutaneous reduction and fixation of displaced phalangeal neck fractures in children. J Pediatr Orthop 2012;32:156–61.
37. Cornwall R, Waters PM. Remodeling of phalangeal neck fracture malunions in children: case report. J Hand Surg Am 2004;29:458–61.
38. Maschke S, Seitz W, Lawton J. Radial longitudinal deficiency. J Am Acad Orthop Surg 2007;15:41–52.
39. Colen D, Lin I, Levin S, et al. Radial longitudinal deficiency: recent developments, controversies, and an evidence-based guide to treatment. J Hand Surg Am 2017; 42:546–63.
40. James M, McCarroll H, Manske P. The spectrum of radial longitudinal deficiency: a modified classification. J Hand Surg Am 1999;24:1145–55.
41. Mo J, Manske P. Surgical treatment of type 0 radial longitudinal deficiency. J Hand Surg Am 2004;29:1002–9.
42. Kotwal P, Varshney M, Soral A. Comparison of surgical treatment and nonoperative management for radial longitudinal deficiency. J Hand Surg Eur 2012;37: 161–9.

43. James MA, Bauer AS. Malformations and deformities of the wrist and forearm. In: Wolfe SW, Hotchkiss RN, Pederson WC, et al, editors. Green's operative hand surgery. 7th edition. Amsterdam: Elsevier; 2017. p. 1328–64.

44. Damore E, Kozin S, Thoder J, et al. The recurrence of deformity after surgical centralization for radial clubhand. J Hand Surg Am 2000;25:745–51.

45. K. C SS. The frequency and epidemiology of hand and forearm fractures in the United States. J Hand Surg 2001;26:908–15.

46. Seymour N. Juxta-epiphysial fracture of the terminal phalanx of the finger. J Bone Joint Surg Br 1966;48:347–9.

47. Bae DS. Hand, wrist, and forearm fractures in children. In: Wolfe SW, Hotchkiss RN, Pederson WC, et al, editors. Green's operative hand surgery. 7th edition. Amsterdam: Elsevier; 2017. p. 1328–64.

48. Jain A, Sierakowski A, Gardiner MD, et al. Nail bed INJury Assessment Pilot (NINJA-P) study: should the nail plate be replaced or discarded after nail bed repair in children? Study protocol for a pilot randomised controlled trial. Pilot Feasibility Stud 2015; 1:29.

49. Abzug JM, Kozin SH. Seymour fractures. J Hand Surg Am 2013;38:2267–70 [quiz: 2270].

50. Reyes BA, Ho CA. The high risk of infection with delayed treatment of open Seymour fractures: Salter-Harris I/II or juxta-epiphyseal fractures of the distal phalanx with associated nailbed laceration. J Pediatr Orthop 2017;37:247–53.

51. Krusche-Mandl I, Kottstorfer J, Thalhammer G, et al. Seymour fractures: retrospective analysis and therapeutic considerations. J Hand Surg Am 2013;38:258–64.

52. Malik S. Syndactyly: phenotypes, genetics and current classification. Eur J Hum Genet 2012;20:817–24.

53. Goldfarb CA, Steffen JA, Stutz CM. Complex syndactyly: aesthetic and objective outcomes. J Hand Surg Am 2012;37:2068–73.

54. Braun TL, Trost JG, Pederson WC. Syndactyly release. Semin Plast Surg 2016;30:162–70.

55. Dao KD, Shin AY, Billings A, et al. Surgical treatment of congenital syndactyly of the hand. J Am Acad Orthop Surg 2004;12:39–48.

56. Tonkin MA. Failure of differentiation part I: Syndactyly. Hand Clin 2009;25:171–93.

57. Upton J. Apert syndrome. Classification and pathologic anatomy of limb anomalies. Clin Plast Surg 1991;18:321–55.

58. Apert M. De l'acrocephalosyndactylie. Bull Soc Med Hop Paris 1906;23:1310–30.

59. Guero SJ. Algorithm for treatment of Apert hand. Tech Hand Up Extrem Surg 2005;9:126–33.

60. Van Wyhe RD, Trost JG, Koshy JC, et al. The duplicated thumb: a review. Semin Plast Surg 2016;30:181–8.

61. Tonkin MA. Thumb duplication: concepts and techniques. Clin Orthop Surg 2012; 4:1–17.

62. Manske MC, Kennedy CD, Huang JI. Classifications in brief: the Wassel classification for radial polydactyly. Clin Orthop Relat Res 2017;475:1740–6.

63. Zuidam JM, Selles RW, Ananta M, et al. A classification system of radial polydactyly: inclusion of triphalangeal thumb and triplication. J Hand Surg Am 2008;33:373–7.

64. Dijkman RR, van Nieuwenhoven CA, Selles RW, et al. A multicenter comparative study of two classification systems for radial polydactyly. Plast Reconstr Surg 2014;134:991–1001.

65. Wolfe S, Hotchkiss R, Pederson W, et al. Green's operative hand surgery. 7th edition. Philadelphia: Elsevier; 2017. p. 1304–15.
66. Larsen M, Nicolai JP. Long-term follow-up of surgical treatment for thumb duplication. J Hand Surg Br 2005;30:276–81.
67. Tada K, Yonenobu K, Tsuyuguchi Y, et al. Duplication of the thumb. A retrospective review of two hundred and thirty-seven cases. J Bone Joint Surg Am 1983;65: 584–98.
68. Soldado F, Zlotolow D, Kozin S. Thumb hypoplasia. J Hand Surg Am 2013;2013:1435–44.
69. Kozin SH. Deformities of the thumb. In: Wolfe SW, Hotchkiss RN, Pederson WC, et al, editors. Green's operative hand surgery. 7th edition. Amsterdam: Elsevier; 2017. p. 1289–327.
70. Goldfarb C, Gee A, Heinze L, et al. Normative values for thumb length, girth, and width in the pediatric population. J Hand Surg Am 2005;30:1004–8.
71. Tonkin M. On the classification of thumb hypoplasia. J Hand Surg Eur 2013;39: 948–55.
72. Kozin S. Pollicization: the concept, technical details, and outcome. Clin Orthop Surg 2012;4:18–35.
73. Netscher D, Aliu O, Sandvall B, et al. Functional outcomes of children with index pollicizations for thumb deficiency. J Hand Surg Am 2013;38:250–7.
74. Lightdale-Mirric N, Mueske N, Lawrence E, et al. Long term functional outcomes after early childhood pollicization. J Hand Ther 2015;28:158–65.

Pediatric Orthopedic Trauma

Jamie Grossman, MD, MS[a,*], Benjamin Giliberti, MD[a],
Robert Dolitsky, MD[a], Gregory Parker, MD[a], Bum Kim, BA[b], Kamen Kutzarov, MD[a],
Evan Curatolo, MD[a,c]

KEYWORDS

• Pediatric • Orthopedic • Trauma • Fracture • Injury • Management • Cast • Surgery

KEY POINTS

• The signs, symptoms, and management of compartment syndrome, one of the most dangerous and serious complications of pediatric orthopedics trauma, are examined.
• The incidence, risk factors, presentation, and diagnosis of nonaccidental trauma are explored so that it can be identified and stopped.
• Upper and lower extremity fractures and injures are reviewed to allow for the detection of injuries that require acute operative intervention.

COMPARTMENT SYNDROME

Compartment syndrome is a serious condition resulting from increased pressures within a compartment limiting blood flow that can end in permanent disability of the affected limb if not diagnosed and treated in a timely manner.

The following are common causes of compartment syndrome[1]:

• Fractures (most associated)
• Soft tissue injuries
• Burns
• Animal/insect bites
• Tight dressings, casts, antishock garments
• Penetrating trauma
• Bleeding disorders

Signs/Symptoms (6 P's):

• Pain (with passive stretch and/or not relieved with pain medication)
• Pressure

---

[a] Department of Orthopedics, Monmouth Medical Center, 300 2nd Avenue Long Branch, NJ 07740, USA; [b] 300 2nd Avenue Long Branch, NJ 07740, USA; [c] Atlantic Pediatric Orthopedics, 1131 Broad Street, Suite 202, Shrewsbury, NJ 07702, USA
* Corresponding author.
E-mail address: jmgrossman2@gmail.com

Pediatr Clin N Am 67 (2020) 101–118
https://doi.org/10.1016/j.pcl.2019.09.010
0031-3955/20/© 2019 Elsevier Inc. All rights reserved.

- Pallor
- Paresthesia
- Paralysis
- Pulselessness

Acute compartment syndrome can be difficult to spot in the younger pediatric population because of their inability to communicate. The following symptoms can be helpful in detecting compartment syndrome in the pediatric population (3 A's)[1]:

- Anxiety (restlessness)
- Agitation (crying)
- Analgesia (increasing dose/frequency)

The most reliable diagnosis requires the direct measurement of compartment pressure with a needle. An absolute compartment pressure of 30 mm Hg or greater or a compartment pressure 30 mm Hg above the diastolic blood pressure/mean arterial pressure is indicative of compartment syndrome and requires emergent treatment.[2]

Treatment

Initial treatment consists of removing all causes of pressure externally and elevation. Surgical treatment with fasciotomy is necessary to relieve the pressure and prevent further damage (**Fig. 1**). Desired outcomes can be achieved if decompression is performed in less than 8 to 12 hours. Complications include functional muscle loss, neurologic impairment, arrest in growth, and infection.[1]

MANIFESTATIONS OF PEDIATRIC ABUSE

Close to 1 million children are victims of abuse each year, and abuse is the second most common cause of death in infants and children.[3] After skin lesions, fractures are the second most common physical presentation of abuse. Fractures are present in 11% to 55% of abused children, and are most common in children younger than

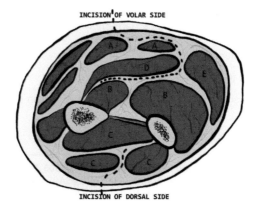

A-SUPERFICIAL FLEXOR COMPARTMENTS
B-DEEP FLEXOR COMPARTMENTS
C-EXTENSOR COMPARTMENTS
D-FLEXOR DIGITORUM SUPERFICIALIS
E-FLEXOR CARPI ULNARIS

Fig. 1. Forearm fasciotomy axial anatomy.

3 years.[3] The younger the child with a fracture, the more likely abuse is the cause. Premature infants are more susceptible to fracture, but are also at higher risk of abuse.

Presentation

A history that does not adequately explain an injury should raise suspicion for abuse.

- Any physical finding should be considered together with the medical and social history
- Acute or subacute fractures may cause local tenderness and swelling
- Chronic fractures may appear swollen from callous formation or deformity but will be nontender
- Skin should be carefully examined for bruises, burns, scars
- Bruises over bony prominences are commonly accidental

Imaging

- Skeletal survey should be performed in children younger than 2 years suspected of child abuse.
- A bone scan can be obtained in addition to skeletal survey to help detect fractures of the diaphysis.[4]
- A follow-up skeletal survey after 2 weeks can increase the sensitivity of identifying occult fractures. Up to 10% of suspected abuse victims that have a negative skeletal survey will have positive findings on a 2-week follow-up survey.[4]
- Children older than 2 years should have specific imaging, instead of a skeletal survey.[4]
- Both anteroposterior (AP) and lateral views should be obtained of the suspected extremity or joint.

Radiographic Findings

The most common fracture patterns seen in abuse are those that are also seen in accidental trauma, including clavicle fractures and long bone fractures, such as femur and humerus fractures. Certain fracture patterns that may be less common, but are highly specific for abuse, include the following[4]:

- Rib fractures
- "Corner" fractures appear on radiographs as metaphyseal avulsion fractures
- "Bucket-handle" fractures have a thin rim of metaphyseal bone centrally and a thicker portion of metaphyseal bone on the periphery, giving it the appearance of a bucket-handle
- Spinous process fractures
- Scapula fractures
- Sternal fractures
- Multiple fractures in various stages of healing
- Femur fractures in infants, especially those who do not ambulate yet

Differential Diagnosis

The following conditions can have similar presentations to the abused child and should be considered in cases of suspected child abuse:

- Osteogenesis imperfecta
- Scurvy
- Rickets
- Osteomyelitis

- Osteopenia of prematurity
- Vitamin deficiencies[3]

DISTAL RADIUS AND ULNA FRACTURES
Presentation

Children with distal radius and ulna fractures will typically present with pain and swelling and sometimes a deformity localized to the distal forearm. In minimally displaced fractures associated with the physis, as well as incomplete, buckle, and greenstick type fractures, deformity may not be present and children may present days after the traumatic insult with unresolved pain and guarding. Patients with more obvious deformity should be examined for skin compromise and neurovascular insult. Fractures involving the diaphysis of the radius and ulna will typically present similarly with pain, swelling, and deformity. It its especially important with displaced diaphyseal fractures to recognize the presence of an open fracture or compartment syndrome.

Radiographic Anteroposterior and Lateral Imaging

- Wrist
- Forearm
- Elbow

Special Considerations

- Galeazzi fracture: distal radius fracture with associated disruption of the distal radioulnar joint
- Monteggia fracture: fracture of the middle or proximal ulna with dislocation of the radiocapitellar joint

Treatment

Minimally displaced fractures or incomplete fractures are inherently stable and are treated with splint or cast immobilization for 3 to 4 weeks.[1] Displaced fractures, fractures involving the physis, and open fractures may require reduction possibly with percutaneous or operative fixation.

RADIAL NECK FRACTURES

In the pediatric population, most fractures that occur at the proximal radius occur at the radial neck. They typically occur after a fall onto an outstretched arm. A valgus stress on the elbow during the trauma can further deform the fracture. Radial neck fractures also can occur in conjunction with an elbow dislocation.

Presentation

Patients will typically present after a fall with pain over the radial head or neck. Examination of the patient should include evaluation of the wrist and elbow, including supination and protonation, which is often painful and limited, along with a complete neurovascular examination, paying particular attention the posterior interosseous nerve function due to its proximity to the proximal radius.

Radiographic Imaging

- AP, lateral, and oblique radiographs of the elbow
- AP and lateral radiographs of the forearm
- Radiocapitellar view of the elbow to remove superimposition of the radial head and neck on the proximal ulna

Treatment

Treatment of radial neck fractures is based on angulation of the neck. Given the large remodeling potential at the proximal radius in a skeletally immature patient, angulation of less than 30° is tolerated in patients older than 10 years and less than 45° in patients younger than 10 years. Angulation greater than 30° to 45° can be treated with closed reduction. Several closed reduction maneuvers have been described, including the Patterson, Israeli, and the Esmarch technique. If closed reduction yields acceptable angulation, long arm casting can be used to hold reduction. If closed reduction fails, then closed reduction with percutaneous pinning or open reduction with internal fixation is necessary.

ELBOW DISLOCATIONS

Elbow injuries are common among children because they tend to protect themselves by falling on an outstretched arm. Emergency room physicians accurately diagnosed elbow fractures in children only 53% of the time. Elbow dislocations are most frequent in adolescents aged 10 to 19 years old and almost half were sustained in sports.[1]

To evaluate fractures of the elbow, the person evaluating the radiographs must understand the age of ossification and fusion of the various ossification centers (**Table 1**). Ossification is the time the bone appears on the radiograph. Fusion is when the ossification center forms a boney connection with the humerus. The medial epicondyle is the last to fuse to the metaphysis.

Presentation

Elbow held in flexed position. The forearm may appear shortened.

Imaging

Radiographs:
- AP and lateral radiographs of elbow
- Posterolateral dislocation is the most common followed by posteromedial and anterior
- The most commonly associated condition is medial epicondyle fracture

Treatment

Treatment consists of a timely closed reduction. Following reduction, post reduction imaging should be obtained to evaluate for boney fragments incarcerated within the

Table 1		
Chart for evaluation of fractures based on ossification age and years a fusion		
Ossification Center	Years at Ossification	Years at Fusion
Capitellum	1	12
Radial head	4	15
Medial epicondyle	6	17
Trochlea	8	12
Olecranon	10	15
Lateral epicondyle	12	12

joint. If there is no limitation, the patient will undergo brief immobilization for 1 to 2 weeks. If the medial epicondyle is incarcerated, the reduction occurs under open direct visualization.

- If "elbow dislocation" occurs in a patient younger than 3 years, there should be concern for a physeal injury.

SUPRACONDYLAR FRACTURE

Supracondylar fractures are one of the most common injuries in pediatric patients, usually occurring between the ages 5 and 7 years old. Injury occurs after a fall onto an outstretched arm.

Presentation

Refusal to move the elbow, gross deformity about the elbow, swelling, ecchymosis in antecubital fossa.

- Neurovascular examination
  - Anterior interosseous nerve neurapraxia: unable to make an A-ok sign (flex interphalangeal [IP] joint of thumb and distal IP of index finger)
  - Median nerve: Loss of sensation over palmar aspect of index finger
  - Radial nerve: unable to extend wrist, metacarpophalangeal joint, thumb IP
  - Assess for radial and ulnar artery pulse and vascular perfusion
    - Well perfused: warm and pink
    - Poorly perfused: cold, pale, arterial capillary refill more than 2 seconds

Imaging

Radiographs: AP and lateral of the elbow.
  Evaluate for "posterior fat pad sign": lucency along the posterior distal humerus on the lateral elbow film

Treatment

Treatment is dependent on the displacement of the fracture. Nondisplaced fractures are treated in cast immobilization for 3 to 4 weeks while displaced fractures require surgical fixation. Emergency operation is required if the hand is poorly perfused.[1]

MEDIAL EPICONDYLE FRACTURE OF THE ELBOW

Medial epicondyle fractures are common among boys between the ages of 9 and 14 years. They are associated with elbow dislocations approximately 50% of the time.[1] The medial epicondyle is usually avulsed anteriorly due to the pull from the flexor pronator mass and the ulnar collateral ligament.

Presentation

Medial elbow pain, valgus instability, 50% with elbow dislocation.

Images

AP, lateral, internal oblique view and distal humeral axial view of the elbow.

Treatment

- If <5 mm of displacement, immobilization in a long arm cast for up to 3 weeks.
- Absolute indications for operative treatment include entrapment in the elbow joint, fracture including the articular surface and open fracture.

- Relative indications for operative fixation include ulnar nerve dysfunction, >5 mm displacement, and displacement in valgus stress athletes, such as throwers and gymnasts.

LATERAL CONDYLE FRACTURE OF THE ELBOW

Lateral condyle fractures of the elbow are the second most common fractures of the elbow after supracondylar fractures. They have a high risk of nonunion, malunion, and avascular necrosis.

Presentation

Lateral elbow pain and swelling, may be subtle.

Imaging

Radiographs:

- AP and lateral views
- Internal oblique views

Treatment

- Depends on amount of displacement
  - If <2 mm displacement, long arm casting is acceptable for 4 to 6 weeks
  - If 2 to 4 mm displacement, patient should undergo closed reduction percutaneous pinning followed by long arm cast
  - If >4 mm displacement or joint incongruity, open reduction with internal fixation

HUMERUS FRACTURES

In the pediatric population, proximal humerus and humeral shaft fractures are relatively uncommon, representing fewer than 5% of all childhood fractures.[1] When they do occur, typical mechanism of injury includes direct or indirect trauma. When a detailed history is not consistent with a traumatic mechanism, pathologic fracture through a primary bone lesion or nonaccidental trauma should be considered.

Presentation

Patients will typically present after an injury with pain localized to the shoulder or arm. Pain can be exacerbated by motion. Deformity can be masked by soft tissues.

Radiographic Imaging

- Shoulder: AP, scapular Y, and axillary view
- Humerus: AP and lateral views
- Elbow: AP, lateral, and oblique views

Treatment

Regardless of the mechanism, most humerus fractures in the pediatric population can be treated nonoperatively given the large degree of motion from the glenohumeral joint as well as the large remodeling potential of the proximal humeral physis. Most nondisplaced or minimally displaced proximal humerus fractures in patients younger than 11 years can be treated with a short period of immobilization with a sling. For birth-related injuries, the extremity sleeve can be pinned to the patient's chest while the fracture heels. After 11 or 12 years of age, radiographic parameters for nonoperative management are less than 30° of varus or valgus, 20° of anterior angulation, and up to 2 cm of shortening. For these fractures, coaptation splinting, functional bracing, or hanging arm casting are acceptable treatment options. Fractures that do not meet these requirements may require operative reduction and fixation.

CLAVICLE/ACROMIOCLAVICULAR/STERNOCLAVICULAR FRACTURES

The clavicle, also known as the collarbone, is the most commonly fractured bone in the pediatric population with midshaft fracture taking up 80% of those involved.[5] Common causes of clavicle fractures range from the natural birth process to falls and high-energy mechanisms.

Presentation

Children typically present with discomfort with shoulder movement. Sometimes there may be noticeable swelling, crepitation, deformity, and ecchymosis. Rarely is there tenting of the skin. Ptosis (droopy eyelid) and miosis (constricted pupil) can indicate that the brachial plexus is involved.[5]

Imaging

- AP and lateral of clavicle

Treatment

Most of the time, treatment of pediatric clavicle fractures consists of nonoperative methods, especially those displaced less than 1.5 cm to 2.0 cm. Immobilization of the shoulder girdle typically with a sling provides support for the upper limb during the healing process. Open fractures, significant skin tenting, and fractures involving neurovascular compromise may require operative treatment.

ACROMIOCLAVICULAR DISLOCATIONS
Presentation

- Pain at the acromioclavicular joint
- Numbness/tingling from swelling or possible brachial plexus injury
- Feels like "bump"

Imaging

- AP and lateral of shoulder and clavicle

Treatment

Depending on the severity of the fracture, if nonoperative treatment is optimal, a sling or a shoulder immobilizer can be used for 2 to 4 weeks. Extreme sports should be avoided for 3 months after the injury.

STERNOCLAVICULAR FRACTURE/DISLOCATIONS

Sternoclavicular (SC) fractures or dislocations are rare and secondary to high-energy mechanisms (motor vehicle/sports).

Presentation

- Pain localized to the SC joint
- Shortness of breath, dyspnea
- Dysphagia, odynophagia, hoarseness
- Paresthesias or weakness if brachial plexus is involved

- Ecchymosis and swelling about the SC joint
  - Anterior dislocation results in accentuated presence of the medial clavicle
  - Posterior dislocation might allow for palpation of the corner of the sternum[1]

Treatment

Closed reduction may be necessary in acute posterior SC fracture dislocations. Recurrent instability can occur following closed treatment requires open treatments. It is essential to have a thoracic surgeon on standby with open reductions of sternoclavicular fractures.[1]

SPINE
Thoracolumbar Trauma

Spine fractures in children are rare, approximately 1% to 2% of all pediatric fractures. Motor vehicle accidents are the most common cause of spine fractures in the pediatric population. There is a high incidence of associated injuries, so a complete physical examination should be performed.[6]

Spinal cord injuries in children are less common than in adults. This may be due to the increased flexibility of the pediatric spine relative to that of adults and therefore allows greater deformation before fracture. This can lead to an entity called spinal cord injury without radiographic abnormality. These patients need close follow-up to monitor neurologic status. Flexion/extension radiographs can help determine instability from ligamentous injuries that would require surgical stabilization.[6]

Imaging

- AP and lateral radiographs.
- Computed tomography (CT) scans are now standard in the evaluation of trauma patients, as they have a sensitivity of close to 100% in detecting spine injuries compared with 70% in plain radiographs.[7]
- MRI is used to evaluate the spinal cord and soft tissue structures and should be obtained when neurologic symptoms are present.

Treatment
Most thoracolumbar spine fractures in the pediatric population are stable and without neurologic deficit. These generally can be managed with symptomatic treatment and gradual return to activity.

Spondylolysis
Spondylolysis is a defect or stress fracture in the pars interarticularis, which is the segment of bone located between the superior and inferior articular processes. The mechanism is usually repetitive hyperextension.

Spondylolysis can eventually lead to spondylolisthesis, which is the translation of a vertebral body on the segment below. The most common spinal level for this to occur is at the L5-S1 segment.[8]

Presentation
Most patients are asymptomatic, but some may present with a dull, ache or discomfort in the low back with occasional radiation to the bilateral buttock or thighs in more severe cases. In mild cases, the examination will be normal.

Imaging

- AP, lateral, and oblique radiographs of the spine
- Flexion/extension radiographs of the spine help determine stability

Treatment

The natural history of spondylolysis with mild spondylolisthesis is generally benign, and patients who are asymptomatic can participate in all activities without restriction.

Patients who are symptomatic are generally treated nonoperatively with observation, activity modification, physiotherapy, and bracing.

Compression fractures

- Angulation less than 10°: symptomatic treatment[6]
- Angulation 10° to 15°, and Risser stage less than 3: treated with hyperextension cast or brace to prevent development of kyphosis
- Angulation greater than 15° or 50% compression of anterior vertebral body: surgical stabilization

Burst fractures

- A type of compression fracture in which the fracture extends to the posterior wall of the vertebral body
- If the alignment is maintained and there is no neurologic injury, can treat without surgery in a cast or brace
- Neurologic symptoms are an indication for surgery

Lap-belt fractures

- These occur when the seat-belt is resting over the abdomen instead of the hips
- A flexion distraction mechanism causes the spine to fracture
- Associated with intra-abdominal injuries
- Unstable injuries typically require surgery[6]

Limbus fractures (apophyseal fractures)

- An avulsion fracture of the apophyseal ring
- Presents with radiculopathy
- Usually requires surgery to remove the bone fragment impinging on the nerve

Cervical Spine Trauma

By 10 years of age, the spine has reached skeletal maturity, and the injuries sustained at that point are similar to those sustained in adults.

Children are more likely to sustain ligamentous injuries of the upper cervical spine. Adolescents and adults more commonly fracture the lower cervical spine.[9]

Atlas (C1) fracture

- Usually treated with a rigid cervical orthosis or halo, and rarely requires surgery.[10]

Transverse atlantoaxial ligament rupture

- This ligament prevents anterior translation of C1 on C2.
- Diagnosed on radiograph with an atlanto-dens interval greater than 5 mm. This interval is measured on the lateral radiograph as the distance between the dens of C2 and the posterior border of the anterior arch of C1.
- Simple immobilization does not provide adequate stability for ligamentous healing, so the recommended treatment is surgical fixation.[9]

Atlantoaxial rotatory displacement

- Rotatory instability of C1 on C2, ranging in severity from mild to severe[10]
- Present with tilted head, neck pain
- Diagnosed with dynamic CT
- Treatment
  - Symptoms less than 1 week: soft collar, nonsteroidal anti-inflammatory drugs
  - Symptoms more than 1 week: halter traction, rigid collar
  - Symptoms more than 3 months: surgery

Odontoid (dens) fractures

- Common pediatric spine fractures.
- Usually a fracture through the physis.
- Rarely presents with neurologic deficits.
- Usually treated in a rigid orthosis or halo.

C3-7 injuries

- More common in older children[10]
- Vertebral body compression fractures, or facet fractures/dislocations
- Physeal fractures of the inferior endplates can occur, usually from hyperextension
  - Heal rapidly and can be treated with simple positioning
- Traumatic ligamentous injuries are treated with surgery if there is instability, or collar for comfort if mild sprain

Pseudosubluxation

- Physiologic subluxation of cervical spine up to 4 mm in children
  - Due to the horizontal facets, which become more vertical as they get older
  - Most common at C2-C3 level
- Treatment is observation

Pelvic Avulsion Fractures

Avulsion fractures occur when a tendon or ligament pulls off a piece of bone.

These fractures result from the forceful contraction of large muscle groups that originate on pelvic apophyses during explosive activities such as sprinting, jumping, or kicking.

They occur predominantly in adolescents during sports activities.

Patients may report a pop at the time of injury, and present with pain and difficulty bearing weight.

Physical findings

Tenderness, swelling, weakness of the involved muscle.

Table 2 lists 6 most common apophyseal avulsion fractures, and their muscular attachment(s).

Imaging

Radiographs
- AP of the pelvis for displacement of the affected apophysis
- A frog-leg lateral of the hip
- CT or MRI may help make the diagnosis if suspicion is high but radiographs are negative

Table 2	
Most common apophyseal avulsion fractures	
Apophysis	**Muscular Attachment**
Ischial tuberosity	Hamstrings
Anterior superior iliac spine (ASIS)	Sartorius, tensor fascia lata
Anterior inferior iliac spine (AIIS)	Rectus femoris
Pubic symphysis	Rectus abdominis
Iliac crest	Abdominal muscles
Lesser trochanter	Iliopsoas

Treatment

- Most patients do well with nonoperative management:
  - Rest, protected weight bearing with crutches for at least 2 weeks, followed by physical therapy for stretching and strengthening
  - Return to sports at 6 to 8 weeks when asymptomatic[11]
- Indications for operative treatment
  - Displacement more than 1.5 to 2.0 cm[12]
  - Persistent pain or disability despite nonoperative treatment

Hip Fractures

Presentation

Children with hip fractures typically present with a history of high-energy trauma and shortened, externally rotated, and painful lower limb. Life-threatening injuries initially must be ruled out. Diagnosis of hip fractures in infants can be difficult, as infection and congenital dislocation of the hip must be considered.[13,14]

Imaging

- AP pelvis (including view with leg held in extension and internal rotation)
- AP and lateral of hip
  - Cross-table lateral
    - Frog-leg lateral may be considered but could cause further displacement of the fracture
- MRI
  - For nondisplaced fractures and stress fractures

Treatment

All hip fractures in children should be treated and closely followed by an orthopedic surgeon because of potential complications including avascular necrosis, coxa vara, and leg length discrepancy. More proximal fractures have higher rates of avascular necrosis and growth arrest. Nondisplaced hip fractures in the very young are generally treated with spica cast immobilization for 6 to 8 weeks with close follow-up. Nondisplaced fractures in older patient or displaced fractures almost always require operative fixation by an orthopedic surgeon.[13]

Traumatic Hip Dislocations

Traumatic hip dislocations in children, although rare, are more common than hip fractures. Younger children (younger than 5 years) can sustain a dislocation with minimal trauma, whereas older children generally require high-energy mechanisms for a dislocation to occur.[14]

Presentation
Children with traumatic hip dislocations present with a painful hip, refusal to ambulate, and abnormal positioning of the extremity. A neurovascular examination is crucial to avoid missing a sciatic or gluteal nerve palsy.

Imaging
- AP pelvis
- Lateral

Treatment
Early closed reduction is crucial to decrease both the need for a possible open reduction in the operating room and the incidence of avascular necrosis. Frequently after reduction, bed rest, spica cast immobilization, or bracing is used anywhere from 4 to 12 weeks.[13]

Femoral Shaft Fractures

Femoral shaft fractures in children are common. The mechanism of injury can range from nonaccidental trauma in a newborn or infant, to a fall in a child younger than 10 years, or a high-energy motor vehicle accident in a teenager.

Presentation
Pediatric femoral shaft fractures typically present with thigh pain, swelling, and deformity. In younger children (younger than 3), and especially in patients before walking age, it is imperative to consider nonaccidental trauma.

Imaging
- AP and lateral radiographs of the femur, hip, and knee

Treatment
Treatments are generally chosen based on the patient's age. From birth until 5 years of age, patients are usually treated nonoperatively with either a Pavlik harness or spica cast immobilization. Beyond 5 years of age, children with femoral shaft fractures frequently require surgical fixation.[15] Aside from the tremendous short-term disability experienced by the patient, most femoral shaft fractures have a good prognosis with few long-term complications.[16]

Distal Femur Fractures

Presentation
Children with distal femur fractures present with a history of trauma, knee pain, and inability to bend the knee or bear weight. On examination, there may be swelling, flexed positioning of the knee, and varus or valgus instability.[17]

Imaging
- AP, lateral, and oblique radiographs of the distal femur
- MRI to confirm physeal fracture

Treatment
Distal femur fractures in children are uncommon injuries that require close follow-up because of the high incidence of limb length discrepancy and angular deformity. The lower limb grows approximately 23 mm per year with up to 40% (9 mm) of growth coming from the distal femoral physis.[17]

Nondisplaced distal femur fractures can usually be treated with cast immobilization in a long leg cast for 4 to 6 weeks. Displaced fractures require reduction and percutaneous or operative fixation.[17]

Proximal Tibia Fractures

Pediatric proximal tibial physeal fractures are rare injures. Epiphyseal fractures are commonly seen in children 12 to 14 years old as the result of high-energy trauma. Metaphyseal fractures are more commonly seen in the 3-year-old to 6-year-old age group and are typically the result of low-energy mechanisms. Unlike distal femur fractures in the previous section, the proximal tibial physis is relatively stable owing to the many ligaments surrounding the knee.[18]

Presentation
Children with proximal tibia fractures will present with pain and refusal to bear weight on the affected extremity. It is crucial to perform a good neurovascular examination, as the physis is in close proximity to the vascular structures. With metaphyseal fractures, it is important to be on the alert for compartment syndrome.

Imaging
- AP and lateral radiographs of the knee
- CT scan of the knee to evaluate fracture displacement

Treatment
Nondisplaced and stable fractures are treated with immobilization in a long leg cast for approximately 4 to 6 weeks. In cases of unstable or irreducible fractures, percutaneous fixation or operative fixation may be required.[19]

Tibial Shaft Fractures

Introduction
Tibial shaft fractures in children can be caused by different mechanisms depending on the age group. In toddlers, they result from low-energy falls or twisting, and are aptly named "toddler's fracture." In older children, they are more commonly the result of high-energy trauma.

Presentation
Children with tibial shaft fractures typically present with pain and swelling and refusal to bear weight on the affected extremity. Treating physicians always should be on the alert for compartment syndrome in these injuries.

Imaging
- AP and lateral radiographs of the tibia and fibula
- AP and lateral radiographs of the ipsilateral knee and ankle

Treatment
Almost all pediatric tibial shaft fractures can be treated nonoperatively with long leg casting. Displaced fractures may be treated with closed reduction and application of long leg cast. In certain fractures (intra-articular extension, unacceptable reduction, lost reduction), operative fixation may be required.[20]

Ankle Fractures

Ankle fractures are one of the most common types of fractures among adolescents, especially those participating in sports activities. Age and bone maturity can offer insight into the type of fracture. Transitional fractures of the distal tibia and fibula occur when the patient is reaching skeletal maturity due to the nature of the closure of the physis. The distal tibia physis closes from central to anteromedial to posterolateral. There are 2 classification systems for ankle fractures; one is dependent on anatomy, Salter-Harris classification, and the other, Dias-Tachdjian, is based off of mechanism of injury. During this transitional period, children commonly have a Tillaux fracture, which is a Salter-Harris type III fracture of the distal tibia, or a Triplane fracture, which is a Salter-Harris III fracture on the AP radiograph and a Salter-Harris II fracture on the lateral radiograph of the ankle.

Physical findings
Pain, ecchymosis, and swelling with inability to bear weight.

Imaging

- AP, lateral, and mortise ankle radiographs
- Full-length tibia/fibula radiograph
- CT scan to evaluate fracture displacement and articular step-off

Treatment
Treatment is dependent on fracture pattern and displacement. Minimally displaced distal fibula fractures can be treated in removable walking boot or a short leg cast for 4 weeks. Other ankle fractures with acceptable alignment are treated nonoperatively as well with a cast for approximately 6 weeks. More displaced or unstable ankle fractures require operative fixation with either closed reduction percutaneous pinning, or open reduction and internal fixation.

Foot Fractures

Pediatric foot radiographs are notoriously hard to read for the generalist because of the abundance of small bones with open physes of various ossification stages, as well as variable presence of accessory bones (**Fig. 2**).

Talus fractures
Talus fractures are very rarely seen in the pediatric foot. They typically result from forceful dorsiflexion, supination, or a combination of the two, with an axial load. Many of these fractures can be seen on plain radiographs but typically warrant a CT scan for complete evaluation. Most minimally displaced talus fractures are amenable to nonoperative treatment with a non–weight-bearing cast below the knee,[21] but any significant displacement warrants rigid operative fixation because of the risk of osteonecrosis[22]

Calcaneus fractures
Calcaneus fractures are rare in the pediatric population and are typically a result of axial loading and falls from height. Most calcaneal fractures warrant imaging with a CT scan for treatment planning. Minimally displaced fractures can be treated in a non–weight-bearing below-the-knee cast for 4 to 6 weeks.[23] Surgical treatment is reserved for displaced intra-articular fractures and tongue-type avulsion fractures.[24]

Midfoot fractures
Fractures of the navicular, cuboid, and cuneiforms are very rare fractures in children. The mechanism is typically a compression or crush injury of the foot. Most of these fractures can be treated in a non–weight-bearing cast for 4 to 6 weeks.

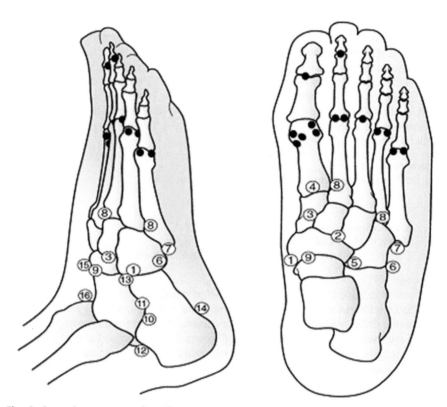

Fig. 2. Secondary centers of ossification and sesamoids of the foot. Sesamoid bones are shaded black. Secondary centers of ossification are 1, is tibiale extemum; 2, porcessus uncinatus; 3, os intercuneiforme; 4, pars peronea merarsalia; 5, cuboides secundarium; 6, os perineum, 7, os vesalianum, 8, os intemetatarseum; 9, os superatalare; 10, talus accessories; 11, is sustentaculum; 12, is trigonum; 13, calcaneus secundarium; 14, os subcalcis; 15, is supranaviculare; 16, is talotibiale. (*From* Keats TE: Atlas if normal roentgen variants that may simulate disease, ed 4, Chicago, 1988, Year Book Medical Publisher, pp xv, 1085.)

First to fourth metatarsal fractures

Metatarsal fractures are the most common type of fracture in the pediatric foot. The mechanisms of injury vary, but include direct and indirect, twisting, loading trauma. Imaging may or may not reveal a cortical break or buckle fracture. In absence of these radiographic findings, immobilization and repeat radiographs out of immobilization in 10 to 14 days will often reveal a more clear fracture line or newly developed callus. Treatment of these fractures consists of a weight-bearing cast or boot for 3 to 4 weeks.[25] Acceptable criteria for angulation and displacement in pediatric patients have not been established, but it is exceedingly rare for this type of injury to require operative treatment.

Fifth metatarsal fracture

The fifth metatarsal is the most commonly fractured metatarsal in the pediatric foot. Most of the fractures occur through the base of the metatarsal, which is divided into 3 zones (**Fig. 3**). Treatment for Zone I fractures is below-the-knee walking cast for 3 to 6 weeks. Treatment for Zone II fractures or Jones fractures consists of a non–weight-bearing cast for 6 weeks. Treatment of Zone III fractures includes

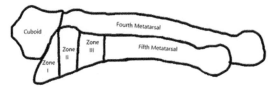

Fig. 3. Zone I fractures: avulsion fractures; zone II fractures: Jones fractures through watershed zone; zone III fractures: diaphyseal stress fractures.

non–weight bearing in a cast for 6 weeks and an additional 4 weeks of protected weight bearing.[26] Zone II fractures are notorious for nonunion because of the poor blood supply of the area and may require surgical fixation if they continue to be symptomatic.

Phalangeal fractures

Phalangeal fractures are some of the most common fractures to be seen by the general pediatrician.[27] The vast majority can be treated with buddy taping and a hard-soled shoe for 3 to 4 weeks. The exception is Salter-Harris injuries of the distal phalanx that involve a nail bed laceration. These injuries are frequently missed and must be treated with debridement and antibiotics because of the increased risk of infection.

DISCLOSURE

The authors have nothing to disclose.

REFERENCES

1. Flynn JM. Rockwood and Wilkins fractures in children. Philadelphia: Wolters Kluwer; 2015. p. 117–30, 349–472, 565–79, 581–628, 807–40.
2. Schaider JJ, Barkin RM. Rosen & Barkins 5-minute emergency medicine consult. Philadelphia: Wolters Kluwer Health/Lippincott Williams & Wilkins; 2015.
3. Schwend RM, et al. The orthopaedic recognition of child maltreatment. In: Rockwood and Wilkins' fractures in children. 8th edition. Lippincott Williams & Wilkins; 2015. p. 231–62.
4. Kocher MS, Kasser JR. Orthopaedic aspects of child abuse. J Am Acad Orthop Surg 2000;8(1):10–20.
5. Flynn JM. Operative techniques in pediatric orthopaedics. Philadelphia: Lippincott Williams & Wilkins; 2011. p. 60–2.
6. Flynn JM. Thoracolumbar spine and lower extremity fractures. In: Sink EL, editor. Lovell and Winter's pediatric orthopaedics. 7th edition. Lippincott Williams & Wilkins; 2014. p. 1773–6.
7. Newton PO, Luhmann SJ. Thoracolumbar spine fractures. In: Rockwood and Wilkins' fractures in children. 8th edition. Wolters Kluwer Health; 2015. p. 901–19.
8. Powers AK, et al. Spondylolysis and spondylolisthesis. In: Lovell and Winter's pediatric orthopaedics. 7th edition. Wolters Kluwer Health/Lippincott Williams & Wilkins; 2014. p. 791–820.
9. Kokoska ER, Keller MS, Rallo MC, et al. Characteristics of pediatric cervical spine injuries. J Pediatr Surg 2001;36:100–5.
10. Loder RT. The cervical spine. In: Lovell and Winter's pediatric orthopaedics. 7th edition. Lippincott Williams & Wilkins; 2014. p. 821–93.

11. McCarthy J, Herman M, Sankar W. Pelvic and acetabular fractures. In: Flynn JM, et al, editors. Rockwood and Wilkins' fractures in children. Lippincott Williams & Wilkins; 2015. p. 921–52.
12. Ghanem IB, Rizkallah M. Pediatric avulsion fractures of pelvis: current concepts. Curr Opin Pediatr 2018;30(1):78–83.
13. Sink EL, Kim Y-J. Fractures and traumatic dislocations of the hip in children. In: Flynn JM, editor. Rockwood and Wilkins' fractures in children. 8th edition; 2015. p. 953–86.
14. Pring M, Rang M, Wenger D. Pelvis and hip. In: Wenger DR, Pring ME, editors. Rang's children's fractures. 3rd edition. Philadelphia: Lippincott Williams & Wilkins; 2005. p. 165–80. Orthopedic surgery.
15. Pring M, Newton P, Rang M. Femoral shaft. In: Wenger DR, Pring ME, editors. Rang's children's fractures. 3rd edition. Philadelphia: Lippincott Williams & Wilkins; 2005. p. 181–200. Orthopedic surgery.
16. Flynn JM, Skaggs DL. Femoral shaft fractures. In: Flynn JM, Skaggs DL, Waters PM, editors. Rockwood and Wilkins' fractures in children. 8th ed.; 2015. p. 987–1026.
17. Herman MJ, Smith BG. Fractures of the distal femoral physis. In: Flynn JM, Skaggs DL, Waters PM, editors. Rockwood and Wilkins' fractures in children. 8th edition; 2015. p. 1027–56.
18. Edmonds EW, Mubarak SJ. Prxoimal tibial physeal fractures. In: Flynn JM, Skaggs DL, Waters PM, editors. Rockwood and Wilkins' fractures in children. 8th edition; 2015. p. 1057–76.
19. Lalonde F, Wenger D. Tibia. In: Wenger DR, Pring ME, editors. Rang's children's fractures. 3rd edition. Philadelphia: Lippincott Williams & Wilkins; 2005. p. 215–26. Orthopedic surgery.
20. Mooney JF III, Hennrikus WL. Fractures of the shaft of the tibia and fibula. In: Flynn JM, Skaggs DL, Waters PM, editors. Rockwood and Wilkins' fractures in children. 8th edition; 2015. p. 1137–72.
21. Eberl R, Singer G, Schalamon J, et al. Fractures of the talus-differences between children and adolescents. J Trauma 2010;68:126–30.
22. Fernandez ML, Wade AM, Dabbah M, et al. Talar neck fractures treated with closed reduction and percutaneous screw fixation: a case series. Am J Orthop (Belle Mead NJ) 2011;40:72–7.
23. Yu GR, Zhao HM, Yang YF, et al. Open reduction and internal fixation of intra-articular calcaneal fractures in children. Orthopedics 2012;35(6):e874–9.
24. Ceccarelli F, Faldini C, Piras F, et al. Surgical versus non-surgical treatment of calcaneal fractures in children: a long-term results comparative study. Foot Ankle Int 2000;21(10):825–32.
25. Owen RJ, Hickey FG, Finlay DB. A study of metatarsal fractures in children. Injury 1995;26(8):537–8.
26. Herrera-Soto JA, Scherb M, Duffy MF, et al. Fractures of the fifth metatarsal in children and adolescents. J Pediatr Orthop 2007;27(4):427–31.
27. Crawford A. Fractures and dislocations of the foot and ankle. In: Green NE, editor. Skeletal trauma in children. Philadelphia: WB Saunders; 1994. p. 449–516.

The Limping Child

Monica Payares-Lizano, MD, FAAOS, FAAP

KEYWORDS

- Limp • Limping child • Gait abnormality • Antalgic gait • Septic arthritis
- Lower-extremity fractures • Leg length discrepancy

KEY POINTS

- Limping is a common complaint in children. Whether it is associated with pain or painless, it can be caused by a multitude of conditions ranging from mild, such as a sprain, to life threatening, such as malignancies.
- Establishing the underlying diagnosis requires a thorough assessment including history, examination, laboratory studies, and imaging if required.
- It is important to recognize orthopedic emergencies such as septic arthritis, vascular compromise, compartment syndrome, and open fractures.

 Video content accompanies this article at http://www.pediatric.theclinics.com.

INTRODUCTION

Evaluation of a limping child can be challenging for both parents and clinicians because of the multitude of potential diagnoses. A thorough understanding of normal gait patterns, accompanied by history and physical examination, can guide clinicians in undergoing efficient diagnostic testing. Evaluation must be done in an organized systematic approach, which can lessen the burden, home in on the underlying cause, and allow management to be started promptly. However, first it is necessary to understand and define what is a normal pattern before undergoing a full work-up.

Defining Normal and Abnormal Gait: What Is a Limp?

Normal gait is a smooth, rhythmic process that requires minimal expenditure of energy. This process changes with age. When children begin ambulating, which occurs most typically between the ages of 12 and 16 months, they show what is commonly referred to as toddler pattern (Videos 1 and 2). This pattern is characterized by short stride lengths, fast cadence, slow velocity, and wide base.[1] They have immature motor planning and coordination and the arm motion is nonreciprocal with legs, and these combined can lead to frequent falls. The fluidity of gait improves between 3 and 5 years

Disclosure: The author has no disclosures.
Orthopaedic Surgery Program, Nicklaus Children's Hospital, 3100 Southwest 62nd Avenue, Miami, FL 33155, USA
E-mail address: Monica.Payares-Lizano@nicklaushealth.org

of age, the arm and leg reciprocity is attained, and the overall coordination is improved (Video 3). By the age of 7 years, the child shows a mature adult gait[2] (Video 4).

The mature gait cycle includes swing and stance phase. Stance phase includes initial contact, loading response, midstance, terminal stance, and preswing and comprises 60% of the gait cycle. In swing phase, the remaining 40% of the gait cycle is spent after toe-off; the foot is advanced in the air to position itself for the next heel strike.[3]

Analyzing the different types of deviations can help clinicians hone down the diagnosis. An antalgic or painful gait is one resulting from pain in the heel, knee, or hip. This pain results in a shortened stance phase on the affected leg as well as a shortened stride length of the normal side to be able to quickly get to the well leg in stance phase again (Video 5: antalgic gait). If it is painful enough, the child may refuse to weight bear altogether.

A limp is a deviation from a normal age-appropriate gait pattern resulting in an uneven, jerky, or laborious gait, and can be caused by pain, weakness, or deformity as a result of a variety of conditions. The exact incidence of limping in children is unknown. One study of children younger than 14 years presenting to an emergency department with an acute atraumatic limp reported an incidence of 1.8 per 1000 children, a male-to-female ratio of 1.7:1, and a median age of 4.4 years (**Table 1**).[3]

Nonantalgic (or nonpainful gait) can also be sign of neurologic issues. Some examples of nonantalgic gait are equinus (toe walking), Trendelenburg, circumduction, and steppage.[1]

In equinus, or toe-walking gait, there is plantarflexion of the ankle joint that can be habitual or idiopathic or can be caused by shortening or tight heel cord, clubfoot, leg length discrepancy, or cerebral palsy. In Trendelenburg gait pattern, children have the appearance of shifting their weight over the affected side during stance phase. This shifting is a sign of weak hip abductors, as opposed to an antalgic gait, in which the stance phase is not shortened. This pattern can be seen in Legg-Calvé-Perthes disease (LCPD), developmental dysplasia of the hip (DDH), slipped capital femoral epiphysis (SCFE), muscular dystrophy, and hemiplegic cerebral palsy. Video 6 shows

Table 1
Age-specific diagnosis in patients presenting with a limp

Toddler (<3 y)	Child (3–10 y)	Adolescent (>10 y)
Developmental dysplasia of the hip	Legg-Calvé-Perthes disease	Slipped capital femoral epiphysis
Congenital limb deficiencies	Stress fractures	Legg-Calvé-Perthes disease
Neuromuscular abnormalities	Tumors	Juvenile idiopathic arthritis
Painful gait	Osteochondrosis	Overuse syndromes
Toddler fracture	Kohler disease	Osteochondrosis
Septic arthritis	Osteochondritis dissecans	Tumors
Reactive arthritis	Osgood-Schlatter disease	Osteochondritis dissecans
Transient synovitis	Transient synovitis	Stress fractures
Osteomyelitis	Osteomyelitis	Tarsal coalition
Foreign object in knee or foot	Leg length discrepancy	Discoid meniscus

From Herman M, Martinek M. The Limping Child. Pediatrics in Review 2015;36;184; with permission.

a 21-month-old boy who has a history of septic arthritis and subsequently developed avascular necrosis of the femoral head. **Fig. 1** shows MRI of the 21-month-old patient consistent with avascular necrosis (AVN).

In circumduction gait there is stiffness at the knee or ankle and the child uses excessive abduction of the hip, pelvic rotation, and hiking to be able to clear the foot during swing phase. This gait can be seen with leg length discrepancy, cerebral palsy, or any other cause that leads to stiffness of the knee or ankle (Video 7).

Children with leg length discrepancy may vault or toe walk with the shorter limb to clear the longer limb.

Children with weak ankle dorsiflexors, such as those with Charcot-Marie-Tooth disease, develop a steppage gait. In steppage gait, they hyperflex the knee to clear the foot in swing and are unable to decelerate the foot between heel strike and foot flat, and thus they end up with a slapping foot on the ground (Video 8). Video 8 shows a 15-year-old boy with Charcot-Marie-Tooth with weak ankle dorsiflexors. Other conditions that can present with this type of gait include myelodysplasia, Friedreich ataxia, and cerebral palsy.

CLINICAL EVALUATION
History

Depending on the age of the child, getting an accurate history can be difficult, and thus being able to interview the parents or primary caregiver is important. If suspecting nonaccidental trauma or possible sexually transmitted disease exposure, it may be beneficial to interview the child or adolescent separately.

A helpful mnemonic that is traditionally used to evaluate pain is OLD CART (onset, location, duration, characteristics, associated/alleviating factors, relieving factors, treatment) to remember what to ask for. This mnemonic can be applied to the evaluation of a limp (**Table 2**). The initial interview helps narrow down the differential (**Table 3**).[3]

Always ask the history of any prior evaluations and attempt to obtain records of prior work-up, if possible. Ask about family history of autoimmune diseases, neuromuscular diseases infection exposure, and recent travel.

Physical Examination

Depending on the age and the acuteness of the presentation, children may not be cooperative with full examination and thus clinicians must take full advantage of every

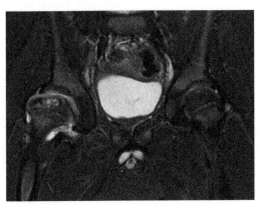

Fig. 1. AVN of the femoral head. Accompanies Video 1 showing Trendelenburg gait in a 21-month-old boy.

Table 2
OLDCART history tips associated with limp

Onset	When did the limp begin? Associated with acute event or overuse?
Location	Ask about possible location; it may not be apparent initially
Duration	Ask about how long the limp has been present and the timing of when it happens; whether it is in the morning or afternoon, after activities, and so forth
Characteristics	Ask about its characteristics; is it constant, intermittent, or transient?
Associated/ Alleviating factors	Associated symptoms; eg, fevers, chills, weight loss, anorexia night sweats. Can also ask about any aggravating symptoms; ie, when putting weight on it, straightening or bending it, after walking for a long time
Relieving factors	Does anything make it better? Hold leg in flex, externally rotated position, medication
Treatment	Have you tried any medications; eg, nonsteroidal antiinflammatory drugs or antibiotics

moment of the interactions. Start with observing as the patient walks into the room if are able to. Patients may change their minds or refuse after being formally introduced. As a general rule, I like to leave the painful extremity last, because the child is likely to be unable to continue the examination if the clinician has hurt them.

Table 3
Pointers from the clinical history to determine diagnosis

History Finding	Possible Cause
Acute trauma	Fracture, sprain
Associated with abdominal pain	Acute abdomen, psoas abscess, appendicitis
Associated with back pain	Vertebral osteomyelitis, diskitis
Associated with neck pain, photophobia	Meningitis
Associated with fevers, chills, weight loss	Septic arthritis, osteomyelitis, rheumatologic disease, or tumor
Insect bite, recent travel	Lyme disease, dengue, chikungunya
Sickle cell	AVN, bone infarcts, sickle cell crisis
Bleeding disorders	Hemarthrosis, hemophilia, von Willebrand
Migratory arthralgias or morning stiffness	Rheumatologic disorders, acute rheumatic fever
Pain at night or intermittent at rest	Malignant tumor
Pain burning or radiating	Neuropathic, peripheral, or spinal
Pain constant	Infection or tumor
Pain localized	Trauma, infection, or tumor
Pain increases with activity	Overuse, stress fracture
Pain decreases with activity	Rheumatologic
Sexually active	Gonococcal arthritis, reactive arthritis
Preceded by diarrhea	Reactive arthritis
Preceded by pharyngitis	Acute rheumatic fever

Data from Sawyer JR, Kapoor M. The limping child: a systematic approach to diagnosis. Am Fam Physician. 2009 Feb 1;79(3):215-24.

In general, look at the appearance of the patient. Does the patient look lethargic, irritable, or in distress despite looking well. Look at the skin. Are there any rashes or skin lesions? If possible, put a gown or shorts on the patient and make sure to check the entire body. It is ideal to examine patients without shoes to make sure the patient was not covering any potentially important signs.

Approach the patient in a systematic way to decrease the chances of missing important information. My preference is to start from the floor going up. Evaluate the feet and ankles, then the knees, then the hip, and try to observe each joint for at least 2 or 3 cycles if possible. If the evaluation is for a more chronic issue or an intermittent one, ask parents whether they have videos on their mobile devices, and if not then ask them to make one during an episode and bring it to a follow-up evaluation. Starting with the feet, see whether the patient is planting the foot on the lateral border or the medial border to avoid putting pressure on a possible entry point for a puncture wound or fracture, and whether the patient is achieving heel strike, flatfoot, or toe strike. Look at the foot progression angle because this helps in assessing rotational issues. When looking at the knee, check whether there is a stiff-knee gait and whether it is crouched, and then look at the hips and pelvis for whether there is any anterior or posterior tilt, Trendelenburg, or out-of-phase abduction. Look at the posture of the spine and upper extremities.

Next focus on a standing examination. For the spine, make sure there is no asymmetry in the coronal or sagittal planes. Note whether there is any shoulder or pelvic obliquity. If concerned for possible leg length discrepancy, use blocks and determine whether the pelvic obliquity is correct. A Trendelenburg test can help assess any hip abductor weakness. Have the child stand on the affected leg with the knee flexed at 90° and the hip extended. If the child is unable to elevate the hemipelvis, this can be another sign of abductor weakness and may indicate hip disorder (Video 9).

If there is suspicion for a possible muscular dystrophy on the history, a Gower test should be performed.

Table examination

Examine the skin for rashes. Again look at the face and notice any abnormal findings; look at the head. Is there any asymmetry, or any signs of plagiocephaly or torticollis? Look at the chest for any asymmetry. Look at extremities for swelling, effusions of the joints, and the resting position of the extremities. For instance, if a child is presenting with a septic arthritis of the hip, the child will be more comfortable with the leg in flexion abduction and external rotation (**Fig. 2**).

Examined the abdomen. It is important to rule out any intra-abdominal issues. It is common to find children with psoas abscesses or even appendicitis that presents initially with a limp.[4]

A psoas sign can help to distinguish between the causes. This sign has pain with passive extension of the hip. Check the sacroiliac joint with the FABER (flexion, abduction, and external rotation) test. In the supine position flex, abduct, and externally rotate the hip joint. This test can indicate sacroiliac disorder.

Going down the lower extremity, look for asymmetry. Palpate the entire extremity and note any grimacing or withdrawal. Even in a nonverbal child it should be possible to observe any discomfort with certain movements or tenderness in the particular region. Check the range of motion in all joints.

Please see orthopedic examination article elsewhere in this issue for more details on the orthopedic physical examination.

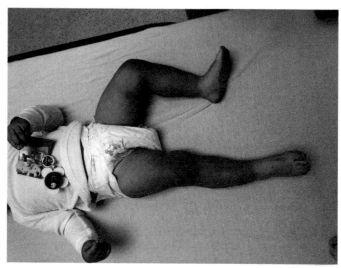

Fig. 2. Position of rest in a patient with septic arthritis. The leg is held in flexion, abduction, and external rotation to decrease intracapsular pressure and allow some relief of pain.

Diagnostic Tests

Laboratory tests are most commonly indicated when the history and physical examination are consistent with possible infections or inflammatory causes. These tests include a complete blood count, erythrocyte sedimentation rate (ESR), C-reactive protein (CRP), and blood cultures.

Titers can be added if there is a suspicion based on history. Rheumatoid factor can also be added as well as antinuclear antibody for an initial rheumatologic work-up. If septic arthritis is suspected, an arthrocentesis is performed urgently and sent for Gram staining, cell count, and culture.[1]

Imaging

The imaging of limping children is based on the patient's age, location of pain, history of trauma, and concern for infection. Plain radiographs should be done first, before any advanced imaging. Bartoloni and colleagues[5] have developed several helpful imaging algorithms to guide diagnostic imaging approach based on age group: toddlers (1–3 years of age), children (3–10 years), and adolescents (11–16 years) (**Figs. 3–5**). If unable to determine the site, initial full-length imaging may be necessary.[6] The most common cause of limp is again minor trauma, and radiographs are a good start. In most situations, anteroposterior (AP) and lateral radiographs of the segment are most helpful. A third view may be helpful; for instance, an oblique of an ankle or a nondisplaced fracture of the tibia seen in a toddler's fracture. Keep in mind that there are several fractures that have negative radiographs initially, as well as early infection. Radiologic evidence of some fractures or infections may not show up for 7 to 10 days. At that time, imaging may reveal a periosteal reaction. If infection is a possibility, then laboratory tests are warranted and ultrasonography is an appropriate initial imaging modality with high sensitivity for detection of joint effusions.[7]

Ultrasonography is especially helpful in determining hip effusions (**Fig. 6**), soft tissue abscesses, and even foreign bodies that cannot be visualized on plain films.

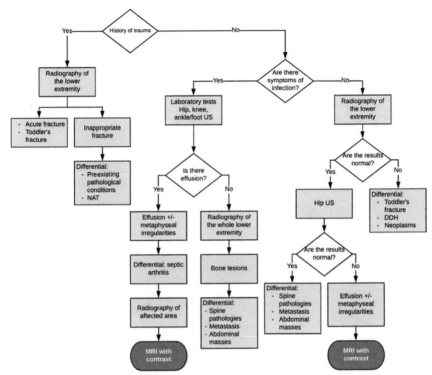

Fig. 3. Diagnostic imaging in toddlers. NAT, non-accidental trauma; US, ultrasonography. (*Adapted from* Bartoloni A, Aparisi Gómez MP, Cirillo M, et al. Imaging of the limping child. Eur J Radiol. 2018;109:155-170; with permission.)

Radiographs have low sensitivity in detecting early osteomyelitis of soft tissue infection.

A bone scan can be helpful in infections and tumors if the site cannot be localized based on history and physical. Although it is sensitive for these, it lacks specificity.[8]

Computed tomography (CT) is used primarily for finer bony details and can be helpful in further evaluating complex or intra-articular fractures and thus has limited value in initial evaluation of limping children.[9]

MRI is helpful in visualizing joints, soft tissues, cartilage, and bone marrow, and is particularly helpful for musculoskeletal infections, neoplasms, vascular abnormalities, and AVN. It is both sensitive and specific. MRI is warranted in cases of negative radiographic findings and can be confirmatory, showing extent of involvement of both the bone and soft tissues. The use of contrast can be considered in specific cases and can help better delineated small abscesses when there is significant edema or a need for more specific location for preoperative planning for possible drainage. It can also help delineate the possibility of osteomyelitis with periosteal abscesses associated with acute septic arthritis.[10,11]

Making the Diagnosis

Making the diagnosis of a limping child is not always straightforward but a good start can be provided by the process shown in **Fig. 7**.

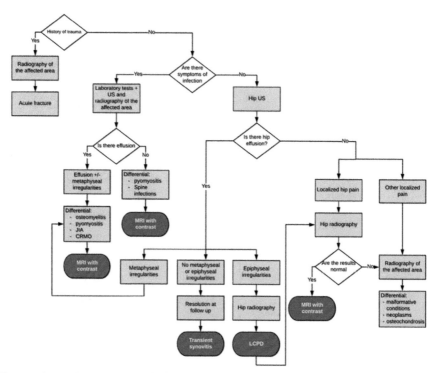

Fig. 4. Diagnostic imaging in children. CRMO, chronic recurrent multifocal osteomyelitis; JIA, juvenile inflammatory arthritis. (*Adapted from* Bartoloni A, Aparisi Gómez MP, Cirillo M, et al. Imaging of the limping child. Eur J Radiol. 2018;109:155-170; with permission.)

Causes
Consideration of some of the common and worrisome diagnoses can help clinicians become aware of the things they should be thinking about and should not miss. As Herman and Martinek[12] state, it is extremely important to consider the main orthopedic emergencies and rule these out because delays can have an effect on the patient's prognosis (**Table 4**).

Traumatic injuries
Vascular compromise Check whether there is an obvious deformity or swelling and nonpalpable pulses, or bluish discoloration likely secondary to venous conditions or paleness from arterial insufficiency. Clinicians may consider realigning the extremity to see whether the process changes. Emergent orthopedic consultation is required (**Fig. 8**).

Open fractures These are fractures in which the integrity of the skin is violated and the underlying bone is exposed to the outside. This fracture requires more aggressive initial management and this should be determined by the orthopedist. It can be as small as a poke hole or can involve extensive soft tissue compromise and loss. The most common open fractures that are missed are the Seymour fractures (**Fig. 9**), which are displaced fractures of the distal phalanx physis. Management may consist of removal of the nail and debridement of the fracture with reduction and nailbed laceration repair as well as antibiotic treatment. These fractures are easily missed in the emergency department because sometimes there is only a small widening seen

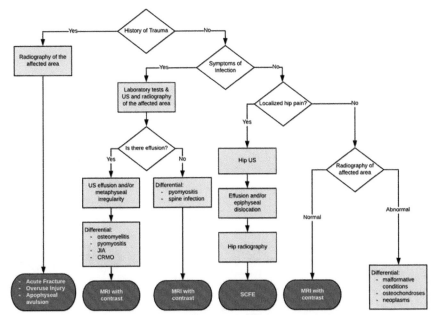

Fig. 5. Diagnostic imaging in adolescents. (*Adapted from* Bartoloni A, Aparisi Gómez MP, Cirillo M, et al. Imaging of the limping child. Eur J Radiol. 2018;109:155-170; with permission.)

through the growth plate and possible small ecchymosis or bleeding from nail bed and fail to recognize this as an open fracture. If this injury is not recognized it can result in significant infection, osteomyelitis, and nailbed issues.

Compartment syndrome Compartment syndrome is an increase in myofascial pressure secondary to swelling or bleeding into the muscle compartments. This increasing pressure prevents adequate blood flow to the compartment, resulting in severe pain, and can lead to muscle nerve damage and tissue necrosis, and even potentially the loss of the limb. This condition is an orthopedic emergency. In adults, clinicians usually refer the 5 Ps for evaluation of compartment syndrome. The 5 Ps are pain out of proportion, pain with passive stretch, paresthesias, pulselessness,

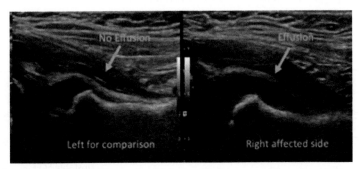

Fig. 6. Ultrasonography of 18-month-old boy with increased laboratory test results and refusal to bear weight. Right side was affected, and the left included for comparison. There is elevation of the capsule with evidence of fluid within the hip joint.

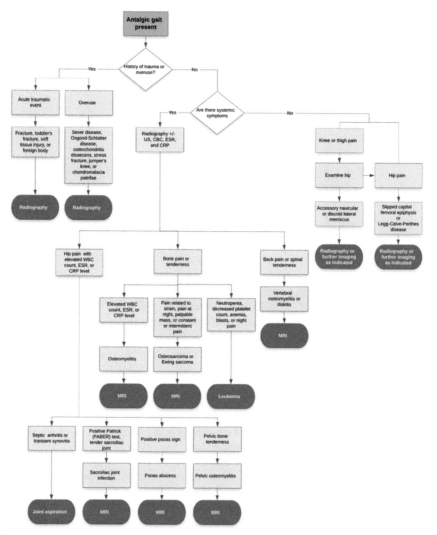

Fig. 7. Antalgic gait evaluation. WBC, white blood cell count.

Table 4	
Orthopedic urgencies and emergencies	
Orthopedic Urgencies	**Orthopedic Emergencies**
Open fractures	Septic arthritis
Stable SCFE	Neurovascular compromise
	Compartment syndrome
	Unstable SCFE

From Herman M, Martinek M. The Limping Child. Pediatrics in Review 2015;36;184; with permission.

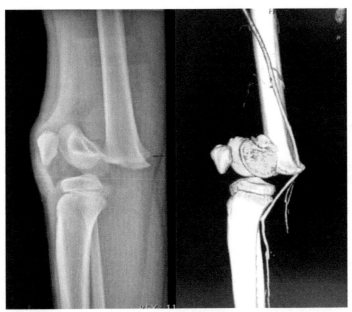

Fig. 8. Radiograph and CT arthrogram showing distal femoral physeal fracture causing vascular compromise. Patient is an 8-year-old whose leg was caught on a pier and lost pulses. The patient was airlifted to our institution after initial manipulation with nonpalpable pulses with some perfusion. Patient had emergent open reduction and percutaneous pinning, and pulses returned after reduction.

and paralysis. However, in children, this can be more challenging to identify. Instead, the 3 As are commonly accepted as the indicators for pediatric compartment syndrome: increase in analgesia requirement, anxiety, and agitation. These signs can be seen after fractures of the tibial tubercle or shaft, supracondylar humerus fractures, or forearm fractures.

Nonaccidental trauma In patients with lower-extremity fractures that are not yet ambulatory or patients with fractures at different stages of healing, this should be immediately suspected (**Fig. 10**). An evaluation by child protective services and a bone survey are warranted.

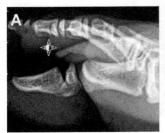
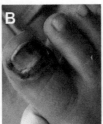
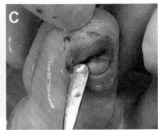

Fig. 9. Seymour fracture. A 6-year-old boy who stubbed his toe on furniture 10 days before presentation. Low-grade fevers and drainage. (*A*) Folded periosteum at the nail bed into the growth plate. (*B*) Purulent collection at the eponychium. (*C*) Removal of nail reveals laceration of the nail bed and the reason why these are considered open fractures.

Other common diagnoses

Toddler's fracture Tibial shaft is a common location for injury in young children. The so-called toddler's fracture can present with limping after a minor fall or twisting injury. There has recently been an increase in these playground injuries with parents holding the children and coming down a slide and the leg getting caught on the side of the slide. More often than not, the initial imaging is negative, only to be positive after 7 to 10 days once the healing has started. Sometimes an oblique radiograph can be helpful (**Fig. 11**).

Management consists of casting in a short-leg walking cast for 3 to 4 weeks. These fractures usually heal uneventfully.

Foot Nondisplaced fractures of the metatarsal and phalanges are very common, and usually present with point tenderness, focal swelling, and ecchymosis. Patients may position the foot to place the weight-bearing pressure away from the injury. For instance, children with first metatarsal base fractures walk on the lateral aspect of the foot.

Puncture wounds and foreign body Children commonly walk barefoot and frequently step on objects such as glass or splinters that puncture the plantar surface, and some of these foreign bodies may be retained, resulting in inflammation and infection. These symptoms are not noticed for several days to weeks until limping begins, when a small area of swelling or drainage may be noticed. Initial evaluation for retained or foreign objects should include radiographs and ultrasonography. If it is decided to treat with antibiotics, consider adding *Pseudomonas* coverage. If there is a foreign body it should be surgically explored and removed if management has not improved

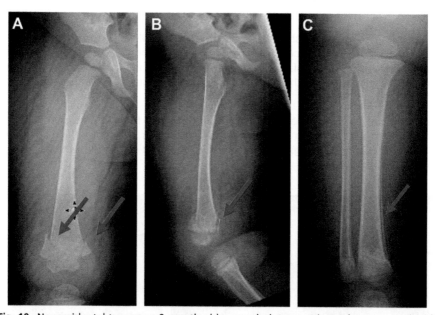

Fig. 10. Nonaccidental trauma: a 9-month old nonambulatory patient who presented with corner fractures of the distal femur and distal tibia and fibular fracture at different stages of healing. (*A*) AP distal femur showing acute metaphyseal corner fractures (*arrows*). (*B*) Lateral of femur with metaphyseal corner fracture (*arrow*). (*C*) Ipsilateral distal tibia fracture with periosteal reaction consistent with healing fracture (*arrow*).

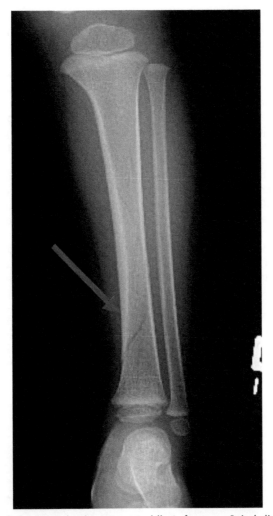

Fig. 11. Tibial shaft fracture also known as toddler's fracture. Spiral distal shaft fracture (*arrow*).

with oral antibiotics. Patients should have close follow-up and, if not improved, consider intravenous (IV) antibiotics.

Infection and inflammatory conditions
There is a wide range of musculoskeletal manifestations for infection, including local cellulitis, myositis, osteomyelitis, inflammatory arthritis, septic arthritis, and these can present with a painful limp, inability to weight bear, and fevers. There may or may not be focal swelling, tenderness to palpation, erythema, joint effusion, or limited range of motion.

If there is concerned about septic arthritis, it is extremely important to recognize this promptly because, again, any delays in treatment could be detrimental.

Herman and Martinek[12] point out that the damage to the cartilage and blood supply to the femoral head begins within 6 to 12 hours of the onset of the infection. This damage can become irreversible after 1 to 2 days. The patient may present with a similar presentation for a mild toxic synovitis with fevers; inability to bear weight; and holding the extremity in flexion, external rotation, and abduction (see **Fig. 2**; **Fig. 12**).

Differentiating between a toxic synovitis and a septic arthritis can be challenging. Kocher and colleagues[13] found a relationship with several clinical factors and the likelihood of having a septic arthritis: temperature more than 38.5°C (101.4°F), white blood count more than 12,000/μL, ESR more than 40 mm/h, and inability to weight bear. The risk of having septic arthritis increases with the number of indicators present (**Table 5**).

Caird and colleagues[14] added CRP to the criteria, with increases greater than 2.5 mg/L also being a sign of possible septic arthritis.

If there is a high suspicion, ultrasonography of the joint is required, with arthrocentesis for confirmation. The arthrocentesis has a positive white blood count of greater than 50,000/μL and greater than 75% polymorphonuclear leukocytes and positive Gram stain. Emergency drainage with irrigation debridement should be done as well as initial empiric coverage of antibiotics. The antibiotics should then be changed to a more targeted treatment based on the cultures and sensitivities. Patients usually start to do better within a few days. Clinicians should observe clinically and follow laboratory tests, trending down with improvement in the ability to weight bear.

Toxic synovitis Toxic synovitis is the most common nontraumatic diagnosis of limping children. It can be diagnosed in as many as 85% of children with atraumatic hip pain and limping. Commonly the synovitis is preceded by an upper respiratory infection, which develop as much as 2 weeks to a month before presentation of the limp.

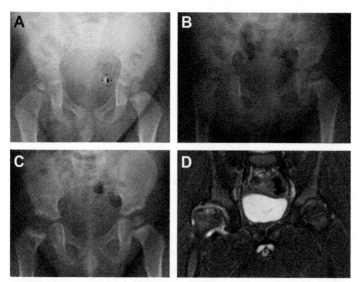

Fig. 12. Sequelae of patient who presented with 7 days of fevers and refusal to weight bear found to have right septic arthritis and managed with emergent irrigation and debridement. (*A*) AP pelvis on initial presentation showing asymmetry of the femoral head. (*B*) Postoperative radiographs at 4 weeks showing early signs of AVN. (*C*) Six-month follow-up AP and frog lateral radiographs showing AVN. (*D*) MRI confirming AVN of the head with collapse of lateral pillar.

Table 5	
Kocher criteria	
Kocher Criteria Factor	**Likelihood of Septic Arthritis by # of Factors**
Inability to bear weight	1 = 3%
ESR>40 mm/h	2 = 40%
WBC>12,000/μL	3 = 93%
Fever >38.5°C (101.4°F)	4 = 99%

Abbreviation: WBC, white blood cell count.
  Data from Kocher MS, Zurakowski D, Kasser JR. Differentiating between septic arthritis and transient synovitis of the hip in children: an evidence-based clinical prediction algorithm. J Bone Joint Surg Am. 1999 Dec;81(12):1662-70.

Radiographs are usually negative. Patients may or may not have any effusion on ultrasonography, and white blood count is low, between 5 and 15,000/μL, with negative Gram stain on arthrocentesis. This condition is usually self-limited and pain can be managed with antiinflammatory medications.

Osteomyelitis and deep soft tissue infections Again, this may be difficult to diagnose early in the process and can be nonspecific or have no detectable clinical markers until a few days after onset. White blood count, sedimentation rate, and CRP are usually increased. MRI can be the best diagnostic test (**Fig. 13**). Treatment requires medical as well as surgical treatment in certain cases; for instance, methicillin-resistant *Staphylococcus aureus* can be a very resistant infection if there is a drainable abscess or periosteal abscess, and it may require multiple debridements. There are pathogens that are more common in particular age groups; **Table 6** lists most common organisms based on age and antibiotics of choice for treatment.

Juvenile inflammatory arthritis open Juvenile inflammatory arthritis (JIA) is the most common rheumatologic illness in children. Its prevalence is 1.6 to 86.1 per 100,000 persons. It is an autoimmune disease characterized by joint swelling that persists in children younger than 16 years old for more than 6 weeks.[15] It can be subclassified into systemic, oligoarthritis with 4 joints or fewer, polyarthritis, psoriatic, enthesitis-related arthritis, and others. Systemic symptoms, including lethargy, loss of appetite, and morning stiffness, are usually seen and this condition needs a diagnosis of exclusion, usually after trauma and infection have been ruled out. MRI shows

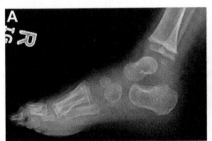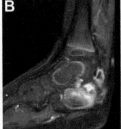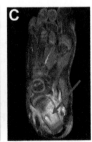

Fig. 13. Calcaneus osteomyelitis. A 4-year-old boy presents with fevers and limping, walking on tiptoes. (*A*) Lateral radiograph of foot with no significant findings. (*B*, *C*) Sagittal and coronal contrast-enhanced MRI showing increased uptake of contrast as well as an abscess (*arrow*). Patient was managed with drilling and IV antibiotics.

Age	Organism	Antibiotics
Table 6 **Septic arthritis: common organisms and antibiotic treatment**		
<12 mo	*Staphylococcus* species, group B *Streptococcus,* and gram-negative bacilli	First-generation cephalosporin
6 mo to 5 y	*S aureus, Streptococcus pneumoniae,* group A *Streptococcus, Haemophilus influenzae*	Second-generation or third-generation cephalosporin
5–12 y	*S aureus*	First-generation cephalosporin
12–18 y	*Neisseria gonorrhoeae, S aureus*	Oxacillin, cephalosporin

contrast-enhanced effusion and, depending on the subtype, some laboratory tests may be negative. Refer to a rheumatologist for further evaluation.

Lyme disease In Lyme disease, the second most common manifestation is arthritis, after erythema migrans. It is transmitted by tick bites caused by *Borrelia burgdorferi*. It is most commonly seen in the northeast of the United States. Other symptoms may include headache, malaise, and fatigue. Arthralgia is seen in the early phase, and arthritis may be delayed for months to years[15]

The knee is the most common joint affected. Diagnosis may be detected by Lyme enzyme–linked immune-absorbent assays titers and Western blot.

DEVELOPMENTAL CAUSES

DDH, LCPD, and SCFE are the 3 most common hip conditions in children and adolescents that present with atraumatic limping.

Developmental Dysplasia of the Hip

DDH is a spectrum of conditions that range from mild formation abnormalities (dysplasia) of acetabulum and/or femoral head to frank dislocation. It mostly occurs in infants and young children, with an incidence of 1 per 1000 live births. It is most common in girls, left side, first born, breech with a strong family history. It can be associated with one of the packing conditions, such as torticollis, metatarsus adductus, and congenital knee dislocation. It is usually diagnosed before ambulatory age; however, it may be recognized at a later date as a leg length discrepancy (**Fig. 14**).

Legg-Calvé-Perthes Disease

Idiopathic AVN of the femoral head has an incidence of 1 per 1200 children, and is usually more common in boys between the ages of 2 and 12 years, most commonly between 6 and 8 years of age. It classically presents with painless limp and limited range of motion at the hip, specifically hip abduction. Outcomes vary based on age of onset, stage at time of presentation, and the resultant femoral head deformity after the remodeling phase (**Fig. 15**).

Slipped Capital Femoral Epiphysis

SCFE is displacement of the capital femoral epiphysis from the metaphysis. Weakness of the physis causes the displacement or slip (**Fig. 16**). This weakness occurs most commonly because of abnormal mechanical stresses or secondary to endocrine or

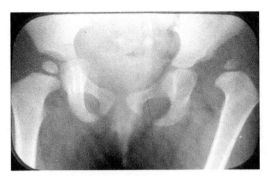

Fig. 14. DDH. Dislocation of the left hip with shallow acetabulum.

metabolic conditions such as hypothyroidism or renal osteodystrophy. It occurs most commonly in prepubertal obese male children between 10 and 14 years old. It occurs during periods of rapid growth and the patients may complain of hip or knee (15%–23%) pain. It can present with external rotation of lower extremity and Trendelenburg gait from limb shortening.

Chronic Recurrent Multifocal Osteomyelitis

Chronic recurrent multifocal osteomyelitis is a recurrent inflammatory condition that can occur in multiple skeletal sites (**Fig. 17**). It was first described by Giedion and colleagues[16] in the early 1970s. It predominantly affects children and adolescents, with a peak age of onset of 10 years and a female/male ratio ranging from 1.7:1 to 4:1. It is frequently associated with other inflammatory disorders, including palmoplantar pustulosis, chronic arthritis, psoriasis, inflammatory bowel disease, pyoderma gangrenosum, Sweet syndrome, and severe acne. Cultures are usually negative and the condition does not respond to antibiotics. Management is conservative with antiinflammatories.[17]

Malignancy

Benign neoplasms and malignancies are uncommon causes of limping but can be the most common reason for anxiety in parents. The clinical picture for these can

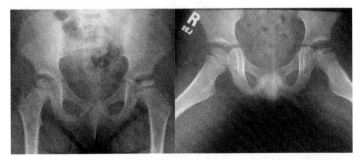

Fig. 15. LCPD. A 9-year-old boy brought in with initially painless limp. Limp worsened and became painful with episodes of hip/knee pain over 6 months. AP (*left*) and frog lateral (*right*) views show left hip with remodeling stage with some collapse of the lateral pillar and flattening of femoral head.

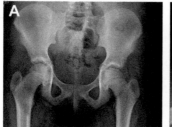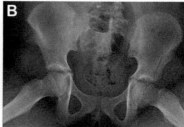

Fig. 16. SCFE. (*A*) AP radiograph and (*B*) frog-leg lateral view showing a left-sided slip (*arrow*).

vary widely and they can occur in all age groups. Nonetheless, a common feature of many bone tumors is pain, especially pain that is worse at night. Lower-extremity neoplasms are also associated with limping and insidious pain with activities, as well as palpable or visible masses. Systemic signs and symptoms, such as lethargy, fever, and weight loss, may be seen in children with malignancies.[12]

Spine

Spinal disorders can manifest as lower-extremity issues and should be considered. Some examples are diskitis, epidural abscess, herniated discs, compression of spine/nerve roots, and spine tumors (**Fig. 18**).

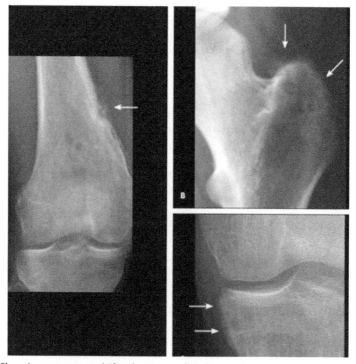

Fig. 17. Chronic recurrent multifocal osteomyelitis (*arrows*).

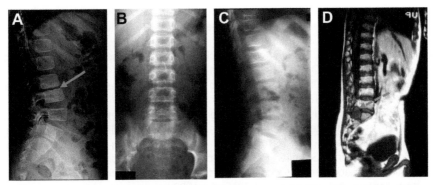

Fig. 18. Spinal causes of limping. (*A*) Diskitis; the arrow point to the affected disk with narrowing of the intervertebral space and end-plate changes. (*B, C*) AP and lateral spine radiographs with mild spondylolithesis L5 to S1. (*D*) MRI revealed mass of L5-S1 disc space behind S1 (*dashed arrow*).

SUMMARY

Limping presents a diagnostic challenge because of the number of possible causes. A careful and systematic evaluation can shorten the long list of potential diagnoses to direct appropriate diagnostic tests to determine the cause of the problem. Trauma and infections are the most common causes of limping. Inflammatory conditions, developmental diagnoses, and overuse injuries are other causes. Although rare, malignancies, such as osteosarcoma and blood cell cancers, must also be considered as potential causes of limping in children and adolescents.

ACKNOWLEDGMENTS

The author would like to acknowledge Cassandra Pino, MS, for her assistance in editing this article and Claire Beimesch for some clinical images.

SUPPLEMENTARY DATA

Supplementary video related to this article can be found at https://doi.org/10.1016/j.pcl.2019.09.009.

REFERENCES

1. Flynn JM, Widmann RF. The limping child: evaluation and diagnosis. J Am Acad Orthop Surg 2001;9(2):89–98. https://doi.org/10.5435/00124635-200103000-00003.
2. Rossiter D, Ahluwalia A. The Limping Child: a systemic approach to assessment and management. Br J Hosp Med 2018;79(10):C150–3.
3. Naranje S, Center FCM, City F. A systematic approach to the evaluation of a limping child. Am Fam Physician 2015;92(10):12.
4. Lifschitz A, Gedalia A, Mares A. Inflammatory irritation of iliopsoas muscle as a reason for the limping in children. Harefuah 1989;(116):464–5.
5. Bartoloni A, Aparisi Gómez MP, Cirillo M, et al. Imaging of the limping child. Eur J Radiol 2018;109:155–70.
6. Safdar N, Rigsby C, Iyer R, et al. ACR Appropriateness Criteria Acutely Limping child up to age 5. J Am Coll Radiol 2018;15(11S):S252–62.

7. Nazarian L. The top 10 reasons musculoskeletal sonography is an important complementary or alternative technique to MRI. Am J Roentgenol 2008;190: 1621–6.

8. Aronson J, Garvin K, Seibert J, et al. Efficiency of the bone scan for occult limping toddlers. J Pediatr Orthop 1992;12:38–44.

9. Cutler L, Molloy A, Dhukuram V, et al. Do CT scans aid assessment of distal tibial physeal fractures? J Bone Joint Surg Br 2004;86:239–43.

10. Nguyen A, Kan J, Bisset G, et al. Kocher criteria revisited in the era of MRI: how often does the Kocher criteria identify underlying osteomyelitis? J Pediatr Orthop 2017;37:e114–9.

11. Monsalve J, Kan J, Schallert E, et al. Septic arthritis in children: frequency of co-existing unsuspected osteomyelitis and implications on imaging work-up and management. Am J Roentgenol 2015;204:1289–95.

12. Herman M, Martinek M. The limping child. Pediatr Rev 2015. https://doi.org/10.1542/pir.36-5-184.

13. Kocher MS, Zurakowski D, Kasser JR. Differentiating between septic arthritis and transient synovitis of the hip in children: an evidence-based clinical prediction algorithm. J Bone Joint Surg Am 1999;81:1662–70.

14. Caird MS, Flynn JM, Leung YL, et al. Factors distinguishing septic arthritis from transient synovitis of the hip in children. A prospective study. J Bone Joint Surg Am 2006;88:1251–7.

15. Syed R. Evaluating the limping child: a rheumatology perspective. Mo Med 2016; 113(2):131–5.

16. Giedon A, Holthusen W, Masel LF, et al. Subacute and chronic "symmetrical" osteomyelitis. Ann Radiol 1972;15:329–42.

17. Herring J. 5th edition. Tachdjian's pediatric orthopaedics: from the Texas Scottish rite Hospital for children, vol. 1. Philadelphia: Elsevier; 2014.

Pediatric Hip and Pelvis

Bertrand W. Parcells, MD

KEYWORDS

- Developmental dysplasia of the hip (DDH) • Femoroacetabular impingement (FAI)
- Slipped capital femoral epiphysis (SCFE) • Legg-Calvé-Perthes disease (LCP)

KEY POINTS

- The most common pediatric orthopedic conditions of the hip and pelvis involve abnormal architecture of the joint leading to pain and dysfunction.
- Developmental Dysplasia of the Hip (DDH) and Femoroacetabular Impingement (FAI) are two common and distinct forms of structural pathology in the pediatric hip.
- Research increasingly shows that some shapes of the hip joint can increase such risks.
- The correlation between anatomic variation and present or future symptoms is rarely straight forward.
- Future investigations are aimed at identifying risk factors to provide pediatric orthopedists tools to risk stratify their patients and understand when conservative approaches such as close observation versus surgical interventions are more appropriate.

HIP DYSPLASIA

Developmental dysplasia of the hip (DDH) is a condition typically in newborns and infants (occasionally in older children) in which the ball and socket (femoral head and acetabulum) of the hip joint are incongruous. When the femoral head and acetabulum fail to properly line up in utero or postnatally, the close proximity and necessary joint pressures are incongruous or missing. These features are necessary for the appropriate development of the hip joint. Without this requisite close contact, the femoral head and acetabulum no longer influence the others' appropriate anatomic normalcy, leading to dysfunction and potential future deformity. This abnormal development of the femoral head and acetabulum may lead to dysplastic structures (underdeveloped acetabulum), resulting in dislocation or subluxation. Besides these mechanical factors, ligamentous and capsular laxity contributes as well. The primary architectural defect leading to pathology is related to the angle of the acetabulum. DDH may be congenital or influenced by postnatal positioning and genetic factors.

DDH may be considered a type of "packaging disorder." One theory describes how the fetus is potentially packaged too tightly within the uterus. This may be brought on by fetal positioning (breech), size, or other conditions such as oligohydramnios. All of

Seaview Orthopaedic & Medical Associates, 1200 Eagle Avenue, Ocean, NJ 07712, USA
E-mail address: bparcells@SeaviewOrthop.onmicrosoft.com

Pediatr Clin N Am 67 (2020) 139–152
https://doi.org/10.1016/j.pcl.2019.09.003
0031-3955/20/© 2019 Elsevier Inc. All rights reserved.

the aforementioned factors may contribute to a decrease in room of the fetus and may cause abnormal bending of the legs and hips ultimately causing DDH. There are other packaging disorders that can be associated with DDH such as metatarsus adductus, congenital muscular torticollis, and congenital knee dislocations. Other contributing factors may be genetic influences, fetal and maternal ligamentous laxity, and postnatal malpositioning.

Female, first born, familial, and breech positioning are commonly quoted as being risk factors for DDH. It is certainly more commonly seen in female infants (6:1) secondary to increased ligamentous laxity and in first born secondary to a smaller and undistended uterus. It has been observed that up to 25% of DDH is bilateral. Although it may be more common in certain ethnicities, DDH is rarely diagnosed in African American children. Additional common influencing factors include gestational diabetes (larger infants); left hip (left occiput anterior positioning most common); Native Americans (cultural swaddling influences); and breech positioning.[1]

The special circumstance of the teratologic hip is worth mention. This occurs when a hip dislocation occurs in utero. This is diagnosed on the first examination with a hip dislocation that is irreducible. The teratologic hip may be associated with neuromuscular, genetic, and syndromic conditions. Such conditions may include spina bifida, arthrogryposis, Larsen syndrome, Ehlers-Danlos syndrome, and associated with other congenital limb deformities. There is a higher likelihood of bilateral hip dislocation.

Diagnosis

As the incidence of DDH can be as common as 1:100, every newborn is examined for hip stability.[1] This is a prominent feature of the musculoskeletal examination of newborns, as an early diagnosis may be successfully treated most often with conservative measures. Instability is tested by stressing the hip with the Barlow test (an attempt to dislocate a reduced hip) and the Ortolani test (an attempt to relocate a dislocated hip) (**Fig. 1**). There are subtleties and variations in the examination that may lead to the diagnosis of a hip click or hip subluxation. Other positive clinical findings would include a positive Galeazzi examination (indicating limb length discrepancy from a dislocated hip), unequal loin folds, and asymmetric hip adduction.

To confirm diagnosis or if there is further concern for hip instability, additional imaging studies are ordered. If the child is younger than 6 months, a dynamic hip ultrasound (**Fig. 2**) is used, as the femoral head and acetabulum have not yet ossified. If the child is older than 6 months, plain radiographs are used. The amount of acetabular deficiency is characterized by the lateral center-edge angle and the acetabular inclination measured on radiograph (**Fig. 3**).

Treatment

Treatment of DDH is based on the severity of deformity and the patient age upon diagnosis. Age is important because the younger the child, the less invasive the treatment. Because a younger child has significant plasticity or, the ability to remodel, both the acetabulum and the femoral head have potential to be molded.

A Pavlik harness is used to treat DDH in children younger than 6 months if the hip remains reduced in a position of hip stability (flexion and abduction). When a child wears a Pavlik harness, the acetabulum and the femoral head are forced into close contact allowing remodeling to occur (**Fig. 4**).

If treatment with a Pavlik harness fails to hold the hip in a stable position, a hip spica cast (which covers the pelvis, hips, and legs) is applied in the operating room.

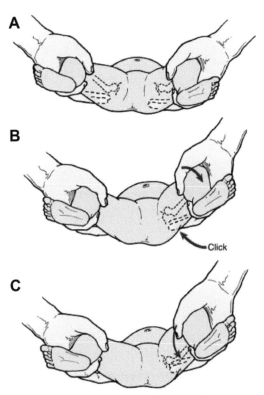

Fig. 1. Example of Ortolani and Barlow maneuvers. (*A*) In the newborn, the 2 hips can be equally flexed, abducted, and laterally rotated without producing a "click." (*B*) Ortolani's sign or first part of Barlow's test. (*C*) Second part of Barlow's test. (*From* Magee DJ. Orthopedic Physical Assessment; Philadelphia, PA: Elsevier; pgs. 689-764; 2014; with permission.)

Reduction of the acetabulum and the femoral head is confirmed with an intraoperative arthrogram and/or and postoperative MRI. Hip spica casting is also used in children aged 6–18 months when a Pavlik harness is insufficient. A spica cast holds the hip in the same position as a Pavlik harness; however, it is rigid and less forgiving. Whether

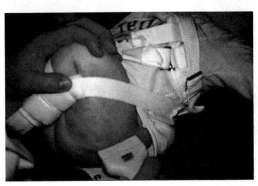

Fig. 2. Dynamic hip ultrasound. (*From* Dare CK, Clarke NMP. Orthopedic Problems in the Neonate. In: Rennie & Roberton's Textbook of Neonatology, Fifth Edition. Philadelphia, PA: Elsevier, 2012.)

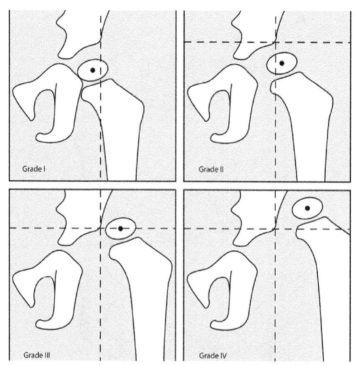

Grade I

Grade II

Grade III

Grade IV

Fig. 3. Example of DDH classification. (*From* Narayanan U1, Mulpuri K, Sankar WN,Reliability of a New Radiographic Classification for Developmental Dysplasia of the Hip. J Pediatr Orthop. 2015 Jul-Aug;35(5):478-84. https://doi.org/10.1097/BPO.0000000000000318.)

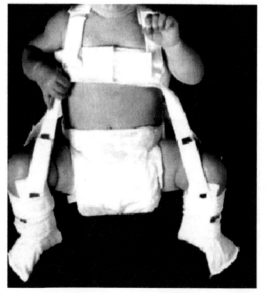

Fig. 4. Pavlik harness. (*From* Orthoinfo. Development of Dislocation (Dysplasia) of the Hip (DDH). Available at: https://orthoinfo.aaos.org/en/diseases–conditions/developmental-dislocation-dysplasia-of-the-hip-ddh/.)

a Pavlik harness or spica cast is used, children are held in this position for a few months to give the bones and surrounding soft tissue time to remodel.

The most challenging cases occur when the child is older than 2 years, as the hip is less plastic and thus surgery is required to reshape the acetabulum and the femoral head. The extent of surgery required to correct DDH becomes progressively greater with increasing age. This type of surgery is referred to as "hip preservation" and the most common procedure is a periacetabular osteotomy (see **Fig. 5**). The goals of hip preservation are to correct the primary deformity, eliminate instability, prevent articular damage, and delay or prevent the onset of degenerative disease and dysfunction.

Natural History

Uncorrected DDH is the most common cause of hip replacement surgery in patients younger than 50 years (accounts for 50% of cases).[2] It leads to osteoarthritis (OA) because the position of the acetabulum causes undercoverage of the femoral head and thus a smaller surface area of contact between acetabulum and the femoral head, which increases forces on the cartilage resulting in early wear.[1]

FEMOROACETABULAR IMPINGEMENT

Femoroacetabular impingement (FAI) is an incongruent ball-and-socket deformity that leads to repetitive contact at terminal hip motion. It is an increasingly recognized cause of hip pain and more controversially, a potential factor for future arthritis.[2–4]

The impingement can be caused by an abnormally shaped femoral head, which is called a cam impingement. The aspherical head (increased anterior-lateral contour) will reduce the head-neck offset and will cause "outside-in" microtrauma, also known as an inclusion-type injury. This refers to the mechanism of injury. Cam impingement is most common in young, athletic men, rarely presents before adolescence, and may be associated with a subclinical slipped capital femoral epiphysis that was missed in childhood.[5–21]

The impingement can also be caused by an abnormal acetabulum, which is called a pincer impingement. This type of impingement is caused by an area of the acetabular rim that overcovers the femoral head and causes repetitive trauma by direct impact of the rim against the femoral neck. The pincer impingement may be caused by

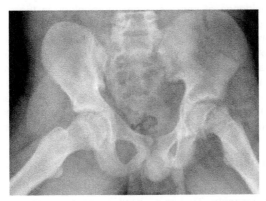

Fig. 5. Radiograph demonstrating left hip SCFE. Image *reproduced* with permission from Medscape Drugs & Diseases (https://emedicine.medscape.com/), Imaging in Slipped Capital Femoral Epiphysis, 2017. Available at: https://emedicine.medscape.com/article/413810-overview.

acetabular retroversion, or general overcoverage, or hip protrusio. The contact between the rim and head-neck junction causes labral separation and cartilage damage of the acetabulum (similar to cam impingement). Pincer deformities are more common in women. The damage created by a pincer deformity is commonly smaller than that caused from cam deformities and, thus, more benign.

FAI is not just caused by abnormal anatomy but also by repetitive athletic activity. It is most commonly seen in athletes, because impingement occurs at the extremes of hip motion, which rarely occurs during activities of daily living. Painful cases of impingement are common to athletes, although painless structural "abnormalities" are commonly seen in the general population, thus blurring the lines between what is considered normal hip morphology.

Diagnosis

Patients complain of groin pain that begins after small trauma or commonly with insidious onset. The pain can be intermittent or caused by exercise, prolonged walking, running, or sitting. On physical examination, patients often have decreased range of motion, particularly with hip internal rotation and hip flexion. Radiographs of FAI can often be normal and only show subtle changes. If FAI is suspected, an MR arthrogram is performed—this is an MRI with intraarticular injection of contrast material. Labral pathology such as tear and cartilage injury can be identified.

Treatment

Nonoperative treatment includes activity modification, physical therapy, cortisone injections to reduce inflammation, or surgical treatment depending on the severity of symptoms. Surgery aims to improve hip motion and prevent impingement by shaving down the area of pathologic morphology. Open surgical treatment is performed using the technique of surgical hip dislocation. More recently, arthroscopic management of these pathologies has increased in popularity. Our ability to diagnose FAI has improved significantly, and hence, improved surgical techniques have led to improved outcomes.

Natural History

The cause and effect of FAI and OA has been proposed in many studies. Some studies suggest a high incidence of cam or pincer morphology in the general population without OA,[22] suggesting FAI may not be a direct cause of OA but rather a result of selection bias. There is controversy about the generally high incidence of FAI. Abnormal morphology in the general population was seen in 15% of men and 7% of women.[22,23] Examining 1000 young men in the Swiss military, there was a 24% incidence of FAI.[24–28] Looking at athletes, the incidence of FAI in hockey is 68%,[29] 50% in youth soccer,[30] and 48% in track and field.[31] This overall high incidence confuses the correlation between clinically relevant FAI and OA. Long-term studies will improve our understanding of the influence of FAI on later degenerative changes.

SLIPPED CAPITAL FEMORAL EPIPHYSIS

Slipped capital femoral epiphysis (SCFE) is a relatively common hip disorder that affects primarily adolescents. The name itself is actually a misnomer—the femoral head actually remains seated within the acetabulum; however, the proximal femoral neck/shaft moves (slips) anteriorly and rotates externally. SCFE is considered a form of epiphysiolysis. The deformity created is a complicated 3-dimensional misaligned shape (**Fig. 5**). Unfortunately, this often leads to dysfunction, deformity, FAI, or degenerative disease.

There are varying presenting ages and incidence—indeed there are differing incidences based on seasonal variation and ethnicity. The overall incidence of SCFE ranges from 0.5 to 18 depending on the source. The overall incidence of SCFE in the United States was 10.8 per 100,000 between 1997 and 2000 (13.35 boys: 8.07 girls for a ratio of 1.65). Average presenting age was 12.7 years for boys and 11.2 years for girls. US geography influences incidence as demonstrated in multiple papers: Northeast 17.15; West 12.70; South 8.12; and Midwest 7.69. Multiple investigators have demonstrated that ethnic incidence varies as well: 40-fold increase in some Polynesian children with the lowest risk in children of Indo-Mediterranean region.[32]

Interestingly, there is a clear relationship among obesity and SCFE. For instance, the number of obese adolescents of Scottish dissent from 1981 to 2005 had doubled with the number of morbidly obese adolescents quadrupled. The incidence of SCFE in that same population increased from 3.78 to 9.66 per 100,000 and the mean age at presentation decreased (from 13.4 to 12.6 in boys and 12.2 to 11.6 in girls). Of children diagnosed with SCFE, 70% are at or greater than the 80th percentile for obesity and 50% are at or greater than the 90th.[33]

The cause of SCFE has been shown to be multifactorial: mechanical, endocrine, and genetic influences. Mechanical factors include increase in acetabular retroversion which changes the contact points and stresses. The inclination of the proximal femoral epiphysis also affects the incidence. Endocrine disorders may also predispose children to developing SCFE—may be as high as 5% to 8% of all patients with SCFE.[33] Common endocrine disorders include hypothyroidism, Down syndrome, Klinefelter and Marfan syndromes, hypogonadism, panhypopituitarism, and renal osteodystrophy. Indeed, endocrine workup should be initiated for patients developing SCFE early (<10 year old) or with bilateral presentation. Lastly, a genetic influence has been suggested but not fully elucidated as yet. For instance, Loder and colleagues have demonstrated an increased incidence in some children of Amish dissent. Scharschmidt and colleagues[34] have demonstrated downregulation of gene expression for type II collagen and aggrecan in children with SCFE.[35–37]

Diagnosis

The most common presentation is an adolescent, prepubescent obese boy: patient will complain of groin, thigh, and/or knee pain episodic and insidious in nature. Patients often present with a limp. There is typically no history of trauma. Physical examination may reveal an antalgic or Trendelenburg type gait pattern with the affected lower extremity externally rotated. There is typically limited painful internal rotation and often obligate external rotation and abduction with attempts at flexion the hip.

All patients with atraumatic knee or hip pain require an anteroposterior and frog-leg lateral view of both hips for complete evaluation. Klein's line (line extending toward femoral head from the femoral neck) will not intersect the lateral capital epiphysis, confirming an SCFE diagnosis (**Fig. 6**). If normal radiographs and the practitioner still has suspicion for SCFE, an MRI may be ordered as it is sensitive for confirming a diagnosis.[33]

Treatment

Ultimately, the goals of treatment are to prevent further displacement, decrease pain, and return of function and to avoid recognized late complications of delayed treatment to include avascular necrosis. Stability of the SCFE dictates the urgency of treatment. Stability is defined by the ability of the patient to bear weight comfortably with or

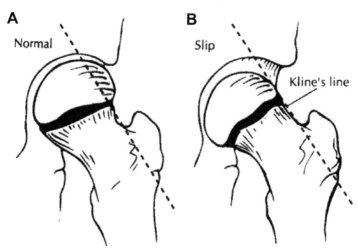

Fig. 6. Diagnostic radiograph picture demonstrating Klein's line. (*A*) Normal hip. (*B*) SCFE—femoral head below Klein's line. (*From* Houghton KM. Review for the generalist: evaluation of pediatric hip pain. Pediatr Rheumatol Online J. 2009 May 18;7:10. https://doi.org/10.1186/1546-0096-7-10; with permission.)

without crutches. Stability also allows for some degree of prognosis as unstable SCFE is related to an increased rate of osteonecrosis (as high as 60%).

For stable SCFE, surgical intervention is typically placement of a single, centrally located cannulated screw (**Fig. 7**). There have been many studies evaluating many different techniques to include multiple screws, reduction maneuvers before fixation,

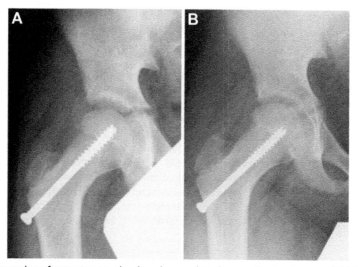

Fig. 7. Examples of percutaneously placed cannulated screw for treatment of SCFE.(*A*) Immediate post-surgical screw position. (*B*) Screw positioning approximately one year postoperatively. (*From* Jarrett DY, Matheney T, Kleinman PK.Imaging SCFE: diagnosis, treatment and complications.Pediatr Radiol. 2013 Mar;43 Suppl 1:S71-82. https://doi.org/10.1007/s00247-012-2577-x. Epub 2013 Mar 12; with permission.)

and percutaneous capsulotomies. Current recommendations suggest that single cannulated screw placement alone is sufficient.

Unstable SCFE surgical intervention is more urgent. In situ fixation with a single cannulated screw is the recommended protocol. Multiple studies have shown a decreased risk of osteonecrosis if in situ pinning is combined with a decompressive arthrotomy/capsulotomy. Much interest and many studies have investigated open procedures to restore the anatomy (**Fig. 8**). These studies have shown excellent results in patients without osteonecrosis. There is also a modest decreased incidence of osteonecrosis with the open method.[38]

Special note should be made for the need for prophylactic pinning in certain cases. Prophylactic pinning is generally recommended if associated with an endocrinopathy with no comorbidities. No such recommendations are made for patients presenting with unilateral SCFE.

Outcomes

Osteonecrosis of the femoral head is a potential complication of SCFE. Recent reviews have revealed an overall risk for osteonecrosis in patients with unstable SCFE treated with urgent operative intervention as high as 25%. Another complication of SCFE is FAI. It has been shown that up to 33% of patients reporting pain after SCFE fixation show signs of FAI. More investigations are needed to improve our understanding.[33]

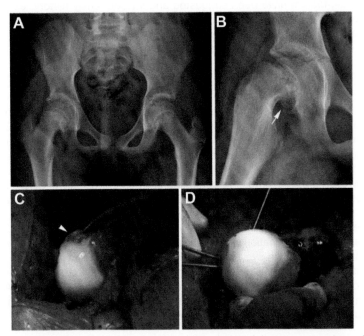

Fig. 8. Open surgical hip dislocation for treatment of SCFE. (*A*) Anteroposterior radiograph showing right hip SCFE. (*B*) Lateral radiograph showing right hip SCFE. *White arrow* showing femoral neck collapse. (*C*) White arrowhead showing ligamentum. (*D*) Femoral head epiphysis mobilized. (*From* Ross JR, Schoenecker PL, Clohisy JC.Surgical dislocation of the hip: evolving indications HSS J. 2013 Feb;9(1):60-9. https://doi.org/10.1007/s11420-012-9323-7. Epub 2013 Jan 24; with permission.)

LEGG-CALVÉ-PERTHES DISEASE

Legg-Calvé-Perthes disease (LCPD) is an idiopathic necrosis of the femoral head and femoral neck in pediatric patients. One of the predisposing factors is the unique vasculature of the proximal femur in children. Specifically, the epiphysis has paltry vasculature, which is for our purposes, relatively fragile. This vascular fragility, or relative vascular watershed area, leaves the epiphysis and physis susceptible to osteonecrosis before skeletal maturity. The disease is known to exist in 4 distinct phases: sclerosis, fragmentation, reossification, and remodeling (**Fig. 9**).[39–41]

LCPD occurs only in the pediatric population, and onset of disease is between 4 and 8 years. The disease typically affects predominantly boys by a 5:1 ratio. The incidence depends on many factors, but overall is between 0.5 and 30 per 100,000 children. The highest incidence is in Caucasians and those with short stature.[42]

There have been many attempts to explain the cause of LCPD, specifically vascular compromise. LCPD is not commonly associated with trauma. This lends credence to the suggestion that a systemic vascular issue or challenge is largely responsible. Typically, symptoms are insidious in nature. There have been many studies that support this vascular fragility theory, as there is an increased risk of cardiovascular disease in adults with a childhood diagnosis of LCPD. Additional studies suggest a hematologic challenge, as there are an increased number of patients with a history of LCPD who exhibit protein S deficiency and factor VIII and V Leiden defects.[39]

Certain risk factors have been suggested and include family history, exposure to secondhand smoke, low birth weight, urban living, Caucasian race, and abnormal birth presentation. Up to one-third of patients with LCPD are also diagnosed with attention deficit hyperactivity disorder.[42]

Diagnosis

The most common presentation of a child with LCPD primarily involves a progressive unexplained limp. The limp typically progresses to complaints of groin, thigh, and/or knee pain. Complaints at presentation will differ depending on the stage of LCPD previously discussed. Overall, patients will have symptoms if episodic and at times worsening limp and vacillating complaints of pain. The typical disease process from sclerosis to remodeling can last 3 to 5 years. LCPD typically presents as a unilateral issue; however, it may progress to contralateral limbs but usually in different stages of disease. If a child is diagnosed with bilateral LCPD in similar stages, one should consider other systemic issues such as hypothyroidism, skeletal dysplasia such as multiple epiphyseal dysplasia, and sickle cell disease.[42]

There are many classification systems used that are beyond the scope of this article. One of the more common systems is the Herring lateral pillar system (**Fig. 10**). This system has the most consistent interobserver predictability. Regardless, these systems (except when suspected very early) use radiographs for classifying. At times, MRI is a study of choice when considering a diagnosis of LCPD with normal radiographs.

Treatment

The goal of treatment is to minimize the late effects of femoral head deformity and joint incongruence. Treatment options, as typical for orthopedics, range from conservative to surgical intervention. They depend on the stage of disease, symptoms, and radiographic features of joint containment.

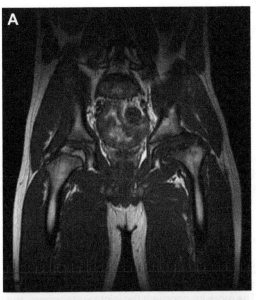

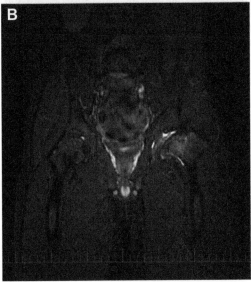

Fig. 9. Radiograph of bilateral LCPD in differing stages. Fifteen-year-old boy with sequelae of LCPD. Coronal T1 (*A*) and coronal STIR (*B*) show bilateral changes of LCPD, mild on the right (linear subchondral signal abnormality) and more advanced on the left, where, in addition to subchondral clefts, coxa plana/coxa magna with superolateral subluxation of the femoral head is also noted. (*From* Carpineta L, Faingold R, Albuquerque PA, et al. Magnetic resonance imaging of pelvis and hips in infants, children, and adolescents: a pictorial review. Curr Probl Diagn Radiol. 2007 Jul-Aug;36(4):143-52; with permission.)

Treatment will typically begin with activity modification, nonsteroidal antiinflammatory drugs, crutches, and brace wear or Petrie casting. If the femoral head begins to lose congruence, surgical intervention becomes more of an effective option. Hip adductor tenotomies to maintain hip abduction, hinged articulated distraction external

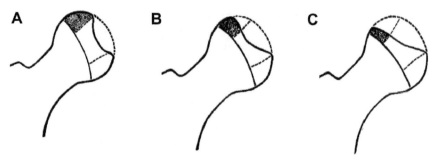

Fig. 10. Herring lateral pillar classification—stages A, B, and C. (*From* Mahadeva D, Chong M, Langton DJ,Reliability and reproducibility of classification systems for Legg-Calvé-Perthes disease: a systematic reviewof the literature. Acta Orthop Belg. 2010 Feb;76(1):48-57.)

fixator application, femoral head osteotomies with surgical hip dislocation, and periacetabular osteotomies are all surgical options.[43]

Natural History and Outcomes

The natural history of LCPD ultimately depends on the residual deformity after the final, remodeling stage. The more incongruent the joints surfaces are, the more likely motion may be limited, dysfunction, and potential limb length discrepancy may occur. Physeal bars (areas of the physics that prematurely fuse), grossly deformed femoral heads, and greater trochanteric overgrowth may all lead to late deformity and dysfunction. Late issues secondary to LCPD may ultimately result in surgical intervention as an adult to include hip replacement or other surgical intervention.

REFERENCES

1. Casteneda P. Developmental dysplasia of the hip. Orthopedic Knowledge Update 5: Pediatrics. Chapter 20. p. 245–258. Copyright 2016 American Academy of Orthopedic Surgeons.
2. Sankar WN, Nevitt M, Parvizi J, et al. Femoroacetabular impingement: defining the condition and its role in the pathophysiology of osteoarthritis. J Am Acad Orthop Surg 2013;21(Suppl 1):S7–15.
3. Sankar WN, Matheney TH, Zaltz I. Femoroacetabular impingement: current concepts and controversies. Orthop Clin North Am 2013;44(4):575–89.
4. Sankar WN, et al. Staging of hip osteoarthritis for clinical trials on femoroacetabular impingement. J Am Acad Orthop Surg 2013;21(Suppl 1):S33–8.
5. Bedi A, et al. Assessment of range of motion and contact zones with commonly performed physical exam manoeuvers for femoroacetabular impingement (FAI): what do these tests mean? Hip Int 2013;23(Suppl 9):S27–34.
6. Bedi A, et al. Elevation in circulating biomarkers of cartilage damage and inflammation in athletes with femoroacetabular impingement. Am J Sports Med 2013; 41(11):2585–90.
7. Bedi A, Kelly BT. Femoroacetabular impingement. J Bone Joint Surg Am 2013; 95(1):82–92.
8. Solomon L. Patterns of osteoarthritis of the hip. J Bone Joint Surg Br 1976;58(2): 176–83.
9. Harris WH. Etiology of osteoarthritis of the hip. Clin Orthop Relat Res 1986;(213): 20–33.

10. Ganz R, et al. The etiology of osteoarthritis of the hip: an integrated mechanical concept. Clin Orthop Relat Res 2008;466(2):264–72.

11. Wagner S, et al. Early osteoarthritic changes of human femoral head cartilage subsequent to femoro-acetabular impingement. Osteoarthritis Cartilage 2003; 11(7):508–18.

12. Reiman MP, et al. Diagnostic accuracy of clinical tests for the diagnosis of hip femoroacetabular impingement/labral tear: a systematic review with meta-analysis. Br J Sports Med 2015;49(12):811.

13. Kowalczuk M, et al. Does femoroacetabular impingement contribute to the development of hip osteoarthritis? a systematic review. Sports Med Arthrosc Rev 2015; 23(4):174–9.

14. Ganz R, et al. Femoroacetabular impingement: a cause for osteoarthritis of the hip. Clin Orthop Relat Res 2003;(417):112–20.

15. Clohisy JC, et al. Radiographic structural abnormalities associated with premature, natural hip-joint failure. J Bone Joint Surg Am 2011;93(Suppl 2):3–9.

16. Lung R, et al. The prevalence of radiographic femoroacetabular impingement in younger individuals undergoing total hip replacement for osteoarthritis. Clin Rheumatol 2012;31(8):1239–42.

17. Ecker TM, et al. Pathomorphologic alterations predict presence or absence of hip osteoarthrosis. Clin Orthop Relat Res 2007;465:46–52.

18. Johnston TL, et al. Relationship between offset angle alpha and hip chondral injury in femoroacetabular impingement. Arthroscopy 2008;24(6):669–75.

19. Pollard TC, et al. The hereditary predisposition to hip osteoarthritis and its association with abnormal joint morphology. Osteoarthritis Cartilage 2013;21(2): 314–21.

20. Zilkens C, et al. Symptomatic femoroacetabular impingement: does the offset decrease correlate with cartilage damage? A pilot study. Clin Orthop Relat Res 2013;471(7):2173–82.

21. Kumar D, et al. Association of cartilage defects, and other MRI findings with pain and function in individuals with mild-moderate radiographic hip osteoarthritis and controls. Osteoarthritis Cartilage 2013;21(11):1685–92.

22. Frank JM, et al. Prevalence of femoroacetabular impingement imaging findings in asymptomatic volunteers: a systematic review. Arthroscopy 2015;31(6): 1199–204.

23. Jung KA, et al. The prevalence of cam-type femoroacetabular deformity in asymptomatic adults. J Bone Joint Surg Br 2011;93(10):1303–7.

24. Reichenbach S, et al. Prevalence of cam-type deformity on hip magnetic resonance imaging in young males: a cross-sectional study. Arthritis Care Res (Hoboken) 2010;62(9):1319–27.

25. Reichenbach S, et al. Association between cam-type deformities and magnetic resonance imaging-detected structural hip damage: a cross-sectional study in young men. Arthritis Rheum 2011;63(12):4023–30.

26. Agricola R, Weinans H. Femoroacetabular impingement: what is its link with osteoarthritis? Br J Sports Med 2016;50(16):957–8.

27. Nicholls AS, et al. The association between hip morphology parameters and nineteen-year risk of end-stage osteoarthritis of the hip: a nested case-control study. Arthritis Rheum 2011;63(11):3392–400.

28. Lohan DG, et al. Cam-type femoral-acetabular impingement: is the alpha angle the best MR arthrography has to offer? Skeletal Radiol 2009;38(9):855–62.

29. Brunner R, et al. Prevalence and functional consequences of femoroacetabular impingement in young male ice hockey players. Am J Sports Med 2016;44(1): 46–53.
30. Johnson AC, Shaman MA, Ryan TG. Femoroacetabular impingement in former high-level youth soccer players. Am J Sports Med 2012;40(6):1342–6.
31. Kapron AL, et al. In-vivo hip arthrokinematics during supine clinical exams: application to the study of femoroacetabular impingement. J Biomech 2015;48(11): 2879–86.
32. Lehmann CL, et al. The epidemiology of slipped capital femoral epiphysis. J Pediatr Orthop 2006;26(3):286–90.
33. Loder R. Slipped capital femoral epiphysis. Paediatric Orthopaedics 2009;473–80. https://doi.org/10.1201/b13489-77.
34. Scharschmidt T, et al. Gene expression in slipped capital femoral epiphysis. J Bone Joint Surg Am 2009;91(2):366–77.
35. Murray AW, Wilson NIL. Changing incidence of slipped capital femoral epiphysis. J Bone Joint Surg Br 2008;90-B(1):92–4.
36. Sankar WN, et al. Acetabular morphology in slipped capital femoral epiphysis. J Pediatr Orthop 2011;31(3):254–8.
37. Loder RT, et al. Idiopathic slipped capital femoral epiphysis in amish children. J Bone Joint Surg Am 2005;87(3):543–9.
38. Sankar WN, et al. The unstable slipped capital femoral epiphysis. J Pediatr Orthop 2010;30(6):544–8.
39. Trueta J. The Normal vascular anatomy of the human femoral head during growth. J Bone Joint Surg Br 1957;39-B(2):358–94.
40. Daniel AB, et al. Environmental tobacco and wood smoke increase the risk of legg-calvé-perthes disease. Clin Orthop Relat Res 2011;470(9):2369–75.
41. Vosmaer A, et al. Coagulation abnormalities in legg-calvé-perthes disease. J Bone Joint Surg Am 2010;92(1):121–8.
42. Herring JA. Legg-calvé-perthes disease. Pediatric Orthopaedic Secrets 2007;349–52. https://doi.org/10.1016/b978-1-4160-2957-1.10061-2.
43. Kim HK, Herring JA. Pathophysiology, classifications, and natural history of Perthes disease. Orthop Clin North Am 2011;42(3):285–95.

The Pediatric Knee and Proximal Tibia

Mark Woernle, MD[a], Joel P. Fechisin, MD[b],*

KEYWORDS

- ACL tears • Patellar dislocation and instability • Meniscal tears
- Osteochondritis dissecans • Osgood-Schlatter disease • Discoid meniscus
- Tibial tubercle fractures

KEY POINTS

- Pediatric knee disorders are various and range from trauma and sports injuries to chronic overuse injuries.
- Because pediatric patients are different from adults, management of pediatric injuries and general knee disorders is also often different.
- Primary treatment regimen goals focus on a return to the previous level of function, preservation of anatomy, and decreasing potential long-term effects.

INTRODUCTION

Pediatric knee disorders are various and range from trauma and sports injuries to chronic overuse injuries. Because pediatric patients are different from adults, management of pediatric injuries and general knee disorders is also often different. Primary treatment regimen goals focus on a return to the previous level of function, preservation of anatomy, and decreasing potential long-term effects. Long-term complications may include damage to the physis with resultant potential limb length discrepancy or deformity.

Anterior Cruciate Ligament Tears

The anterior cruciate ligament (ACL) is a semielastic collagenous structure that runs from the lateral femur to the medial tibia and is the primary stabilizer of anterior translation of the tibia as well as rotation of the knee joint. The incidence of ACL tears in the pediatric population has increased dramatically in recent decades, with most experts citing the increase in youth sports participation as the cause (**Fig. 1**).

Other than an increase in pediatric sports participation and with specialization in single sports, there are other risk factors for ACL tears. Other risk factors include an

[a] Monmouth Medical Center, 300 2nd Avenue Long Branch, NJ 07740, USA; [b] Seaview Orthopaedic & Medical Associates, 1200 Eagle Avenue, Ocean, NJ 07712, USA
* Corresponding author.
E-mail address: jpfech@hotmail.com

Pediatr Clin N Am 67 (2020) 153–167
https://doi.org/10.1016/j.pcl.2019.09.012
0031-3955/20/© 2019 Elsevier Inc. All rights reserved.

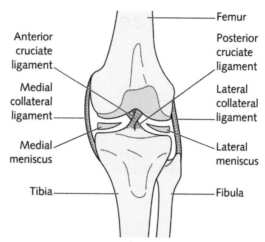

Fig. 1. Basic knee anatomy. (*From* Aitken, M, Gibson A. Crash Course: Rheumatology and Orthopaedics, Fourth Edition. Elsevier: Philadelphia, PA; 2018; with permission.)

increase in posterior tibial slope, increase in Q angles, and a smaller intercondylar notch width. There is a statistically increased risk of ACL rupture in adolescent female athletes compared with their male counterparts. Although ACL tears can occur in almost any activity, increased incidence of ACL tears occur in particular sports, such as football, soccer, lacrosse, basketball, and field hockey.[1]

To combat the increased risk of ACL tears, multiple techniques have been developed. Most programs, such as the Knee Injury Prevention Program, focus on neuromuscular and proprioceptive training. There is significant effort to decrease potential ACL tears for high-risk athletes and also athletes at risk for noncontact tears.[1]

Mechanism/symptoms

The histories of athletes with suspicion for ACL tears typically include a twisting injury to the knee. Patients report hearing or feeling a pop, significant swelling within 24 hours, inability to continue the current activity, and difficulty ambulating with an avoidance of extending the knee. Female athletes are at particular risk for noncontact injuries, particularly in sports such as basketball.

The physical examination is often challenging because patients typically autoprotect the knee; they are unwilling or unable to relax enough for an examination. Typical findings include positive anterior drawer and Lachman tests. There is often limited active and passive range of motion, particularly at the end range of motion, and especially extension. It is important to be vigilant with the remainder of the physical examination because concomitant injuries, such as meniscal or collateral ligament injuries, are common.

Although ACL tears can be diagnosed clinically, MRI is recommended to confirm ACL rupture and to rule out meniscal tears or concomitant ligamentous damage. The initial diagnostic evaluation begins with plain radiographs. Findings on plain films typically reveal an effusion. Occasionally, Segond fractures (capsular small avulsion fractures) and tibial spine fracture are appreciated. It has been shown that there is an increased risk of lateral meniscal tears with ACL ruptures.

Treatment

Current literature suggests increased chance of meniscal injury and chondral disorder in ACL tears treated nonoperatively.[2] The medial meniscus is a secondary anterior stabilizer of the knee. ACL-insufficient patients rely on the medial meniscus as a stabilizer;

this leads to medial meniscal tears with chronic insufficiency. Many additional studies have shown that ACL injuries left untreated surgically can lead to chronic instability and poor functional outcomes.[3] Most pediatric orthopedic surgeons strongly recommend surgical reconstruction in the setting of complete ACL rupture or in partial ACL injuries with knee instability (**Fig. 2**).

Surgical intervention for ACL tears is performed with ACL reconstruction. Surgical repair of ruptured ACLs has been reported to result in high failure rates and chronic instability. Surgical reconstruction in the pediatric population has many challenges. First of these is potential for growth and the presence of growth plates.

Skeletally mature or near-mature patients are candidates for autograft transphyseal reconstruction, which is performed by harvesting the gracilis and semimembranosus hamstring tendons. These tendons are doubled, creating a quadrupled autograft. Bone tunnels are created in the tibia and femur via varying techniques. The autograft is shuttled through these tunnels and tensioned appropriately. The new ACL is then affixed with hardware to create a reconstructed ACL. During any ACL reconstruction, additional abnormalities, such as meniscal tears, are surgically addressed.[4]

However, ACL injuries in skeletally immature patients pose many challenges. The technique used depends on remaining growth potential. Adolescent patients are treated with physical-sparing techniques. The bone tunnels created are confined to the epiphysis. Varying hardware techniques are available. Patients with a significant amount of remaining growth require a different technique.

ACL-insufficient patients with a significant amount of growth remaining are candidates for physeal-sparing techniques. This technique uses a swathe of iliotibial band that is kept attached to the tibia at the Gerdy tubercle, tunneled over the lateral femoral condyle, and eventually sutured to the anterior tibial periosteum (**Fig. 3**).[4]

Tibial Eminence Fractures

Tibial eminence fractures are ACL rupture–equivalent injuries in children. They are avulsion fractures of the anterior tibial eminence. Avulsion fracture of the origin of the ACL, the medial aspect of the lateral femoral condyle, are rare. The anterior tibial eminence is the insertion of the ACL, the ACL footprint. In such injuries, the bone fails before ligamentous failure. Older adolescents experience a midsubstance ACL rupture. These

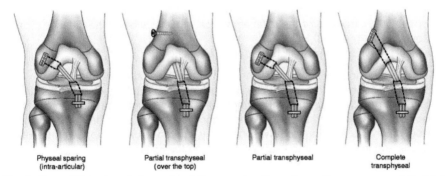

Physeal sparing   Partial transphyseal   Partial transphyseal   Complete
(intra-articular)   (over the top)   transphyseal

Fig. 2. Four different techniques for ACL reconstruction, depending on age and skeletal maturity. (*From* Gagliardi AG, Albright JC. Pediatric Anterior Cruciate Ligament Reconstruction. Orthopedics. 2018 May 1;41(3):129-134. https://doi.org/10.3928/01477447-20180501-06; with permission.)

A

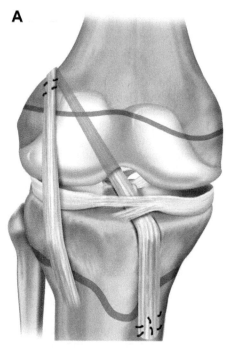

B

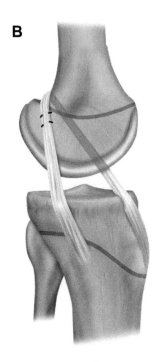

Anterior view   Lateral view

Fig. 3. Physeal-sparing Kocher ACL reconstruction using a bundled slip of the iliotibial band tunneled around the lateral femoral condyle and sutured under the intermeniscal ligament to the tibial periosteum. (*From* Ardern CL, Ekås G, Grindem H, et al. 2018 International Olympic Committee consensus statement on prevention, diagnosis and management of paediatric anterior cruciate ligament (ACL) injuries. Knee Surg Sports Traumatol Arthrosc. 2018 Apr;26(4):989-1010. https://doi.org/10.1007/s00167-018-4865-y. Epub 2018 Feb 17.)

injuries typically occur as a result of a rotational stress with a valgus load on the knee. Collateral ligament and meniscal tears are common associated injuries.

The classification scheme for tibial eminence fracture is the McKeever classification:

Type I (15%): no or minimal displacement of the tibial eminence
Type II (39%): fracture of the tibial eminence with elevation of the anterior aspect only
Type III (45%): completely displaced tibial eminence

This classification scheme assists in treatment options primarily (**Fig. 4**).

The physical examination of patients with a McKeever fracture is similar to that for patients with ACL injury. Physical examination reveals a significant effusion, diffuse tenderness to palpation, and positive anterior drawer and Lachman examinations. Pathognomonic is a history of a twisting injury with an audible pop, swelling within 24 hours, and inability to ambulate or fully extend the knee.

Nonoperative treatment with casting or brace wear is appropriate for nondisplaced McKeever fractures, type I only. Type II and III McKeever fractures require operative intervention to include arthroscopic reduction and fixation with either suture or hardware (screw) (**Fig. 5**). Failure to obtain appropriate reduction may result in malunion or interposition of the insertion of the ACL underneath the anterior horn of the medial

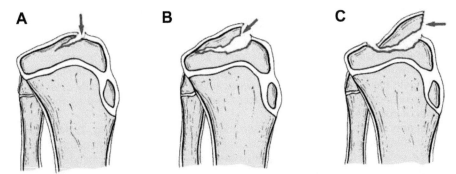

Fig. 4. Meyers and McKeever's classification of fractures of the anterior tibial spine. (*A*) Type I fracture with no displacement of the fracture (*arrow*). (*B*) Type II fracture with elevation of the anterior portion of the anterior tibial spine, but with the fracture posteriorly reduced (*arrow*). (*C*) Type III fracture that is totally displaced (*arrow*). (*From* Zionts, LE. Fractures and Dislocations About the Knee. In Green, NE, Swiontkowski, MF. Skeletal trauma in children, 4e. Philadelphia, PA: Saunders/Elsevier; 2009; with permission.)

meniscus or the intermeniscal ligament. Despite excellent results with either technique, most patients have asymptomatic increased laxity postoperatively.[5]

Meniscal Tears

The menisci are 2 fibroelastic structures within the knee joint involved in force transmission and stability. Tears are often the result of a twisting injury, with lateral tears

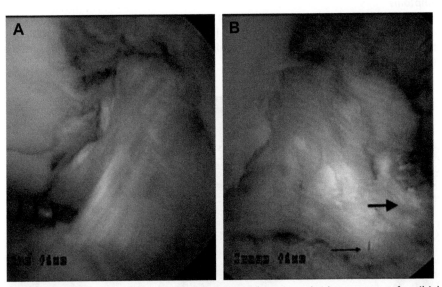

Fig. 5. Arthroscopic views of a patient after use of a suture bridge construct for tibial eminence fracture fixation. (*A*) Assessment of ACL tension with a hook showing appropriate tension and a healed fracture. (*B*) Small and large arrows point to the suture ends from both anterolateral and anteromedial suture anchors from the suture bridge construct. (*From* Mann MA, Desy NM, Martineau PA. Suture bridge fixation for tibial eminence fractures. Arthroscopy. 2013 Mar;29(3):401-2. https://doi.org/10.1016/j.arthro.2012.12.014; with permission.)

more common than medial. Isolated tears are more common in the younger pediatric population, whereas older adolescents are more likely to have concomitant ligamentous injury. Joint line tenderness is the most sensitive finding on examination.

Although the clinical examination is superior to MRI in predicting arthroscopic findings in children with injured knees, MRI examination is performed for confirmation and to delineate the type and location of meniscal tear as well as to identify other intra-articular disorders (**Fig. 6**). Meniscal tears heal better in children and all should be repaired if possible.[6]

Knee arthroscopy is used to surgically address meniscal tears (**Fig. 7**). All effort is made to attempt to repair meniscal tears. There is a significant amount of data to suggest the potential for early degenerative disease with partial meniscectomies performed at early ages. Various techniques are used that take advantage of the significant healing potential in young patients.

Medial Patellofemoral Ligament Tears and Patella Instability

The medial patellofemoral ligament (MPFL) is a condensation of capsular fibers that inserts on the patella and helps resist lateral migration of the patella. Although congenital laxity of the MPFL can lead to patella instability, rupture of the ligament is common following traumatic lateral dislocation of the patella. This condition can occur with an eccentric contraction of the quadriceps or direct trauma.[7] Risk factors for patella dislocation include an increased Q ankle, hypoplastic trochlea, and ligamentous laxity. Of note, certain syndromes or disorders with notable ligamentous laxity place patients at risk, such as Down syndrome and Ehlers-Danlos syndrome.

Symptoms

Complaints during the evaluation consist of pain along the medial aspect of the knee capsule and often lateral femoral condyle. In the setting of an acute patellar femoral dislocation, there is typically a complaint of a large effusion or hemarthrosis and the inability to bear weight.

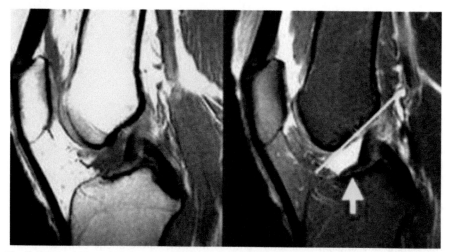

Fig. 6. Sagittal T1 and T2 imaging showing an ACL tear depicted by yellow line. Yellow arrow shows torn ACL stump. (*From* Rubin D and Smithuis R. Knee—Non-Meniscal Pathology. *Radiology Assistant.* Available at: http://www.radiologyassistant.nl/en/p42764e8fe927e.)

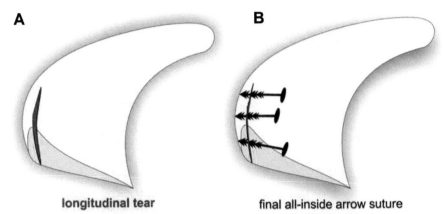

Fig. 7. Meniscal tear and repair technique. (*From* Piedade SR, Pereira da Silva Nunes R, Kaleka CC. All-Inside Meniscal Repair: Updates on Technique. The Menisci. 22 Feb 2017; p. 103-8; with permission.)

Examination

Immediately recognized is a large hemarthrosis and diffuse tenderness to palpation about the anterior aspect of the knee as well and medial and lateral poles of the patella and often lateral femoral condyle. Because the condition is more common in patients with genu valgum, an increased Q ankle is often recognized. Other features of the examination include an apprehension sign: fear of impending dislocation with a laterally directed force about the patella. Common findings also include a positive J sign consistent with maltracking of the patella.

Radiographs are performed both before and after reduction; however, it is more common for autoreduction to occur than the need to physically reduce a dislocated patella. Findings common in radiographs include osteochondral fractures or loose bodies and evidence of a hemarthrosis[8](**Fig. 8**).

Treatment

For most first-time dislocators, nonsteroidal antiinflammatory drugs, activity modification, physical therapy, and patellar stabilizing sleeves are first-line treatment. Because only 15% to 20% of patients have an additional patellar dislocation, conservative treatment is warranted with a history of 1 dislocation. However, the risk of redislocation approaches 90% to 95% for additional patella dislocations if a second event occurs.[9] In these cases, operative intervention to include a medial patella femoral ligament reconstruction or attempt at direct repair is suggested. These procedures are also recommended in patients in whom conservative measure fail and they remain symptomatic.

Operative intervention currently includes an MPFL reconstruction using gracilis allograft or autograft (**Fig. 9**). The gracilis hamstring graft is preferred secondary to its size (typically 4 mm in width) and availability. In addition, a vastus medialis obliquus imbrication (detaching the medial aspect of the quadriceps tendon and advancing it onto the medial aspect of the patella) is an adjunctive technique to provide more postoperative patella stability.[9]

Osteochondritis Dissecans

Osteochondritis dissecans (OCD) is a pathologic lesion affecting articular cartilage and subchondral bone, most often found in the posterolateral aspect of the medial

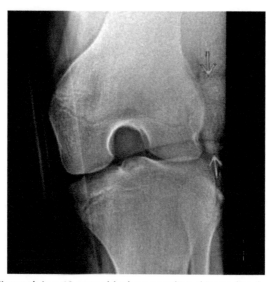

Fig. 8. Tunnel radiograph in a 12-year-old who was splinted immediately after a knee injury shows lateral dislocation of the patella (*arrows*). Typically, the patella reduces spontaneously with knee extension before radiographic evaluation. (*From* Merrow, ACJ. Diagnostic imaging: Pediatrics. Philadelphia, PA: Elsevier; 2017.)

femoral condyle of the knee. The juvenile form occurs between the ages 10 and 15 years when the physes are still patent. The cause is uncertain but likely related to hereditary, traumatic, or vascular insults. The challenges related to diagnosing and treating OCD are multiple. The incidence of OCD is low in the general population but may be higher in athletes and in certain age groups, notably adolescents. Although the most common location is the medial femoral condyle, OCD in other locations, such as the patella, lateral femoral condyle, and trochlea, does occur.

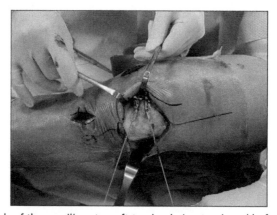

Fig. 9. Two strands of the gracilis autograft tendon being tensioned before fixation. (*From* Kim TS, Kim HJ, Ra IH, et al. Medial Patellofemoral Ligament Reconstruction for Recurrent Patellar Instability Using a Gracilis Autograft without Bone Tunnel. Clin Orthop Surg. 2015 Dec;7(4):457-464.)

The feature of OCD, regardless of the causative factors, is a disruption of cartilage overlying a subchondral bone defect. Cartilage has poor regenerative properties and a disruption has many significant long-term effects, such as degenerative disease.[10]

Presentation
Patients with an OCD, regardless of location, have varying complaints. Often, symptoms of diffuse, ill-defined pain with activity and eventually at rest are typically insidious. Some patients with unstable OCDs complain of mechanical symptoms such as episodes of locking, clunking, giving way.

Examination
The physical examination can be challenging as well. Often an OCD is discovered serendipitously when imaging and investigations are performed for other complaints or injuries. Tenderness to palpation overlaying the affected area is common as well as episodic effusions exacerbated by increased activity levels. Patients may complain of recurrent effusions without trauma and episodes of stiffness.

Radiographs, including tunnel (notch) view, are the initial diagnostic tool when OCD is suspected. As previously mentioned, OCD is often discovered when looking for other disorders for different complaints. If an OCD is identified on plain films, MRI is ordered to understand the extent of disease. In particular, the extent of underlying bony edema and stability of the lesion is evaluated.

Treatment
As with most orthopedic issues, treatment options include conservative or nonoperative and operative interventions. If an OCD lesion is considered stable on MRI, conservative treatment is first initiated. This treatment includes restricted weight bearing with use of crutches for a period of 4 to 6 weeks and use of stabilizing braces to limit joint forces. Often, repeat diagnostic imaging to include radiographs and/or MRIs are performed following cessation of symptoms. Children with open physes have greater potential to heal.

If an OCD lesion is considered stable and conservative treatment fails, several operative techniques exist. Arthroscopic-assisted and radiographic-assisted retrograde drilling of a lesion is one such option. The theory is to allow vascular channels to develop to induce a healing response similar to the response in a healing fracture.

However, if an OCD lesion is deemed unstable, attempts must be made surgically to restore the chondral surface. This surgery is performed by arthroscopic-assisted reduction and stabilization with various hardware to include screws and bioabsorbable chondral darts[11] (**Fig. 10**). If unable to achieve stable, appropriate reduction, there are several techniques to address cartilage loss that are outside of the scope of this article.

Osgood-Schlatter Disease (Tibial Tubercle Apophysitis)

Osgood-Schlatter disease is a type of traction osteochondritis that refers to partial avulsion of the tibial tuberosity. It is the most common chronic overuse syndrome in children. It is a traction apophysitis at the anterior aspect of the tibial tubercle. The peak incidence is between 8 and 15 years of age and it is seen earlier in girls. It is more common in young men and is often noted bilaterally. A precursor to Osgood is often tight hamstrings and quadriceps, and 70% to 80% of lower extremity growth occurs around the knee. It is often seen in jumpers and runners and may be common in almost any sport. As focus on single-sport specialized training increases, chronic overuse syndrome is becoming more common.[12]

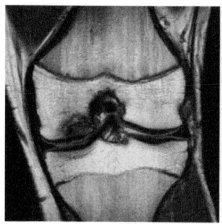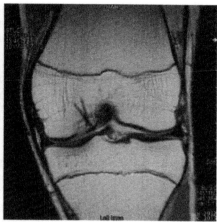

Fig. 10. MRI showing OCD before (*left*) and after (*right*) bioabsorbable dart fixation. (*From* Schindler OS. Current concepts of articular cartilage repair. Acta Orthop Belg. 2011 Dec;77(6):709-26; with permission.)

Examination

Symptoms of Osgood-Schlatter disease consist of complaint of a painful prominence overlying the midaspect of the proximal tibia. Symptoms are exacerbated with attempts to kneel and the resisted knee extension. The pain is activity related and may result in persistent pain with high-impact running or jumping sports, kneeling, and walking up and down stairs.

Physical examination reveals significant tenderness to palpation overlying the tibial tubercle and pain with resisted knee extension. The remainder of the physical examination for the knee is normal. However, hamstring and quadriceps contractures are typically evident.

Diagnostic evaluation is with radiographs. Fragmentation of the prominent anterior tibial tubercle is often evident. No further imaging is required to make the diagnosis (**Fig. 11**).

Treatment

The disease is usually self-limiting, and complaints and symptoms completely resolve when the patient achieves skeletal maturity. Management is supportive and consists of increasing flexibility and strengthening of hamstrings and quadriceps with physical therapy, activity modification, ice, and antiinflammatory use.

Rarely, patients complain of a painful ossicle after skeletal maturity (**Fig. 12**). If conservative measures do not alleviate the pain or the prominence enlarges, surgical excision is performed with excellent results.[13]

Discoid Lateral Meniscus

A discoid lateral meniscus is a congenital abnormal meniscal variant. Normally, menisci are C-shaped fibrocartilaginous structures that serve multiple functions but, most importantly, cushion and appropriately distribute joint forces across the femoral and tibial articulation. The incidence of discoid meniscus may be as high as 1.5% to 16% depending on the source. Interestingly, the contralateral knee is involved in approximately 20% of patients with a confirmed discoid lateral meniscus. It can be symptomatic in children as young as 4 to 5 years old.[14]

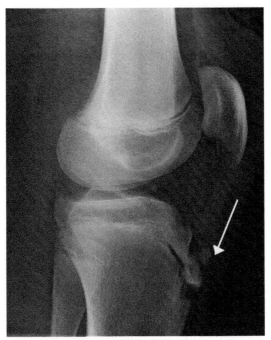

Fig. 11. Radiograph showing fragmentation (*arrow*) of the tibial tubercle consistent with Osgood-Schlatter disease. (*From* Wikimedia.org. Available at https://commons.wikimedia.org/wiki/File:Radiograph_of_human_knee_with_Osgood%E2%80%93Schlatter_disease.png.)

There are different classifications depending on the amount of tibial plateau pathologically overcovered by the discoid meniscus. One type, the Wrisberg type, can be troublesome because it has no posterior horn meniscal attachments and can be pathologically mobile and challenging to treat (**Figs. 13** and **14**).

Examination
Typical complaints include insidious lateral knee pain . Patients may also complain of mechanical symptoms such as locking and giving way. Intermittent and recurrent knee effusions may also be noted, often exacerbated by activity. Parents often report children limping without complaint of pain or decrease in activity levels.

Physical examination reveals lateral joint line tenderness to palpation and decreased active and passive range of motion, with a large effusion usually present. There is often quadriceps atrophy. Most importantly, there is usually a positive McMurray test (pivoting the lower leg with flexion resulting in joint line pain) with pain laterally.

Diagnostic imaging typically begins with radiographs, which are usually not very revealing. The radiographs may show a widened lateral joint space with squaring of the lateral femoral condyle, as opposed to its normal curvilinear shape. After a period of conservative treatment, MRI is usually ordered to identify intra-articular disorder secondary to continued complaints. MRI is the modality of choice and shows an anterior to posterior meniscal horn in continuity on 3 or more consecutive sagittal images.

Treatment
Treatment of a discoid lateral meniscus entirely depends on symptoms and response to conservative measures. Asymptomatic patients are simply observed

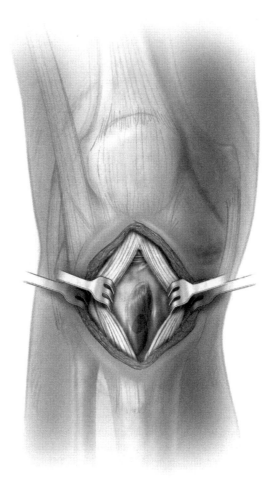

Fig. 12. Area to be excised for a symptomatic bony protuberance after skeletal maturity. (*From* Pihlajamäki HK, Visuri TI. Long-term outcome after surgical treatment of unresolved osgood-schlatter disease in young men: surgical technique.J Bone Joint Surg Am. 2010 Sep;92 Suppl 1 Pt 2:258-64. https://doi.org/10.2106/JBJS.J.00450; with permission.)

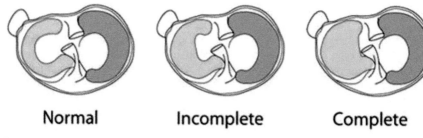

Fig. 13. Normal versus incomplete and compete discoid lateral meniscus. (*From* OrthoInfo. Discoid Meniscus Available at: https://orthoinfo.aaos.org/link/c6adf8e73ba24bd7b38ca30 690fd2604.aspx.)

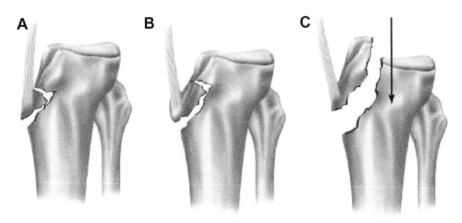

Fig. 14. The different types of tibial tubercle avulsion fractures. (*From* Mostofi S.B. Fractures in Children. In: Fracture Classifications in Clinical Practice 2nd Edition. Springer, London; 2012; pg. 89-102; with permission.)

with frequent office visits. Symptomatic patients are first treated with activity modification, rest, ice, antiinflammatories, and physical therapy for quadriceps and hamstring strengthening. If conservative measure fail symptomatic patients, surgical intervention is warranted.

Surgical intervention is also indicated for patients with significant mechanical symptoms. Surgical techniques include knee arthroscopy with saucerization of the discoid meniscus to resemble a normal C-shaped meniscus. Wrisberg type of discoid lateral meniscus requires advanced techniques to secure the posterior horn to the posterior aspect of the tibial plateau.[14]

Tibial Tubercle Fractures

Tibial tubercle fractures are devastating injuries that occur from eccentric contractions of the quadriceps with a stationary foot and ankle. They typically occur in older adolescents who are approaching skeletal maturity. Typical age is 13 to 16 years for boys and 12 to 14 years for girls. It is much more common in boys. The reason this fracture occurs typically only at these ages is that the proximal tibial physis begins to close posterior to anterior. The anterior aspect of the tibial physis, in which the patellar tendon attaches, is a weak point. It is commonly associated with jumping sports such as basketball.[5]

Technically, the fracture is considered an avulsion of the tibial tubercle. This fracture often extends in the proximal tibial physis, which is significant in that it is an intraarticular fracture that usually requires prompt intervention (see **Fig. 13**).

The Ogden classification scheme was developed and is largely academic. It is rare to treat tibial tubercle fractures conservatively. There is an increased likelihood of additional soft tissue disruption, to include ACL, meniscal, collateral, and patellar tendon ruptures with increasing displacement of the fracture.

Examination

Examination of a patient with a tibial tubercle fracture can be dramatic. Patients complain of significant pain, often deformity, and an inability to bear weight. A thorough neuromuscular examination is mandatory because this type of fracture has a high risk of developing compartment syndrome and potentially vascular injury.

Physical examination reveals a large hemarthrosis with a palpable defect about the tibial tubercle. Diagnostic imaging begins with radiographs, which are sufficient to diagnose the tibial tubercle fracture; however, if accessible, MRI is obtained to evaluate for additional injury because it is common with this type of injury.

Treatment

Assuming no other soft tissue injury, treatment is operative. Open reduction and internal fixation with cannulated screws is the mainstay of treatment. Always surprising is the amount of periosteal disruption observed with these fractures. It is common to observe 10 to 12 cm of periosteal stripping while surgically fixing this fracture.

A high suspicion should be maintained for vascular injury if a displaced Slater-Harris 1 fracture is observed with tibial tubercle fractures. These types of fracture pattern are considered surgical emergencies because there is a high risk of associated popliteal artery pseudoaneurysm.

Patients with tibial tubercle fracture are admitted after fixation, with a typical length of stay of 2 to 3 days, so continuous neurovascular and compartment checks may be performed and documented. If compartment syndrome is suspected, compartment pressure measurements may be obtained with potential compartment releases planned emergently.

REFERENCES

1. Mall NA, Paletta GA. Pediatric ACL injuries: evaluation and management. Curr Rev Musculoskelet Med 2013;6(2):132–40.
2. Lohmander LS, Englund PM, Dahl LL, et al. The long-term consequence of anterior cruciate ligament and meniscus injuries: osteoarthritis. Am J Sports Med 2007;35:1756–69.
3. Øiestad BE, Engebretsen L, Storheim K, et al. Knee osteoarthritis after anterior cruciate ligament injury: a systematic review. Am J Sports Med 2009;37:1434–43.
4. McConkey MO, Bonasia DE, Amendola A. Pediatric anterior cruciate ligament reconstruction. Curr Rev Musculoskelet Med 2011;4(02):37–44.
5. Starkey M. Ligamentous knee injuries. orthopedic knowledge update 5: pediatrics [Chapter 41]. Rosemont (IL): American Academy of Orthopedic Surgeons; 2016. p. 521–36.
6. Bellisari G, Samora W, Klingele K. Meniscus tears in children. Sports Med Arthrosc Rev 2011;19(01):50–5.
7. Warren LF, Marshall JL. The supporting structures and layers on the medial side of the knee: an anatomical analysis. J Bone Joint Surg Am 1979;61A:56–62.
8. Guerrero P, Li X, Patel K, et al. Medial patellofemoral ligament injury patterns and associated pathology in lateral patella dislocation: an MRI study. Sports Med Arthrosc Rehabil Ther Technol 2009;1(1):17.
9. Hinton R, Krishn S. Acute and recurrent patellar instability in the young athlete. Orthop Clin North Am 2003;34:385–96.
10. Zanon G, DI Vico G, Marullo M. Osteochondritis dissecans of the knee. Joints 2014;2(1):29–36.
11. Pascual-Garrido C, McNickle AG, Cole BJ. Surgical treatment options for osteochondritis dissecans of the knee. Sports Health 2009;1(4):326–34.

12. Yen YM. Assessment and treatment of knee pain in the child and adolescent athlete. Pediatr Clin North Am 2014;61(6):1155–73.

13. Circi E, Atalay Y, Beyzadeoglu T. Treatment of Osgood–Schlatter disease: review of the literature. Musculoskelet Surg 2017;101:195.

14. Starkey M. Meniscal tears in children and adolescents. Orthopedic knowledge update 5: pediatrics [Chapter 42]. Rosemont (IL): American Academy of Orthopedic Surgeons; 2016. p. 537–44.

The Pediatric Foot and Ankle

Aron Green, MD

KEYWORDS

- Salter-Harris fractures • Triplane and Tillaux fractures • Sprains • Lisfranc injuries
- Sesamoiditis • Sever disease • Club foot • Tarsal coalitions

KEY POINTS

- Paramount in the initial evaluation of the pediatric foot and ankle patient is a thorough clinical history.
- Toddlers may manifest issues by a refusal to bear weight or significant limping.
- Older children have the ability to isolate their pain and provide a good history of injury.
- As part of history collection, there should be thorough descriptions and classification of pain location and longevity.

INTRODUCTION

Paramount in the initial evaluation of the pediatric foot and ankle patient is a thorough clinical history. Toddlers may manifest issues by a refusal to bear weight or significant limping. Older children have the ability to isolate their pain and provide a good history of injury. As part of history collection, there should be a thorough description and classification of pain location and longevity. Additionally, a history of injury or trauma should be sought and whether there is night pain or a history of recent systemic illness (looking for transient tenosynovitis or joint inflammation) should be determined. Noises (eg, clicking or catching), symptoms of instability, and weakness are all important; however, location of pain is most telling.

ANATOMY OF THE FOOT AND ANKLE

The foot and ankle can be divided into 3 basic zones. The most distal part of the body is the forefoot containing the toes, metatarsals, sesamoids, and metatarsophalangeal (MTP) joints. The midfoot includes the 3 cuneiforms, the navicular, and the cuboid. The forefoot and the midfoot are divided by the tarsometatarsal joints, also known as the Lisfranc joints. The strong plantar Lisfranc ligament provides significant stability to the foot and helps support the medial longitudinal arch. The hindfoot is composed of the calcaneus and the talus. Chopart joints separate the midfoot from the hindfoot. The hindfoot has 1 large joint called the subtalar joint, which is composed of 3 facets. Finally, the ankle joint is composed of the articulation between the hindfoot composed

Seaview Orthopedic & Medical Associates, 1200 Eagle Avenue, Ocean, NJ 07712, USA
E-mail address: shoreorthopod@yahoo.com

Pediatr Clin N Am 67 (2020) 169–183
https://doi.org/10.1016/j.pcl.2019.09.007
0031-3955/20/© 2019 Elsevier Inc. All rights reserved.

pediatric.theclinics.com

of the talus and the 2 leg bones, the tibia and fibula. The ankle is a simple hinge-type joint. Static stability is provided by the lateral ligamentous complex and by the medial deltoid complex. The syndesmosis is the ligamentous complex between the tibia and the fibula. Dynamic stability is provided by the peroneal brevis and longus laterally and the posterior tibial tendon medially.

EXAMINATION OF THE FOOT AND ANKLE

Initial examination of the foot and ankle requires removal of shoes and socks. Assuming there is no trauma or injury that precludes weight bearing, the examination should be done with both feet flat on floor with the patient standing. If able, the patient should be asked to walk, and gait should be assessed. Any antalgia, steppage, or thrusting gait pattern should be noted. Heel walking and toe walking should be evaluated. The gait cycle is composed of stance phase, which includes heel strike, foot flat, heel rise, and toe off. The stance phase of gait should be approximately 60% of the cycle, whereas 40% is swing phase and double stance approximately 25% of the cycle.[1] General observations should include pelvic height or tilt, overall lower extremity alignment (valgum or varum), position of ankle and hindfoot, forefoot and midfoot position, cavus or planus structure, forefoot position, and abnormalities or any skin lesions that may be present. After this initial observation, range of motion of the ankle and foot should be observed. Ankle range of motion should be from approximately 20° of dorsiflexion to 50° plantarflexion, eversion is approximately 15°, and inversion is 35°. Forefoot adduction is 20° with abduction 10°. First MTP joint dorsiflexion is approximately 90° whereas flexion is 45°.

After the foot is taken through a range of motion, the structures of the foot should be palpated. All bony prominences, growth plates, joints, tendons, and ligaments should be evaluated. An effusion or swelling also should be palpated and noted. It is critical to palpate point of maximal tenderness or pain and correlate it with the undersurface anatomy to recognize the structure at risk. Strength then should be tested. This should be done in all 4 quadrants of ankle range of motion—dorsiflexion, plantarflexion, inversion, and eversion all should be tested. The first MTP joint should be tested in both dorsiflexion and plantarflexion.

A vascular examination is essential. Palpation and documentation of the popliteal artery, posterior tibial artery, and dorsalis pedis pulses should be performed. Neurologic examination should include evaluation of the common, superficial, and deep peroneal nerves and sural and tibial nerves. Patellar and Achilles reflexes also should be recorded.

Special testing is done lastly. Stability of the ankle is tested with both the anterior drawer and talar tilt tests. Syndesmotic squeeze and external stress testing of the syndesmosis may be performed to test for additional instability. If there is concern for Achilles contracture, Silfverskiöld testing can be done.

WORK-UP

Initial work-up should include weight-bearing radiographs of either the foot or the ankle, depending on what structure is being examined. A standard series of radiographs includes anterior-posterior, lateral, and oblique views. Specialized views looking at the sesamoids, calcaneus, and subtalar facets can be ordered as needed. Higher-level imaging can be used in select cases as needed. CT scanning is optimal for 3-dimensional imaging of bone structures because it provides for better evaluation of bony anatomy. Magnetic resonance imaging (MRI) is ideal for evaluating soft tissue structures, including tendons and ligaments. MRI also can clearly image cartilage and evaluate areas of bone marrow edema. Care should be taken because normal marrow signal may be confused with trauma in MRI imaging in children.[2] Nuclear medicine scans can be used to identify areas of bone turnover, such as stress fractures or tumor, and also can be used for work-up of an infectious process. Routine blood work is almost never needed, unless an infectious process is suspected. In those cases, complete blood cell count, sedimentary rate, and C-reactive protein should be obtained. If an autoimmune process is suspected, targeted blood work (ie, antinuclear antibodies, human leukocyte antigen B27, and rheumatoid factor) can be obtained.

ACUTE INJURIES
Fractures

Growth plate or Salter-Harris fractures are unique to the pediatric population. In their seminal study, Salter and Harris[3] showed that the pediatric growth plate is in general weaker than tendons and ligaments in growing children and that injuries usually occur to the epiphyseal growth plate. Salter-Harris fractures are graded from I to V depending on severity and what portion of the epiphyseal plate is injured (**Fig. 1**). Ankle fractures in children are the third most common fracture involving the growth plate.[4] A majority of these fractures are from low-energy mechanisms, generally sports related. They are the most common growth plate injury in the lower extremity.[5] There can be complications from growth plate fractures, including growth arrest, deformity, or leg length discrepancy, depending on how much remaining growth. Fractures of the distal tibia have the greatest rates of complications postfracture because of the growth potential of that bone.[6] Depending on gender, the distal tibial and fibular growth plates may remain open until the age of 20. Additionally, the closure of the distal tibial growth plate is slow and eccentrically based. This leads to unique fracture patterns in the adolescent called triplane and Tillaux fractures. CT scans often are used to better assess these and other intra-articular fractures.

Overall goals of treatment are anatomic to near anatomic reduction. Growth plate fractures can damage physeal cells with repeat manipulation or delayed treatment. Physeal damage also may lead to deformity or limb length discrepancy.[7] Nondisplaced fractures can be treated with immobilization. Displaced fractures can be reduced by manipulation and casted—more unstable fracture patterns are placed in a long leg casts with stable fracture patterns treated in short leg casts. Complex fractures, especially intra-articular fractures, are treated with open reduction and internal fixation with partially threaded screws or wires that do not violate the growth plate. Overall, fracture

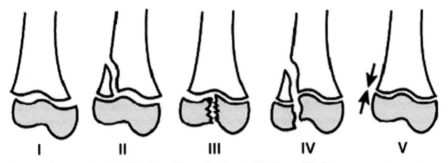

Fig. 1. Salter Harris Classification. (*From* Benjamin HJ, Hang BT. Common acute upper extremity injuries in sports. Clinical Pediatric Emergency Medicine 2007;8(1):15–30. Available at: https://doi.org/10.1016/j.cpem.2007.02.003; with permission.)

healing typically requires 6 weeks with some form of restricted weight bearing. The higher the energy involved with the mechanism of injury, the more likely growth plate damage and ultimately complications may occur.[7] Patients with growth plate injuries should be followed for at least 2 years to 3 years to be assured no complications develop.

Sprains

Despite the perception that tendons and ligaments are strong in children and the growth plate is the failure point in all injuries, ankle sprains may occur. There are more than 10 million ankle sprains in the United States every year[8] and a significant number of those occur in children.[9] Ankle sprains are graded 1 to 3 based on severity of the injury and the number of anatomic structures damaged. Additional types of sprains include high ankle sprains that involve injury to the syndesmosis and medial sprains that injure the deltoid. To diagnose a ligament sprain, there should be no bone or growth plate tenderness on examination. There also should be no pain with palpation of the base of the fifth metatarsal. There typically is anterolateral ankle swelling as well as tenderness over the anterior talofibular and possibly the calcaneofibular ligaments. There also can be pain over the anterior and lateral aspects of the ankle mortise. Drawer testing and talar tilt testing are essential on examination. If there is concern for more significant injury, evaluation of the syndesmosis with squeeze and external rotation stress testing can be done.

Initial treatment of a lateral ankle sprain is immobilization and protected weight bearing. Physical therapy has been shown the most efficacious way to rehabilitate a sprain, allowing rapid return to activity. My general protocol for a significant grade 3 sprain is 2 weeks immobilization in a controlled ankle movement boot with weight bearing as tolerated followed by transition to a lace-up ankle brace for an additional 4 weeks to 6 weeks. Physical therapy is started immediately, focusing on return of range of motion, strength, and proprioception. A high ankle sprain (syndesmotic injury) takes significantly longer to rehabilitate and return to full activity. Multiple ankle sprains may lead to chronic instability.

Chronic instability is categorized into functional versus mechanical instability. Mechanical instability is chronic incompetence of the lateral ligamentous complex. This type of instability typically requires operative intervention to avoid posttraumatic arthritis.[10] Surgical treatment includes the modified Broström-Gould ligament reconstruction and can be done open or arthroscopically. Functional instability is failure of the secondary stabilizers of the ankle.[11] The peroneals are the secondary stabilizers of the ankle. If their strength is not regained, this may lead to continued sensation of giving way, leading to a sense of instability. Physical therapy focusing on strengthening and proprioception helps correct this instability. High ankle sprains are particularly problematic. Forceful external rotation of the foot and ankle is the general mechanism of injury and can account for up to 17% of ankle sprains in an athletic population.[8] Tenderness at the level of the syndesmotic ligament and swelling at the level of the ankle are pathognomonic for high ankle sprain diagnosis. Surgery for these injuries is indicated when there is florid instability with complete loss of normal tibiofibular relationships on radiographs. With normal anatomic relationships, a physical therapy rehabilitation program can restore function. General return to activity is twice as long as a grade 3 lateral ankle sprain.

First Metatarsophalangeal Joint

Turf toe is an injury of the first MTP joint. It is a sprain of the joint capsule as well as the ligaments of the first MTP joint. Like most injuries, this can range from simple sprains to complete ligamentous disruption. Turf toe was named as such because artificial turf has become commonplace in football and currently most sports. It occurs via hyperextension to the MTP joint with injury to the plantar plate and sesamoid complex. Sprains, like ankle sprains, come in types 1 to 3. Treatment options are the same for all sprains, essentially starting with rest, ice, compression, and elevation (RICE) and taping or bracing. Therapy may also be utilized. Surgery is indicated only in severely unstable grade 3 injuries in which there is significant capsular damage.[12]

Sesamoiditis is pain at the level of the sesamoid complex. There are 2 sesamoids encased in the tendon of the flexor hallucis brevis. There are tibial and fibular sesamoids. These small bones act as pulleys to augment the efficacy of the tendon in which they are encased.[13] The tibial sesamoid is the most frequently injured.[14] The blood supply to the complex is variable and tenuous, which may lead to uncertain healing potential.[15] There are no radiographic changes noted with sesamoiditis because this is a clinical diagnosis. Treatment is by taping, padding, or orthotic management with a Morton extension built into the orthosis.

Osteochondritis of the sesamoid also may occur. It is more common in the tibial sesamoid but can occur in either bone. There are radiographic changes with lytic areas ultimately appearing on radiograph. Fractures can occur and are difficult to treat secondary to the variable and tenuous blood supply of the sesamoid. Bipartite sesamoids also occur. They tend to occur in up to 33% of patients and there is debate in the literature as to bilateral occurrence. Some investigators find 25% bilateral bipartite sesamoids whereas others find 85% bilateral.[15] The nature of the bipartite sesamoid may be secondary to a vascular etiology. In general, bipartite sesamoids are asymptomatic; however, acute trauma may inflame the synchondrosis and cause transient symptoms that can be managed with RICE and shoe wear with activity modification.

Lisfranc Injuries

Lisfranc injuries in children are rare.[16] Injuries can be bony with fractures of the cuneiforms or metatarsal bases, or they can be ligamentous with dislocation of the tarsometatarsal joints. A high index of suspicion is necessary because these injuries frequently are missed. These injuries are named after Lisfranc de Saint-Martin. He was a French field surgeon who described a traumatic amputation at the level of the tarsometatarsal joints secondary to having a foot caught in the stirrups of a horse while being dismounted. These generally are high-energy injuries. In the pediatric population, these can be known as bunk bed fractures.[17] There are multiple classification schemes for this injury; however, the direction of dislocation is the most used system (**Fig. 2**). Nondisplaced fractures can be treated with immobilization. Displaced fractures or dislocations require reduction and fixation. In a skeletally immature population, they can be treated with percutaneous pinning with smooth wires. In a skeletally mature patient with a displaced fracture, formal open reduction and internal fixation is performed.

Tendinopathy

Tendonitis in the pediatric population is unusual but can occur secondary to chronic overuse. With the recent increased participation in high-level sports requiring single-sport commitment, tendonitis is more commonplace. Treatment generally consists of cessation of the offending activity. RICE also is a mainstay of treatment. Traumatic injuries of tendons, such as lacerations. are treated with immediate surgical repair with excellent outcomes.[18] Lawn mower injuries generally are problematic secondary to

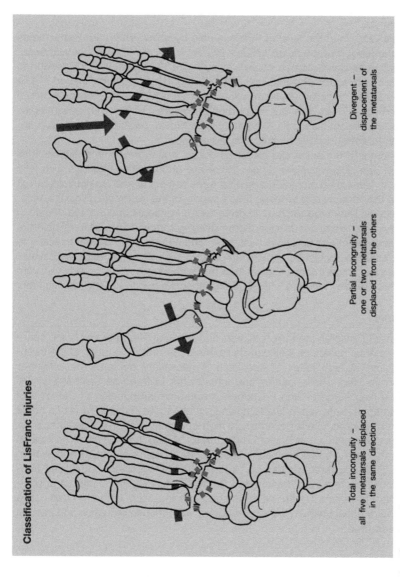

Fig. 2. Lisfranc Classification. (*From* Aiyenuro O, Goldberg AJ. Fractures of the foot and ankle. Surgery (Oxford) 2016;34(9):460–7; with permission.)

the extensive soft tissue defect associated with the injury and they require a multidisciplinary approach for successful limb salvage.[19]

Tendonitis of the posterior tibial tendon is unusual in the general pediatric population; however, it is more common in certain sports, such as ballet. The posterior tendon inserts onto the navicular. A common symptomatic condition is the accessory navicular. Approximately 14% of all feet develop an accessory navicular bone.[20] There are 3 types of accessory navicular bones. Type 1 is a very small accessory bone and is rarely symptomatic. Type 2 is a larger bone and presents with a fibrocartilaginous synchondrosis and may be symptomatic. Type 3 has an osseous fusion with the navicular proper and is rarely symptomatic. Mechanical symptoms may occur with improper shoe wear and are particularly symptomatic in type 2 accessory navicular. There may be an association with a pes planus or flat foot as well.[20] If symptomatic, there is pain with palpation of the accessory navicular and its associated prominence. There also is difficulty initiating and completing a single-leg unassisted heel rise. Treatment includes a period of rest and padding of the accessory navicular. If there is an associated pes planus, an orthotic with a medial longitudinal arch may be useful. If conservative methods fail over a period of weeks to months, more surgical treatment may be required.[21]

Achilles

As opposed to the adult population, Achilles tendonitis is unusual in the pediatric population. If it does occur, it is usually secondary to chronic overuse.[22] Treatment generally is supportive with RICE. Physical therapy, including eccentric stretching and over-the-counter nonsteroidal anti-inflammatory drugs (NSAIDS), can augment treatment.

Sever Disease

The most common cause of pediatric heel pain is Sever disease. This is inflammation of the calcaneal growth plate or apophysis. This generally occurs either in children with tight tendo-Achilles complexes and hamstrings or with participation in sports that use cleats with a negative rise. This generally is seen at the beginning of each sporting season. Soccer, baseball, lacrosse, and field hockey all use negative rise cleats. It is a clinical diagnosis. Patients express an acute onset of heel pain associated with sporting activity. On physical examination, there is focal tenderness at the level of the calcaneal growth plate. It is important to assess flexibility by asking patients to touch their toes with their knees straight. Radiographs may show sclerosis at the level of the apophysis (**Fig. 3**). Treatment is also generally supportive. Use of 1 cm cork or felt heel lift to lessen Achilles stretch, physical therapy for stretching and flexibility, and sport activity rest is the typical treatment regimen. Once the apophysis is closed, symptoms completely resolve. Interestingly, 48% of patients have Osgood-Schlatter disease, osteochondrosis of the tibial tubercle, as well.[22]

Osteochondral Defects of the Talus

Osteochondral defects of the talus are acquired idiopathic lesions of the subchondral bone of the talus. These can cause delamination of the articular cartilage with underlying bone necrosis and variable involvement of the articular cartilage.[23] In many cases, these are considered prearthritic lesions and can progress to frank osteoarthritis of the ankle if not treated. There is significant debate as to how these lesions occur. Some lesions do occur with trauma. An example of such trauma is an ankle fracture or sprain. It has been documented that osteochondral defects may occur in 17-70% of patients with associated ankle fracture.[24] Medial talar dome lesions are

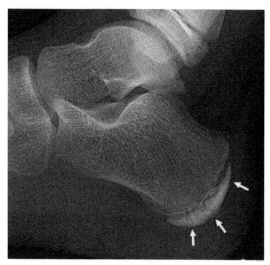

Fig. 3. Sever disease (lateral radiograph). (*From* Wikimedia Commons. Available at: https://upload.wikimedia.org/wikipedia/commons/thumb/2/24/Sclerosis_and_fragmentation_of_the_calcaneal_apophysis.jpg/300px-Sclerosis_and_fragmentation_of_the_calcaneal_apophysis.jpg.)

more common and usually are not associated with a history of trauma. They tend to be larger, deeper, and more posterior in nature. Lateral lesions tend to have an associated history of trauma. These tend to be more superficial in nature and smaller and located more anterior on the talar dome. Lateral lesions tend to be displaced and symptomatic and have a lower likelihood of healing. Lesions can be bilateral in 10% to 25% of cases.[25,26] On examination, there generally is an effusion and point tenderness over the affected part of the talar dome. It is important to establish if there is any instability present as well. Initial work-up is with plain radiographs and MRI and CT are useful higher-level imaging modalities.

There is a fundamental difference between the outcomes of juvenile and skeletally mature defects. Adult defects or those that become symptomatic after skeletal maturity have a worse prognosis and a lower probability of healing conservatively. In the pediatric population (and to a lesser extent the adult population), the initial treatment is conservative.[25] Conservative treatment in this population is 6 weeks of short leg non–weight-bearing casting. The younger the patient, the more probable spontaneous healing occurs. The only exception to initiating conservative treatment is if there is a loose or unstable fragment. This necessitates more urgent surgical intervention. If conservative treatment fails, operative treatment is indicated. Higher-level imaging should be obtained to help guide treatment. The larger the lesion, the more problematic successful healing. Lesions with intact cartilage can be treated by retrograde drilling. Small lesions with damaged cartilage can be treated with microfracture. Unstable fracture pieces can be treated by formal open reduction and internal fixation using absorbable or metallic fixation devices.

CONGENITAL AND DEVELOPMENTAL CONDITIONS
Club Foot

Club foot, or congenital talipes equinovarus, is relatively rare, with fewer than 200,000 cases per year in the United States. It is, however, the most common musculoskeletal birth defect. Club foot generally occurs more frequently in male and has an overall incidence ranging between 1:1000 and 1:250. There is evidence suggesting some genetic influence. It can be bilateral in 30% to 50% of cases.[27] Investigations support a significant genetic component linked to PITX1 gene. Most cases are considered idiopathic; however, there is association with other packaging disorders. A tethered cord or spinal bifida can lead to a neurogenic club foot. Some syndromes also are associated with a club foot.

The pathophysiology of club foot can be remembered with the acronym, CAVE: cavus, adductus of forefoot, varus, and equinus. The foot is clinically rotated inward and downward. The bony deformity is as follows: the talar neck is medially and plantarly rotated, the calcaneus is rotated medially and in varus, and the cuboid and navicular are rotated medially (**Fig. 4**). Physical examination is relatively easy. Position of the foot should be evaluated as well as the relative flexibility and ability to correct the foot.

Initial treatment is generally nonoperative. The gold standard is the Ponseti method. The Ponseti method involves weekly casting for the first 2 months to 4 months. Surgical tendo-Achilles lengthening may be required in 80% to 90% of cases. This is followed by a foot abduction orthosis from months 4 to 8 full time followed by nighttime use for 2 years; 30% to 50% of the time, delayed split anterior tibialis transfer with repeat tendo-Achilles lengthening is required.[28] Overall, the Ponseti method has a 90% success rate. If there is failure of nonoperative treatment, traditional operative correction is warranted. Surgical treatment of club foot can be accomplished by posteromedial soft tissue and capsular release with flexor tendon lengthening only if performed by 12 months. Occasionally, medial column lengthening or lateral column shortening osteotomies may be required if not addressed by the age of 3. Talectomy may be required if not addressed by age 10.[29,30]

Late complications from club foot and club foot treatment may occur. Because the talus in club foot tends to be dysmorphic, it may not articulate normally. This can lead to premature degenerative disease. Initial management of this complication as an adult is conservative; however, surgical correction ultimately may be required.

Congenital Vertical Talus

Congenital vertical talus is a rare deformity, with a reported incidence between 1 in 10,000 and 1 in 150,000 births. There is a slight association with club foot and it occurs

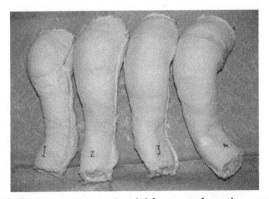

Fig. 4. Club Foot Casting Series. Consecutive clubfoot casts from the same patient, showing correction of all deformities (except equinus), with the foot abducted on the talus 50° to 60° by the fourth casting. The casts were applied weekly. (*From* Colburn M, Williams M. Evaluation of the treatment of idiopathic clubfoot by using the Ponseti method. J Foot Ankle Surg 2003;42(5):259–67; with permission.)

more frequently in males. Half of cases are associated with neurologic disorders and other genetic defects and syndromes. A careful neurologic examination is paramount in the initial evaluation. Up to half can be bilateral.[31] This malady is a rigid foot deformity resulting in a vertical orientation of the talus and reluctant abnormal articulation with the surrounding bones. Soft tissue contractures of the Achilles and peroneals occur quickly. There is a recognized genetic component, with commonly positive family history that may be associated with alterations in the HOXD10 gene. Physical examination demonstrates a significant rocker bottom foot with an equinovalgus deformity that differentiates it from club foot. The altered gait pattern abnormality is considered a calcaneal gait pattern that resembles someone walking with a peg leg. Treatment begins with serial manipulation and castings, ending with percutaneous tendo-Achilles tenotomy and pinning. Surgical management frequently is needed and should be performed at a young age. Surgery is indicated in most cases. Surgery can be quite invasive; however, minimally invasive correction techniques are being developed and successfully used.[32] Salvage for missed or recalcitrant cases can be addressed with triple arthrodesis or talectomy.

Pes Planus

Flat foot deformity, or pes planus, is a frequent complaint. Flat foot deformity is divided into flexible and rigid variants.[33] A vast majority of flat feet resolve by the end of adolescence.[34] Flat foot generally is considered a decrease in the medial longitudinal arch and valgus hindfoot, often with associated forefoot abduction. This can lead to the appearance of having too many toes visible when observing a patient from behind. The incidence in the pediatric population is unknown but its prevalence in the adult population is approximately 20% to 25%. Flexible pes planus is generally well tolerated even in adults and can be strictly observed if asymptomatic. There is a possibility of a pes planus causing late complications, specifically tearing of the spring ligament and posterior tibial tendon. Rigid flat feet generally are associated with tarsal coalition and require some form of treatment.

Physical examination is relatively straightforward with evaluation of the deformity. It is important to identify specific areas of tenderness. Evaluation for an Achilles contracture should be done because this is commonly associated with a flat foot. Standing radiographs should be taken to asses for an accessory navicular or a tarsal coalition. For most cases, observation is the best course of action. Reassurance that this is a normal variant is helpful. Flat feet tend to be very flexible and absorb shock and impact well and have a much greater longevity than a high arched or cavus foot, which tends to be inflexible and develop arthritis at a relatively young age (40s and 50s). There is no well recognized study that supports the theory that conservative treatment may mold the flat foot and correct the deformity.[34]

Treatment of a symptomatic flexible flat foot begins with physical therapy that focuses on stretching routines. Activity-related pain can be treated with RICE, NSAIDS, and activity modification. Additionally, orthotics with a medial longitudinal arch can be prescribed, either custom or over-the-counter varieties. If symptoms persist or are associated with slight weakness, use of an lace-up ankle-stabilizing orthosis can provide relief as well. If there is a severe flat foot that is associated with symptoms, use of a University of California Berkeley Laboratory (UCBL) orthotic can be effective (**Fig. 5**). UCBL orthotics are tolerated well in the pediatric population. There is an association among severe flat foot deformity and the development of knee and lower back pain. Failure of conservative treatment may necessitate surgical intervention. Standard surgical correction for pes planus begins in a stepwise fashion. Initially, a medially displacing calcaneal osteotomy is performed. If flat foot deformity remains, an Evans

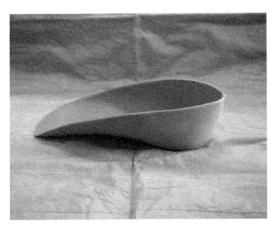

Fig. 5. Example of UCBL orthotic. (*From* Baldwin KD, Esquenazi A, Keenan MA. Rehabilitation and Neuro-Orthopedic Surgery. In Namdari S, Pill SG, Mehta S. Orthopedic secrets. Philadelphia, PA: Elsevier/Saunders; 2015.)

lateral column lengthening can be performed. Additional techniques include posterior tendon tenodesis and Achilles lengthening. Ideally, surgical correction of the foot should be performed close to skeletal maturity to prevent recurrence of the flat foot from remaining growth.

Tarsal Coalition

Tarsal coalition occurs when 2 or more tarsal bones fail to separate. This is due to a failure of mesenchymal segmentation. This can develop into a fibrous coalition or into a more solid coalition with transformation into cartilage and bone. Symptoms generally develop as patients are nearing skeletal maturity because this is when fibrous tissue begins to ossify. Tarsal coalition can affect up to 13% of the population.[35] There generally is a flattening of the foot or a pes planus that is rigid. There can be spasm of the peroneals (also known as peroneal spastic flat foot). There is an increased amount of stress and range of motion of other joints in the foot to accommodate for the loss of motion from the coalition. There are increases in sprains and instability of the foot and these may be presenting chief complaints.

The most common coalition is a calcaneonavicular coalition. This becomes symptomatic at a younger age. Another common location of coalition is a talocalcaneal coalition, which tends to become symptomatic later. Tarsal coalition can occur with various syndromes.[36] Nonsyndromic tarsal coalition is thought to be autosomal dominant in nature. These coalitions occur in 3 different types: fibrous, cartilaginous, and osseous in nature. A vast majority of patients with coalitions are asymptomatic and the coalition is discovered while evaluating other complaints and conditions.

Physical examination focuses on the flat foot deformity, muscle contractures, and sutbtalar range of motion. Radiographs are important in the initial work-up. Radiographs of a calcaneonavicular coalition reveal an anteater sign and talar beaking for a talocalcaneal coalition. If an osseous coalition is present, a computed tomography (CT) scan is useful for assessing size as well as evaluating if there are other coalitions present in the foot. If the coalition is fibrous, an MRI is the modality of choice.

Initial treatment is always conservative. Orthotics with a medial longitudinal arch may be utilized. Use of a lace-up ankle brace also can be used, especially if there is history of instability associated with the coalition. Activity modification is essential and immobilization can be used to see if this eliminates symptoms. For coalitions that fail conservative treatment, operative intervention is warranted. Coalition resection with sparing of the joint is indicated if there is less than 50% involvement of the joint. The goal is to try to preserve or increase motion at the level of the joint. To decrease risk of recurrence of the coalition, some material is interposed into the joint. This could be fat grafting, bone wax, extensor digitorum brevis tendon, or split flexor hallucis longus tendon. If greater than 50% of the joint is involved or the patient is older and skeletally mature with little to no subtalar range of motion, arthrodesis (fusion) of the subtalar joint can be considered. Because there is no motion present at the joint, the concept of replacing painful stiffness with painless stiffness is attractive. The immobility of the joint, whether it is from the coalition or the fusion, predisposes to adjacent joint degeneration in the future. Greater than 70% of patients do well with surgery and are not limited by pain in the future.[37]

Pediatric Bunions

A bunion is a complex deformity of the first ray. There is valgus of the phalanx with varus of the metatarsal. The sesamoid complex remains in place and is displaced from the metatarsal head. Generally, there are 2 forms: adult and adolescent. Adolescent bunions generally are considered congenital and often hereditary.[38] They tend to be bilateral and familial. They also can be associated with a pes planus deformity. Surgical correction has been associated with a very high risk of recurrence historically but with newer techniques this may be decreasing.[39] Initial management always should be conservative with shoe wear and activity modification. Orthotics can be tried to see if they eliminate pain. If at all possible, surgery should be postponed until all growth plates are closed to decrease risk of recurrence.

Evaluation of radiographs should focus on the hallux valgus angle, the intermetatarsal angle, congruency of the first MTP joint, sesamoid position, hallux valgus interphalangeus angle, and distal metatarsal articular angle. There is almost no need for any further imaging. Bunions can be separated into mild, moderate, and severe. Bunion severity dictates the surgical plan. In skeletally immature patients, surgery should avoid the epiphysis to prevent growth arrest. The more severe the deformity, the more invasive the procedure. It should be emphasized to both patient and parents that it is optimal to wait until skeletal maturity for correction.

Osteochondritis

Freiberg disease is avascular necrosis of a metatarsal head. It most frequently affects the second metatarsal. It occurs mostly in females and onset of symptoms usually is during adolescence.[40] The cause is generally thought to be a combination of traumatic and vascular insults, eventually leading to avascular necrosis. Symptoms generally are present while weight bearing and exacerbated with heeled shoes. Nonsurgical treatment always is initiated first. Immobilization is important in the initial stages of the disease. NSAIDS, bone stimulators, and physical therapy all can be used as well. Off-loading the metatarsal head with an orthotic with a metatarsal pad may help as well.[41] If skeletally mature, a corticosteroid injection can be done as well. In a majority of cases, supportive care is enough to decrease symptoms so that function is not compromised. Surgical treatment includes osteotomies, drilling, chilectomy, resection arthroplasty, and interpositional arthroplasty.

Köhler disease is rare and is caused by loss of blood supply to the navicular, leading to avascular necrosis. Ultimately, this results in destruction and fragmentation of the navicular. It is much more common in males than in females and tends to manifest between the ages of 6 years and 9 years old. Treatment generally is supportive, with revascularization of the navicular the rule. Initial off-loading and NSAIDS are helpful. Radiographs tend to improve for up to 4 years after onset. There is no surgical indication for Köhler disease because this is self-limiting.

Congenital Curly or Crossover Toe

Congenital curly, or crossover, toe is a common congenital deformity. Congenital curly toe generally affects the lateral 3 toes and is frequently bilateral. Initial treatment is always conservative and focuses on shoe wear modification. If conservative treatment fails, surgery may be indicated. Surgical intervention is either tenotomy or tendon transfer. Outcomes are universally good with either method.

Tumors

Tumors in the foot and ankle are rare but there are some that occur in the pediatric population with some frequency. Nonossifying fibromas frequently occur in the lower extremity. They generally occur in the metaphysis of long bones. These defects are common in children between the ages of 5 years and 15 years old. A vast majority of them are discovered incidentally with work-up for other issues.[42] They almost always are painless and asymptomatic. They generally enlarge with growth. If there is concern for fracture, a CT scan can be performed; however, plain radiographs generally are sufficient. Observation is the gold standard unless there is a pathologic fracture. If there is concern for pathologic fracture, curettage and bone grafting can be considered.

Unicameral bone cysts frequently occur in the calcaneus and can be a cause of heel pain in a pediatric patient. These lesions usually are found in patients under the age of 20. In the calcaneus, these lesions generally occur at the angle of Gissane. If large enough, they can increase the risk of a pathologic fracture. A calcaneal pathologic fracture can be problematic to treat in the pediatric population. If pain is a symptom, immediate immobilization should decrease the risk of fracture. Imaging with both radiographs and MRI is warranted if there is pain to assess fracture risk. If these lesions are large, they should be curettaged and bone grafted to decrease fracture risk. Patients recover well with this treatment, especially when autograft bone grafting is utilized.[43]

REFERENCES

1. Fry A. Normal and Abnormal Gait. University of Washington Board Review Course, March 6, 2017. Available at: https://uw.cloud-cme.com/assets/uw/Presentations/2781/2781.pdf.
2. Shabshin N, Schweitzer ME, Morrison WB, et al. High-signal T2 changes of the bone marrow of the foot and ankle in children: Red marrow or traumatic changes? Pediatr Radiol 2006;36(7):670–6.
3. Salter RB, Harris WR. Injuries involving the epiphyseal plate. J Bone Joint Surg 1963;45(3):587–622.
4. Niehaus S. Rethinking salter–Harris type I ankle fractures in kids: are they really fractures? Podiatry Today 2016. Available at: https://www.podiatrytoday.com/blogged/rethinking-salter-harris-type-i-ankle-fractures-kids-are-they-really-fractures.
5. Su AW. Pediatric ankle fractures: concepts and treatment principles. Foot Ankle Clin 2015;20(4):705–19.
6. Beals RK, Skyhar M. Growth and development of the tibia, fibula, and ankle joint. Clin Orthop Relat Res 1984;182. https://doi.org/10.1097/00003086-198401000-00038.

7. Leary JT, Handling M, Talerico M, et al. Physeal fractures of the distal tibia: predictive factors of premature physeal closure and growth arrest. J Pediatr Orthop 2009;29(4):356–61.
8. Williams G, Allen EJ. Rehabilitation of syndesmotic (high) ankle sprains. Sports Health 2010;2(6):460–70.
9. Boutis K, Plint A, Stimec J, et al. Radiograph-negative lateral ankle injuries in children: Occult Growth Plate Fracture or Sprain? JAMA Pediatr 2016;170(1). https://doi.org/10.1001/jamapediatrics.2015.4114.
10. Delco ML, Kennedy JG, Bonassar LJ, et al. Post-traumatic osteoarthritis of the ankle: a distinct clinical entity requiring new research approaches. J Orthop Res 2016;35(3):440–53.
11. Tropp H. Commentary: "functional ankle instability revisited. J Athl Train 2002; 37(4):512–5.
12. Williams BE. How to treat turf toe injuries. Podiatry Today 2008;21(9):38–43.
13. Sims AL. Painful sesamoid of the great toe. World J Orthop 2014;5(2):146.
14. Saro C, Bengtsson AS, Lindgren U, et al. Surgical treatment of hallux valgus and forefoot deformities in Sweden: a population-based study. Foot Ankle Int 2008; 29(3):298–304.
15. Gerbor M, et al. Sesamoids. In: Hallus valgus and forefoot surgery. 2002. p. 153–62.
16. Hill JF, Heyworth BE, Lierhaus A, et al. Lisfranc injuries in children and adolescents. J Pediatr Orthop B 2017;26(2):159–63.
17. Johnson GF. Pediatric lisfranc injury: 'Bunk Bed' fracture. Am J Roentgenol 1981; 137(5):1041–4.
18. Wicks MH, Paterson DC. Tendon injuries about the foot and ankle in children. ANZ J Surg 1980;50(2):158–61.
19. Branch LG, Crantford JC, Thompson JT, et al. Pediatric lower extremity lawn mower injuries and reconstruction: retrospective 10-year review at a level 1 trauma center. Ann Plast Surg 2017;79(5):490–4.
20. Nihau's S. Treating the accessory navicular in young athletes. Podiatry Today 2017. Available at: https://www.podiatrytoday.com/blogged/treating-accessory-navicular-young-athletes.
21. Ugolini PA, Raikin SM. The accessory navicular. Foot Ankle Clin 2004;9(1): 165–80.
22. Elengard T, Karlsson J, Silbernagel KG, et al. Aspects of treatment for posterior heel pain in young athletes. Open Access J Sports Med 2010;1:223–32.
23. Zanon G, DI Vico G, Marullo M. Osteochondritis dissecans of the talus. Joints 2014;2(3):115–23.
24. Syed F, Nunag P, Pillai A, et al. Management of recurrent multiple osteochondral lesions of the talus (OCLT) in a young active patient. J Clin Orthop Trauma 2014; 5(2):99–102.
25. Hermanson E, Ferkel RD. Bilateral osteochondral lesions of the talus. Foot Ankle Int 2009;30(8):723–7.
26. Vannini F, Cavallo M, Baldassarri M. Treatment of Juvenile osteochondritis dissecans of the talus: current concepts review. Joints 2014. https://doi.org/10.11138/jts/2014.2.4.188.
27. Roy D. Clubfoot. In: Pediatric clinical advisor. Elsevier; 2007. p. 119. https://doi.org/10.1016/b978-032303506-4.10066-5.
28. Radler C. The Ponseti method for the treatment of congenital club foot: review of the current literature and treatment recommendations. Int Orthopaedics 2013; 37(9):1747–53.

29. Ashby ME. Surgical management of idiopathic clubfoot deformity. J Natl Med Assoc 1976;68(1):31–3.
30. Miller M, Dobbs MB. Congenital vertical talus. J Am Acad Orthop Surg 2015; 23(10):604–11.
31. Abdel-Razzak MY. Surgical Correction of Congenital Vertical Talus by One-stage Peritalar Reduction and Tibialis Anterior Transfer. Alexandria Journal of Pediatrics 2002;16(2):309–25.
32. Chauhan P, Gajjar S. Management of congenital vertical talus: comparison between mini invasive reduction and extensive surgical technique in early age. International Journal of Research in Orthopaedics 2017;3(2):197.
33. Halabchi F. Pediatric flexible flatfoot; clinical aspects and algorithmic approach. Iran J Pediatr 2013;23(3):247–60.
34. Carr JB, Yang S, Lather LA, et al. Pediatric Pes Planus: a state-of-the-art review. Pediatrics 2016;137(3). https://doi.org/10.1542/peds.2015-1230.
35. Lawrence DA, Rolen MF, Haims AH, et al. Tarsal coalitions: radiographic, CT, and MR imaging findings. HSS J 2014;10(2):153–66.
36. Agochukwu NB, Solomon BD, Benson LJ, et al. Talocalcaneal coalition in muenke syndrome: report of a patient, review of the literature in FGFR-related craniosynostoses, and consideration of mechanism. Am J Med Genet A 2013;161(3): 453–60.
37. Mahan ST, Spencer SA, Vezeridis PS, et al. Patient-reported outcomes of tarsal coalitions treated with surgical excision. J Pediatr Orthop 2015;35(6):583–8.
38. Piggott H. The natural history of hallux valgus in adolescence and early adult life. J Bone Joint Surg Br 1960;42-B(4):749–60.
39. Harb Z, Kokkinakis M, Ismail H, et al. Adolescent hallux valgus: a systematic review of outcomes following surgery. J Child Orthop 2015;9(2):105–12.
40. Baravarian B. Key insights on treating Freiburg's infarction. Podiatry Today. 2014; 27(3):84–6.
41. Mah C. Freiberg's disease. The Podiatry Institute; 2008. p. 13–5.
42. Blaz M. Cortical fibrous defects and non-ossifying fibromas in children and young adults: The analysis of radiological features in 28 cases and a review of literature. Pol J Radiol 2011;76(4):32–9.
43. Levy DM, Gross CE, Garras DN, et al. Treatment of unicameral bone cysts of the calcaneus: a systematic review. J Foot Ankle Surg 2015;54(4):652–6.

Pediatric Spine Disorders

Kristen DePaola, MS[a,b,c,1], Laury A. Cuddihy, MD[a,b,c],*

KEYWORDS

- Back pain • Spondylolysis • Spondylolisthesis • Scheurmann kyphosis
- Early onset scoliosis • Juvenile scoliosis • Congenital scoliosis
- Adolescent idiopathic scoliosis

KEY POINTS

- Pediatric spine disorders are numerous and are quite different when compared with the adult population.
- One of the most common causes of back pain in children and adolescents is lower-back muscular strain.
- Common disorders are pediatric spondylolisthesis and spondylolysis, Scheuermann kyphosis, and scoliosis among others.

INTRODUCTION

Pediatric spine disorders are numerous and are quite different when compared with the adult population. This article focuses on some of the more common pediatric spine disorders. This article summarizes such disorders and discusses typical treatment options in the pediatric orthopedic armamentarium.

Common Causes

Muscle strain or overuse

One of the most common causes of back pain in children and adolescents is lower-back muscular strain. This is most commonly associated with chronic overuse typically from sports activities or overtraining. Almost any sport, football, soccer, rowing, cheerleading, dance, may be associated. In addition, children who are not particularly active may have complaints of pain secondary to weak core musculature and/or tight hamstrings. Core muscle imbalance may also be a contributing factor.

Treatment Typical treatment options would include conservative measures, such as activity modification to include ceasing the aggravating activity. Acute strains usually resolve after a period of rest and activity modification. In addition, nonsteroidal

[a] Spine Surgery, Institute for Spine and Scoliosis, Lawrenceville, NJ, USA; [b] Orthopedics, Mount Sinai Hospital, New York, NY, USA; [c] Orthopedics, St Peters University Hospital, New Brunswick, NJ, USA
[1] Present address: 3100 Princeton Pike, Lawrenceville, NJ 08648.
* Corresponding author. 3100 Princeton Pike, Lawrenceville, NJ 08648.
E-mail address: laury.cuddihy@gmail.com

Pediatr Clin N Am 67 (2020) 185–204
https://doi.org/10.1016/j.pcl.2019.09.008
0031-3955/20/© 2019 Elsevier Inc. All rights reserved.
pediatric.theclinics.com

anti-inflammatories, if not medically contraindicated, and ice may be beneficial as well. The aforementioned typically resolves the acute symptoms. If after 4 to 5 days the symptoms continue, warm compresses may be preferred because heat may help relax muscles and decrease muscle spasm.

For children with more chronic symptoms, physical therapy may be used to improve hamstring flexibility. Core strengthening and exercises to improve core imbalance are a typical strategy in physical therapy as well. For children who lead more of a sedentary lifestyle, a regular program of low-impact walking with a goal of 30 to 45 minutes a day can help increase conditioning as initial pain improves. A home exercise program of hamstring stretches and core strengthening would also be beneficial.[1]

Pediatric spondylolisthesis and spondylolysis

Persistent lower-back pain in children and adolescents may suggest other entities. One may think of spondylolysis and spondylolisthesis. These 2 issues exist on a continuum, starting with spondylolysis and progressing to spondylolisthesis. Typical presentation includes complaints of indolent, insidious, idiopathic lower-back pain; however, it may be asymptomatic and found incidentally on radiographs. Additional complaints may include sciatic-like pain, buttock pain, or a bandlike distribution of pain. Hamstring tightness, diagnosed with knee contractures, may also be clinically recognized. Core and lower-back weakness may ensue. It is uncommon for there to be complaints of motor or sensory nerve deficits, bowel and bladder symptoms, or cauda equina syndrome. Initially, this is difficult to distinguish from muscular strains or overuse syndromes; however, the length of symptoms provides suggestions, spondylolysis and spondylolisthesis typically have prolonged course.[2]

Spondylolysis refers to a defect or stress fracture in the pars interarticularis of a vertebral body. Spondylolysis is a defect that is not present at birth and develops over time; this may be seen in 4% to 6% of the adolescent population. The mechanism of injury is typically from repetitive hyperextension. This may commonly occur in the lumbar spine especially at L5 because there is significant motion at that segment. There are many activities that allow for repetitive hyperextension. The prevalence may be as high as 47% in certain athletes, such as gymnasts, weightlifters, and football linemen. Additional sports, as they gain more popularity, such as cheerleading and dance, show increased incidence of spondylolysis as well.

Spondylolisthesis refers to the syndrome when 1 vertebral body translates with respect to the vertebral body below. This most commonly occurs with bilateral spondylolysis that has been present for some time. Patients present with complaints similar to those of spondylolysis because it is a continuum. Complaints of spondylolisthesis are typically idiopathic, insidous, indolent lower-back pain, which may include sciatic-like pain and/or a bandlike distribution of pain.

There are 5 types of spondylolisthesis: dysplastic, isthmic, degenerative, traumatic, and pathologic. Most spondylolisthesis occurs from a progression of spondylolysis. Approximately 15% of individuals with a pars interarticularis lesion (spondylolysis) have progression to spondylolisthesis. Of patients with spondylolisthesis, 90% will have so at L5-S1 levels.[2]

Spondylolisthesis, or a translation of 1 vertebral body on a lower one, may be considered a "slip." There is a risk of any slip progressing. The larger a slip or translation on presentation, the higher the likelihood of progression. Dysplastic slips, which are congenital insufficiencies of the facet joints and the disc complex, have a higher probability of progression as well.

Imaging studies to diagnose spondylolysis begin with plain radiographs. The radiographic views include anteroposterior (AP), lateral, and oblique views. The lateral view will be enough to diagnose 80% of pars defects or sclerosis (stress reaction). An additional 15% of defects will be identified with the oblique views; they will reveal sclerosis and a defect or elongation in the pars, which is recognized as the "scotty-dog sign."

If radiographs are normal and there is high suspicion for spondylolysis, single-photon emission computed tomography (SPECT) is the most sensitive imaging modality when plain radiographs are negative. Bone scans are also useful and an excellent screening tool for lower-back pain in children or adolescents with lower-back pain. However, inactive lesions may be "cold" and have lower sensitivity than SPECT scanning. Computed tomographic (CT) scanning is the most useful imaging tool to delineate the anatomy of a lesion if operative intervention is being considered. MRI is an extremely sensitive tool especially for diagnosing early disease and has the advantage of no radiation exposure.[3]

Spondylolisthesis is also initially evaluated with plain films. In addition to AP and lateral views, flexion and extension views are used to evaluate for instability. The lateral view is used to measure the slip angle and to provide a grade of spondylolisthesis (**Fig. 1**). The Meyerding classification is a grading regime that can be used to

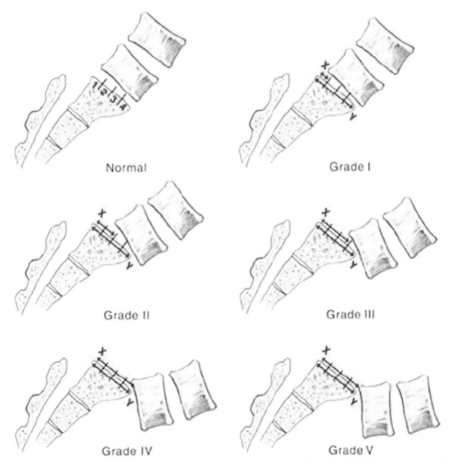

Fig. 1. Meyerding classification of spondylolisthesis. (*From* Mai HT, Hsu WK, Management of Sports-Related Lumbar Conditions. Operative Techniques in Orthopaedics, 25(3), 164-176; with permission.)

provide guidance for treatment. Lower-grade slips, grade I and II, are often treated conservatively, whereas high-grade slips (III, IV, and V spondyloptosis) are treated operatively (**Table 1**).

Slip angles are measured between a line drawn on the endplate of L5 and the endplate of the sacrum. The pelvic incidence is the sum of the pelvic tilt and sacral slopes and is also used to guide treatment. CT scans may be used in particular if a pars defect is considered with normal oblique radiographs. It also is the best study to evaluate the 3-dimensional views of the pars defect. MRI is indicated if neurologic symptoms are clinically recognized. It is also extremely useful to diagnose associated central and foramina stenosis.

Treatment Treatment focuses initially on nonoperative treatments like most orthopedic diagnoses. Observation with no activity limitations is recommended for symptomatic patients with low-grade spondylolisthesis or spondylolysis. If indeed no pain, these children may participate in contact sports.

Symptomatic patients with symptomatic isthmus spondylolysis and/or low-grade spondylolisthesis are treated with physical therapy and activity restrictions. Physical therapy is continued for 6 months and focuses on hamstring stretching and core strengthening. Care must be used when treating patients with low-grade dysplastic spondylolysis because there is a higher chance of progression. Activity modification includes cessation of all sporting activities and certainly includes contact sports. Return to activities depends on severity of disease and type of activity wanting clearance. High-level and contact sports may require an extensive amount of restriction if return is possible at all.

Thoracic-lumbar-sacral orthosis (TLSO) bracing is used as an adjunct to physical therapy and activity modification for patients in certain scenarios. TLSO bracing is useful with acute onset spondylolysis, and low-grade spondylolysis that has failed to improve with physical therapy and activity modification. TLSO bracing is typically used for 6 to 12 weeks. Outcomes of brace immobilization are superior to activity restriction alone for acute spondylolysis.

There are clinical scenarios that require operative intervention. In the case of spondylolysis, operative intervention is suggested if a defect has failed nonoperative management in symptomatic patients and those with multiple pars defects. L5-S1 in situ posterolateral fusion with bone grafting is the typically suggested treatment; however, pars repair has gained more recent attention. Most think that, with isolated spondylolysis and no evidence of spondylolisthesis, pars repair has similar surgical outcomes without the need to fuse a level (**Fig. 2**).

L5-S1 in situ posterolateral fusion with bone grafting is also used for low-grade spondylolisthesis (Meyerding grade I and II) patients who have failed nonoperative management or is progressive or the patient presents with neurologic deficits.

Table 1 Meyerding spondylolisthesis classification	
Grade I	<25%
Grade II	25%–50%
Grade III	50%–75%
Grade IV	75%–100%
Grade V	Spondyloptosis

The percentage refers to the amount of width of the vertebral body that slips on the 1 below.
Data from Ref.[3]

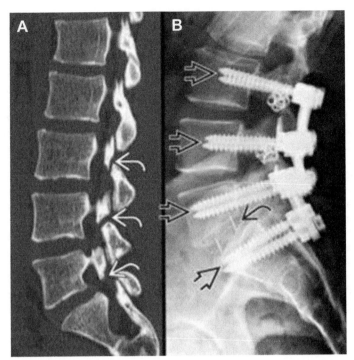

Fig. 2. (*A*) (*left*) Pars interarticularis defects are seen at L3-L4, L4-L5, and L5-S1. (*B*) (*right*) Repair of multiple-level spondylolysis by pedicle screws. An interbody disc spacer is seen. (*From* Ross JS, Bendok BR., McClendon J. Imaging in Spine Surgery. Philadelphia, PA: Elsevier; 2017; with permission.)

L4-S1 posterolateral fusion with bone grafting is suggested for high-grade spondylolisthesis (Meyerding grade III, IV, V). Much controversy surrounds the technique of reducing high-grade slips. There are multiple studies suggesting good results; however, most studies lack enough power to make general guidelines at this point.

Complications of surgical intervention may include neurologic deficits or injury, hardware failure, progression of slippage, and pseudoarthrosis. Overall, surgical outcomes are excellent. Return to activities is the norm; however, permanently avoiding high-level contact sports may be ultimately suggested.[4]

Scheuermann kyphosis

Scheuermann kyphosis is a rigid, pathologic hyperkyphosis that can cause back pain and deformity in children and adolescents. It most commonly occurs in the thoracic spine, which has a better prognosis opposed to the thoracolumbar deformity, which is more painful and more likely to be progressive.

Scheuermann kyphosis is diagnosed with a Cobb ankle greater than 45° of kyphosis measured on a lateral plain radiograph. For an appropriate diagnosis, it must also show anterior wedging of greater than 5° across 3 consecutive vertebrae. Narrowed disc spaces in the affected levels are also recognized. Included in the differential diagnosis is postural kyphosis. Scheuermann kyphosis may be differentiated from postural kyphosis by rigidity of the hyperkyphosis recognized on hyperextension lateral radiographs; Scheuermann kyphosis will not reduce.

The exact pathophysiology is unknown, but the most widely accepted theory suggests that the kyphosis and vertebral wedging are caused by a developmental error, which results in abnormal endplates and the resultant rigid hyperkyphosis. The incidence of Scheuermann kyphosis is 0.4% to 8.3%. It is the most common type of structural kyphotic deformity in adolescents. The typical age of onset is from 10 to 12 years of age, with a small subset of patients with adult onset. The male:female ratio is between 2:1 and 7:1 with an obvious male preponderance.

Associated nonorthopedic conditions include pulmonary compromise or issues with curves exceeding 100°. Associated orthopedic conditions include spondylolysis in the lumbar region (33%), scoliosis (33%), lumbar hyperlordosis and anterior shoulder, and hamstring and iliopsoas contractors.

The prognosis of Scheuermann kyphosis depends on the degree of deformity; —the higher the Cobb ankle, the more likely long-term issues such as back pain may occur. Mild curves with a mean of 71° typically result in occasional back pain in adulthood that very rarely limits activities of daily living. Curves greater than a mean of 75° may result in severe thoracic back pain. Studies suggest some progression in nearly 80% of patients; however, this does not guarantee severe deformity. Long-standing compensatory lumbar hyperlordosis may lead to lumbar spondylolysis in some patients.

Patients typically present with complaint of thoracic and/or lumbar back pain. Cosmetic concerns are also very common. The physical examination reveals increased thoracic kyphosis, which has a sharper angulation when bending forward. A complete neurologic examination is always performed but rarely reveals neurologic deficits. Commonly recognized are hamstring, iliopsoas, and anterior shoulder contractures.

Imaging begins with plain radiographs, and they are typically all that are needed for diagnosis in the neurologically intact patient. AP and lateral plain films typically reveal anterior wedging across 3 consecutive vertebrae of greater than 5°; endplate irregularities; Schmorl nodes (herniation of disc into vertebral body endplates); scoliosis; compensatory hyperlordosis; and spondylolysis. Hyperextension lateral radiographs assist in differentiating from postural kyphosis. MRI is warranted for any patient with neurologic symptoms or deficits and will typically show vertebral wedging, dehydrated discs, and Schmorl nodes.

Treatment Treatment of Scheuermann kyphosis depends on the amount of deformity. Nonoperative treatment to include stretching, physical therapy, nonsteroidal anti-inflammatory drugs (NSAIDs), and observation is recommended for kyphotic deformities less than 60° in asymptomatic patients or those with mild symptoms. Bracing with an extension-type orthosis (Jewitt type, with high sternal chest pad or "cow horns") is an adjunctive treatment. Bracing is most effective in patients with kyphosis between 60° and 80° and with growth potential remaining. The most favorable patients who have good results with Jewitt brace wear are those with curves less than 65° and those who show greater than 15° of correction on radiographs with brace wear.

Operative intervention is generally recommended for patients with kyphosis greater than 75°, severe pain in adolescents and adults, patients with neurologic deficits or signs of spinal cord compression. Surgical technique is typically posterior spinal fusion with instrumentation with osteotomies. Surgical outcome studies show 60% to 90% improvement of pain; interestingly, there is no correlation with amount of correction to improvement in symptoms. Additional studies suggest residual curves greater than 75° lead to worse functional outcomes. Surgical complications may include neurologic (0.6%–0.8%); distal junctional kyphosis (20%–30%); proximal junctional kyphosis; pseudoarthrosis; hardware failure; and loss of correction.[5–7]

Scoliosis

Scoliosis is defined as a pathologic curvature of the spine. There are many ways to categorize scoliosis but may include adolescent idiopathic scoliosis (AIS); early onset scoliosis (juevenile, infantile); congenital scoliosis, and neuromuscular scoliosis.

Adolescent idiopathic scoliosis AIS is defined as idiopathic scoliosis in children diagnosed at 10 to 18 years of age. (**Fig. 3**) AIS is the most common type of scoliosis. AIS has an incidence of 3% for curves between 10° and 20° and 0.3% for curves greater than 30°. For smaller curves that typically require no treatment, there is a 1:1 male-to-female ratio. This ratio shows a remarkable increase to 10:1 female-to-male ratio for curves greater than 30°. The most typical type of curve recognized is a right-sided

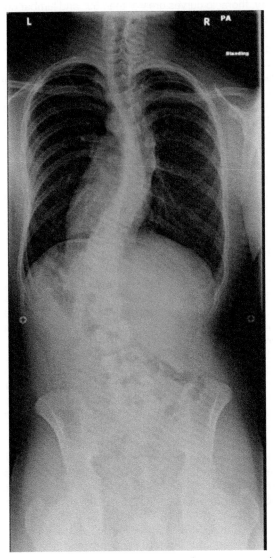

Fig. 3. PA radiograph of a right-sided thoracic curve and compensatory left-sided thoraco-lumbar curve consistent with AIS.

thoracic curve with a compensatory left-sided thoracolumbar curve. Indeed, left-sided thoracic curves are rare and require an MRI to rule out syrinx, dural ectasias, or intraspinal abnormalities. Although an exact genetic predisposition is currently undefined exactly, approximately 10% to 30% of AIS is genetically related, clearly most of AIS is spontaneous, and hence, idiopathic.

Prognosis of AIS depends on many factors. An increased incidence of acute and chronic back pain is recognized in adults for untreated curves that progress greater than 60°. Curves greater than 90° are associated with cardiopulmonary dysfunction, early death, pain, and decreased self-image. There are multiple risk factors for curve progression at presentation. As one would imagine, curve magnitude has a major impact. Curves greater than 25° before skeletal maturity will continue to progress. After skeletal maturity, thoracic curves greater than 50° and lumbar curves greater than 40° will continue to progress 1° to 2° per year.

Curve type also has an impact on prognosis. Generally, thoracic curves are more likely to progress than lumbar curves as are double versus single curves. Factors that predict for significant remaining skeletal growth potential include younger age (<12 years at presentation); Tanner stage (<3 for girls and women); Sanders stage (1–8 and is based on maturing growth plates in the hand); Risser (0–1, which correlates with the greatest velocity of skeletal linear growth); open triradiate cartilage; and peak growth velocity. The best predictor for curve progression is the peak growth velocity period. In girls, this occurs just before menarche and before Risser 1 (girls typically reach skeletal maturity 1.5 years after menarche). The peak growth velocity most closely correlates with the Tanner-Whitehouse III RUS method of skeletal maturity determination. In fact, if a patient has a curve greater than 30° before peak height velocity, there is a strong likelihood of the need for surgical intervention.[8]

The typical patient presents with no complaints. Patients are usually referred to a pediatric orthopedist after the diagnosis is suggested by the pediatrician identified on a well visit or by screening examinations. The physical examination reveals a positive Adams forward bending test (**Fig. 4**), which accentuates the axial plane deformity, which indicates a structural curve. The forward-bending sitting test is also used and eliminates limb length inequality as a contributing factor to scoliosis. Other important physical examination findings include limb length inequality; midline skin defects (hairy patches, dimples, nevi); shoulder height differences; truncal shifts; rib rotational deformities (rib prominence); waist asymmetry; cafe-au-lait spots (neurofibromatosis); foot deformities (cavovarus); and asymmetric abdominal reflexes.

Imaging is an obvious requirement for the diagnosis of and to guide the treatment of AIS. Standing, full-length posteroanterior (PA) and lateral radiographs are initially obtained. AIS is defined as a Cobb angle greater than 10°; —an intrainterobserver error of 3 to 5° has been recognized. It is important to establish coronal balance, which is determined by alignment of a C7 plumb line to the central sacral vertical line. Sagittal balance is determined on a C7 plumb line from the center of C7 to the posterior-superior corner of S1. Some important landmarks when evaluating and treating AIS include table vertebra (most proximal vertebra that is most closely bisected by the central sacral line); neutral vertebra (rotationally neutral vertebra); end vertebra (the vertebra that is most tilted from the horizontal apical vertebra); and apical vertebra (the vertebra or disc that is deviated the farthest from the center of the vertebral column).

Additional imaging, such as MRI, is performed to rule out dural ectasias, intraspinal abnormalities, and tethered cord. An MRI should extend from the posterior fossa to beyond the conus (typically L1). Logistically, the MRI is ordered as a cervical, thoracic, and lumbar/sacral MRI, and owing to the length of each study, may have to be broken

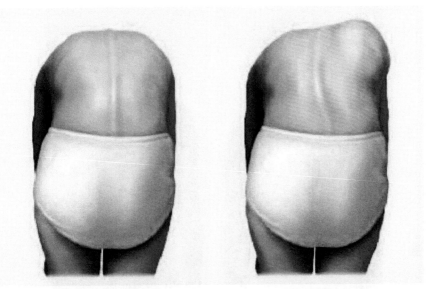

Fig. 4. Forward-bending Adam test: (*left*) normal; (*right*) abnormal. (*From* Altaf F1, Gibson A, Dannawi Z, Noordeen H. Adolescent idiopathic scoliosis. BMJ. 2013 Apr 30;346:f2508. https://doi.org/10.1136/bmj.f2508; with permission.)

up into multiple sessions; each examination can be between 30 and 45 minutes. Absolute indications to perform an MRI include atypical curve pattern (left thoracic, short angular curve, apical kyphosis); rapid progression; excessive kyphosis; structural abnormalities; neurologic symptoms; pain; foot deformities; and asymmetric abdominal reflexes (would suggest a syrinx).

Treatment Treatment of AIS is based on the skeletal maturity of the patient, magnitude of deformity, and curve progression. Nonoperative treatment includes observation and bracing. Observation is indicated for patients with a Cobb angle less than or equal to 25°. If there is a strong family history, nighttime bracing should be considered for those with a Cobb angle less than 25°. Patients are followed at 4 to 6 monthly visits with serial PA full-length scoliosis films.

Bracing (**Fig. 5**) is indicated for skeletally immature patients with a Cobb angle of 25° to 45°. The intention of bracing is to decrease the progression of the curvature; it does not decrease the curve. Bracing is continued until skeletal maturity. It is most effective for a flexible deformity in skeletally immature patients (Risser 0, 1, 2). The outcomes of brace wear are an approximately 50% reduction in the need for surgical intervention with complaint brace wear of at least 12 hours a day for the traditional Boston brace. Other types of bracing are becoming more commonplace and have largely replaced the typical Boston brace (intended to be worn 23 hours a day). Nighttime bending braces (Charleston) and Providence braces are more common now because they tend to lead to increased levels of brace wear compliance; indeed, braces only potentially work if worn. Of note, poor outcomes are related to poor in-brace correction, and in male, obese, and noncompliant patients.[9]

Operative intervention is considered for patients with a Cobb angle greater than 45°. Posterior spinal fusion with instrumentation (**Fig. 6**) is the gold standard and may be used for all types of idiopathic scoliosis. In addition, other emerging techniques are available for certain patient populations. Tethering or guided-growth corrective

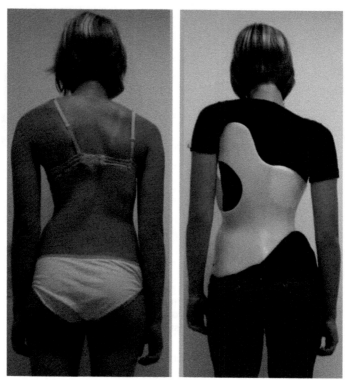

Fig. 5. Application of orthosis for AIS. (*From* Weiss HR. Scoliosis. "Brace technology" thematic series - the Gensingen brace in the treatment of scoliosis. 2010 Oct 13;5:22. https://doi.org/10.1186/1748-7161-5-22; with permission.)

scoliosis surgery is intended to be a fusionless option for particular patients. Anterior spinal fusion may be considered for some patients with a normal sagittal profile (uncommon). Anterior and posterior spinal fusion with instrumentation is indicated for some patients with a curve magnitude greater than 75°. It may also be indicated

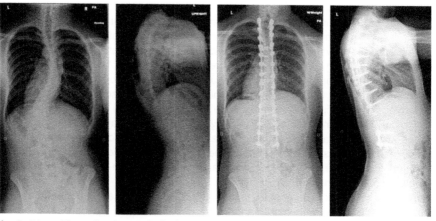

Fig. 6. PA and lateral radiographs before and after posterior spinal fusion with instrumentation for AIS.

for young patients (Risser grade 0, girls <10 years, boys <13 years) in order to potentially prevent crankshaft phenomenon.

There are many potential surgical complications that require mention. The risk of neurologic injury using current techniques is approximately 1 in 1000. The risk is diminished with use of somatosensory and motor-evoked potential with surface electromyography, neuromonitoring. Neurologic injury risk is increased in patients with concomitant kyphosis, need for excessive correction, and use of subliminal wires (one needs to enter the spinal canal to use). Pseudoarthrosis is also a potential complication (1%–2%) that may present as pain, deformity progression, and hardware failure. A symptomatic pseudoarthrosis requires repeat surgical intervention; however, an asymptomatic pseudoarthrosis requires observation alone. This may be more common if hardware failure (rod breakage) is encountered.

Postsurgical infection is always a concern and has an incidence of 1% to 2%. Patients with a postoperative infection may present asymptomatically typically with a healed incision. If encountered, a surgical site infection is treated with incision, irrigation, debridement, and drainage with maintenance of hardware if not proven loose within the first 6 months postoperatively. Of note, *Propionibacterium acnes* is the most commonly found organism when delayed infection is considered.

Crankshaft phenomenon is a rotational deformity of the spine created by continued anterior spinal growth in the setting of a posterior spinal fusion with instrumentation. This complication occurs more commonly in very young patients with which a posterior-only approach is used. This potential complication can be avoided by performing anterior discectomy and fusion with posterior fusion and instrumentation in very young patients.

Another potential postsurgical complication includes superior mesenteric artery syndrome (SMA syndrome). This complication is secondary to compression of the first part of the duodenum because of narrowing of the space between the SMA and the aorta. Indeed, the first part of the duodenum is retroperitoneal and may become kinked during correction of scoliosis. The SMA arises from the anterior aspect of the aorta at the level of the first lumbar vertebra. SMA syndrome presents with symptoms of bowel obstruction in the first postoperative week. It may be associated with general symptoms of an obstruction and may result in electrolyte abnormalities, nausea, bilious vomiting, and weight loss. Risk factors for SMA syndrome include height and weight percentile of less than 50% and less than 25%, respectively. Treatment of SMA syndrome is supportive and includes electrolyte imbalance correction and nasogastric tube insertion. SMA syndrome typically resolves with supportive treatment.[10–12]

Early onset scoliosis

Juvenile idiopathic scoliosis Juvenile idiopathic scoliosis is defined as idiopathic scoliosis diagnosed in children 4 to 10 years of age. Juvenile idiopathic scoliosis is approximately 15% of all idiopathic scoliosis cases. There is a clear preponderance in female patients. There is a high incidence (18%–25%) of neural axis abnormalities. Such abnormalities may include syringomyelia, which is a cyst or tubular cavity recognized within the spinal cord. Other abnormalities include spinal cord tumor, dysraphism, tethered cord, and Arnold-Chiari syndrome in which the cerebellar tonsils are elongated and may protrude through the opening of the base of the skull, which ultimately blocks cerebral spinal fluid flow. Of special note, juvenile idiopathic scoliosis has a high risk of progression; indeed, 70% require some form of treatment, with 50% requiring surgical intervention.

Patients with juvenile idiopathic scoliosis often present as any typical idiopathic scoliosis. However, it is important to determine when the deformity was first noticed and any observed progression. An appropriate perinatal history is obtained. Failure to develop bowel and bladder control by age 3 or 4 may indicate neurologic involvement. The physical examination is identical to AIS; however, special attention to the neurologic examination and other associated orthopedic and nonorthopedic conditions should be made.

Imaging for patients diagnosed with juvenile idiopathic scoliosis is the same as for AIS. The important difference is the use of MRI. All children are indicated for an MRI of the cervical, thoracic, and lumbar/sacral spine if diagnosed at less than 10 years of age or with a curve greater than 20° or rapid progression of a curve because it may indicate neurologic involvement. Even in the absence of neurologic symptoms, the practitioner must rule out neural axis abnormalities, such as dural ectasia and syringomyelia.

Treatment Treatment of juvenile idiopathic scoliosis is nonoperative and operative. Nonoperative treatment is appropriate for patients with a curve less than 20°. This would include observation with frequent, 4 to 6 monthly office visits with appropriate standing PA scoliosis films to evaluate for potential curve progression. Bracing is indicated for curves between 20° and 50°. Similar to AIS, bracing is intended to prevent curve progression, not correct the curve. Brace wear is indicated for 16 to 23 hours a day until skeletal maturity or surgery is indicated.

Operative intervention depends on curve magnitude, age, and potential for growth. Nonfusion procedures (growing rods, vertical expandable prosthetic titanium rib, anterior vertebral body tethering) **(Fig. 7)** are indicated for curves greater than 40 in smaller children with significant growth potential. These methods allow for continued spinal growth over the unfused segments. Once growth potential decreases or skeletal maturity is achieved, posterior and/or anterior spinal fusion with instrumentation is performed. If one fuses a patient prematurely, before skeletal maturity, complications may occur from the decreased thoracic volume from limited thoracic growth. If a child is diagnosed with a curve greater than 50°, combined anterior and posterior spinal fusion is indicated to prevent potential crankshaft phenomenon from occurring. Posterior-alone spinal fusion is indicated for patients with a curve greater than 50° and who are near skeletal maturity. Postoperative complications are similar to those of AIS.

Infantile idiopathic scoliosis Infantile idiopathic scoliosis is defined as idiopathic scoliosis that presents in a patient 4 years or younger. This accounts for only 4% of idiopathic scoliosis and is more common in boys. It is typically diagnosed with a left-sided thoracic curvature. Infantile idiopathic scoliosis may adversely affect growth of alveoli and normal development of the thoracic cage, leading to restrictive lung disease. There is a genetic association, which is autosomal dominant with variable penetrance. Other associated conditions include plagiocephaly; congenital defects; neural axis abnormalities (22% of patient with curves >20° and of which 80% of such patients will require neurosurgical intervention); and thoracic insufficiency syndrome (characterized by decreased thoracic growth and lung volume, curves >60°, and may lead to pulmonary hypertension and cor pulmonale for curves >90°).[13]

The prognosis for infantile idiopathic scoliosis is typically good, with most cases resolving spontaneously. If, however, the curve is progressive by the age of 5, greater than 50% of these children will have a curve greater than 70°, requiring intervention. The Mehta predictors of progression are used to guide treatment and include Cobb angle greater than 20°; rib-vertebral angle difference (RVAD) greater than 20°; and phase 2 rib-vertebral relationship (rib-vertebral overlay). Curves that meet the Mehta criteria are considered to have significant potential to progress and have poorer outcomes and must be treated.

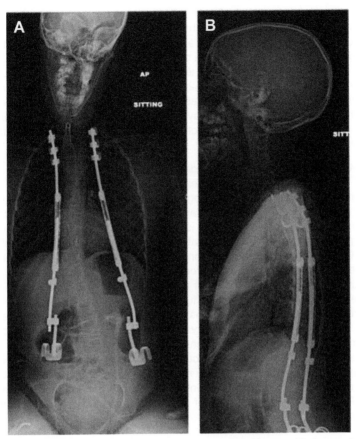

Fig. 7. Radiographs showing growing rods. (*From* Lee MC, Eberson CP. Congenital Myopathy with Early-Onset Scoliosis. In El-Hawary R., Eberson CP. Early onset scoliosis: A clinical casebook. Cham, Switzerland : Springer; pp. 197-210.; 2018.)

Patients do not present with pain. They do, however, typically present with a deformity recognized on physical examination. Some patients' parents are aware of the genetic predilection and seek evaluation by a pediatric orthopedist at the direction of their pediatrician. It is important to note when any family history, developmental milestone achievements, excessive drooling, perinatal history, or age deformity was first noticed and any observed progression. Additional findings on physical examination may include cafe-au-lait spots (neurofibromatosis); sacral hairy patches (spina bifida); sacral dimpling; nevi or other tumors indicative of spinal dysraphism; plagiocephaly; or cavovarus feet. Examination should also include notation of abnormal abdominal reflexes, which may be a sign of a syrinx. Clonus, positive Hoffman sign, and abnormal Babinski testing all may support a suspicion for neurologic involvement.

Imaging to evaluate patients with infantile idiopathic scoliosis begins with PA and lateral radiographs. It is uncommon to be able to obtain standing films, so supine radiographs suffice; however, it should be noted that supine films will underestimate the significance of the curve. Special notice should be made of congenital vertebral defects. Any Cobb angle greater than 20° is associated with a risk of progression. The rib phase, which is the convex rib head position with respect to the apical vertebra, is evaluated. A phase 1 rib shows no overlap, whereas a phase 2 rib shows overlap with the apical vertebra; patients with phase 2 ribs have a higher risk for curve progression. The Mehta angle or the RVAD begins with evaluating a measured angle between the endplate of the apical vertebra and rib (line between midpoint of rib head and neck). RVAD is the difference between 2 consecutive rib-vertebral angles. RVAD greater than 20 is associated with a high risk of curve progression, whereas less than 20 is associated with spontaneous recovery. MRI evaluation of the spine is almost always performed because there is a high incidence of neurologic comorbidities, such as tethered cord, tumor, cyst, and syrinx (20% incidence).[13]

Treatment Again, treatment of infantile idiopathic scoliosis is dictated by curve magnitude and patient age. Nonoperative treatment predominates. Observation alone is appropriate for patients with a Cobb angle less than 20° and an RVAD less than 20° because that is associated with spontaneous resolution in 90% of patients. Serial Mehta casting (**Fig. 8**) or use of TLSO is indicated for patients with flexible curves, Cobb angle greater than 30°, RVAD greater than 20°, and a phase 2 rib-vertebra relationship. Casting or orthotic use functions to straighten the spine in the younger patient opposed to prevention of curve progression in older patients.

Operative intervention is complex but typically revolves around fusionless surgical techniques. The goal is to delay spinal fusion as long as possible to give the patient an opportunity to reach as close as possible to skeletal maturity. Fusion before the age of 10 typically results in pulmonary compromise. Potential surgical techniques include growing rod constructs. This technique allows for spinal growth of the affected part of the spine up to 5 cm before replacement. Serial lengthening, which now may be done in the office, is required every few months. Patients indicated for surgical intervention have a Cobb angle greater than 50° to 60° or have failed Mehta casting or bracing. There are much higher rates of complications associated with infantile idiopathic scoliosis surgical treatment.[13]

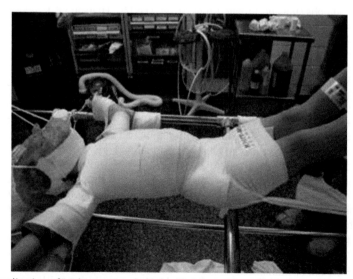

Fig. 8. Application of Mehta casting for infantile idiopathic scoliosis. (*From* Sanders JO. Casting for Infantile Idiopathic Scoliosis. Operative Techniques in Orthopaedics. 2016;26(4):218–221; with permission.)

Congenital scoliosis Congenital scoliosis is defined as the failure of normal vertebral development during the fourth to sixth week of gestation. This is caused by a failure of formation, segmentation, or both (**Fig. 9**). The prevalence of congenital scoliosis in the general population is estimated at 1% to 4%. Most cases occur spontaneously as opposed to a genetic predisposition. Congenital scoliosis may be associated with maternal exposure to alcohol, valproic acid, hyperthermia, or an existing condition of diabetes. There are myriad associated conditions with congenital scoliosis, up to 61% of patients. Spinal cord malformations are common especially with a history of underlying syndromes or chromosomal abnormalities. Cardiac and genitourinary defects may occur in 10% and 25% of patients with congenital scoliosis, respectively.

Of patients, 38% to 55% present with VACTERL syndrome, which is characterized by vertebral malformations, anal atresia, cardiac malformations, tracheoesophageal fistula, renal and radial anomalies as well as limb defects. Hemifacial microsomia, epibulbar dermoids, and congenital scoliosis are associated with Goldenhar/oculoauriculovertebral syndrome. Jarcho-Levin syndrome, or spondylocostal dysostosis, is a syndrome associated with short-trunk dwarfism, multiple vertebral and rib defects, and fusions. This syndrome is typically autosomal recessive and presents with a shortened thorax secondary to the rib fusions and the association with congenital scoliosis, which together may cause thoracic insufficiency syndrome, this combination may

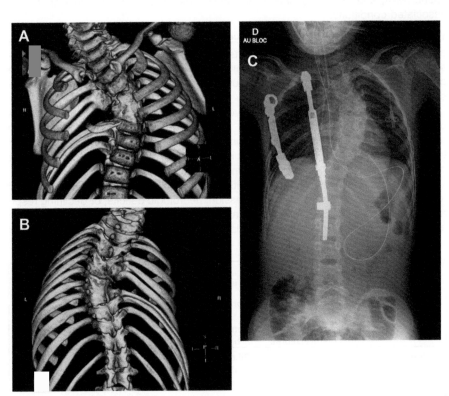

Fig. 9. (*A, B*) Congenital scoliosis showing vertebral body deformities and (*C*) vertical expandable prosthetic titanium rib application. (*From* Dayer R, Ceroni D, Lascombes P. Treatment of congenital thoracic scoliosis with associated rib fusions using VEPTR expansion thoracostomy: a surgical technique. Eur Spine J. 2014 Jul;23 Suppl 4:S424-31. https://doi.org/10.1007/s00586-014-3338-3. Epub 2014 May 14; with permission.)

result in respiratory decompensation and an inability to support appropriate lung growth. Last, congenital scoliosis may be associated with Klippel-Feil syndrome, which presents with a short neck, low posterior hairline, and cervical vertebral fusions.

The prognosis of congenital scoliosis is varied and determined by the morphology of the vertebral body deformity and is expressed typically within the first 3 years of life (**Table 2**). The rate of progression is greatest with a unilateral unsegmented bar with a contralateral hemivertebra. This deformity has the greatest potential for rapid progression and is estimated at 5° to 10° per year. Other vertebral body deformities also show potential for progression as follows from greatest to least: unilateral unsegmented bar; fully segmented hemivertebra; and unsegmented hemivertebra. The deformity with the lowest possibility of curve progression is a block vertebra at less than 2° per year unless associated with rib fusions. Outcomes of congenital scoliosis depend on potential for progression and intervention timing.

Radiographs, to include AP and lateral views, are typically adequate for an initial diagnosis. Follow-up CT scans are important for surgical planning to appropriately evaluate bony anatomy. All patients with congenital scoliosis require MRI evaluation of the entire spine because neural axis deformities are recognized in 20% to 40% of patients. Associated neurologic abnormalities include Chiarl malformations; tethered cord; syringomyelia; diastematomyelia; and intradural lipomas. In addition, renal ultrasound, MRI, and echocardiograms are considered to evaluate for nonorthopedic-associated conditions.

Treatment Treatment is nonoperative initially. Observation with serial examinations and radiographs is considered in patients with an absence of documented progression. Bracing is not commonly used for the structural curve because it has been proven to be ineffective. Bracing may be used to decrease the progression of a flexible compensatory curve, however.

Operative technique depends on the vertebral deformity and curve progression. A posterior spinal fusion with or without osteotomies and correction attempts are used for patients with hemivertebra and unilateral bars because they have been shown to progress without surgical treatment. It is also used in older patients with significant progression, neurologic deficits, or declining respiratory function.

Anterior and posterior spinal fusion with or without a vertebrectomy is considered for young patients with significant progression, neurologic deficits, or declining respiratory function. The typical age for surgical intervention in girls is less than 10 years old and in boys is less than 12 years old. It is also considered for patients with failure of

Table 2		
Classification of vertebral body deformities in congenital scoliosis		
Failure of formation	Fully segmented hemivertebrae	Normal disc above and below
	Semisegmented hemivertebrae	Hemivertebrae fused to adjacent segment above OR below
Failure of segmentation	Block vertebrae	Bilateral bony bars
	Bar vertebrae	Unilateral failure of segmentation of 2 or more vertebrae
Mixed	Unilateral unsegmented bar with contralateral hemivertebrae	Most rapid progression

formation with contralateral failure of segmentation at any age that requires hemivertebrectomy and/or significant correction. Distraction-based growing rod constructs may be used in an attempt to control deformity during spinal growth and delay arthrodesis (see **Fig. 9**). This type of surgical technique requires lengthening approximately every 6 months for best results. Rib osteotomies are considered for patients who have greater than 4 ribs fused because there is significant potential for thoracic insufficiency syndrome in such a setting.

Complications after surgical intervention for congenital scoliosis can be more common. Crankshaft phenomenon is a common complication when performing posterior fusion alone. Complications of short stature and or short trunk are common because the spinal column is affected by fusion and is more common in the younger patient. Neurologic injury may occur with overdistraction or shortening, overcorrection or during harvesting of segmental vessels. Somatosensory and motor-evoked potentials recorded and evaluated intraoperatively are extremely important to avoid neurologic complications.[13]

Neuromuscular scoliosis Neuromuscular scoliosis is defined as an irregular spinal curvature caused by disorders of the brain, spinal cord, and/or muscular system. Associated scoliosis tends to be more rapidly progressive after skeletal maturity. Neuromuscular scoliosis is often associated with pelvic obliquity, and the curves are typically longer because they involve more vertebral bodies (including the cervical spine). Neuromuscular scoliosis has a much higher rate of pulmonary complications with surgical intervention.

Classification and treatment Bracing and observation for progressive neuromuscular scoliosis are ineffective. Surgical correction with spinal fusion is the only treatment that has a documented beneficial impact on deformity (**Table 3**). Indeed, parents and caretakers report excellent improvement in the child's quality of life after deformity correction. There are however well-documented increased risk of wound complications with poor nutritional status (serum albumin <3.5 g/dL), immunocompromised status (white blood cell [WBC] <1500 cell/μL), and the presence of a ventriculoperitoneal shunt.[14]

Disc herniation
Disc herniations rarely occur in children and adolescents. There are, however, certain activities that increase the risk of herniations, such as weightlifting. Because children and adolescents still have viable growth plates at the ends of each vertebral body, disc

Table 3		
Classification and treatment suggestions for neuromuscular scoliosis		
Upper motor neuron	Cerebral palsy	Spastic quadriplegic at highest risk, especially if no ability to sit independently
	Rhett syndrome	>50% will develop scoliosis
Muscle weakness	Spinal muscle atrophy	Progressive; loss of motor neurons in anterior horn of spinal cord
	Muscular dystrophy	95% of patients after becoming wheelchair bound
Paralytic syndromes	Spina bifida/ spinal cord injury	Higher the functional level, the higher the risk for scoliosis
	Polio	Similar to SMA

herniations are unique compared with the adult population. Disc herniations in children and adolescents may avulse a portion of the vertebral body growth plate and may cause spinal nerve root or spinal cord stenosis. This is typically one of the only circumstances in which surgical intervention is necessary. Most commonly, disc herniations in children and adolescents are treated supportively and may include activity modification, ice, NSAIDs, and physical therapy for core strengthening and hamstring stretching (**Fig. 10**).[1]

Infection

Infection in the pediatric spine is uncommon but may affect vertebral bodies (osteomyelitis) or discs (discitis) (**Fig. 11**). Discitis tends to affect younger children compared with vertebral body osteomyelitis. Discitis may present as back pain, fever of unknown origin, lower-back stiffness or spasming, and refusal to walk or bend at the waist. Laboratory tests, such as WBC, C-reactive protein, erythrocyte sedimentation rate, blood, and urine cultures are important for appropriate diagnosis. Radiographs are the first step, but ultimately, MRI is the most useful diagnostic test for confirmation of discitis and/or vertebral body osteomyelitis. The mainstay of treatment is prolonged antibiotic treatment.[1]

Tumor

Spinal tumors in children and adolescents are quite rare. Tumors may be considered in patients with complaints of constant or progressively worsening pain, particularly night pain. Pain associated with fever of unknown origin or weight loss requires

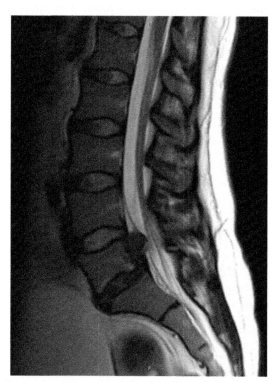

Fig. 10. Sagittal MRI showing L5 herniated disc. (*From* Moore, D. Lumbar Disc Herniation.Orthobullets. 30 July 2019. Available at: https://www.orthobullets.com/spine/2035/lumbar-disc-herniation.)

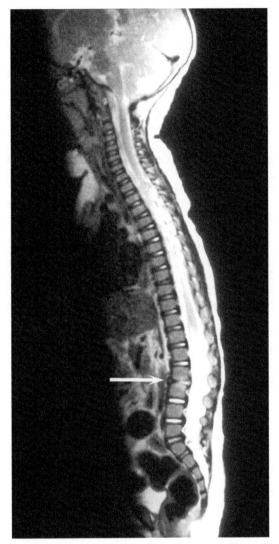

Fig. 11. MRI depicting L2/3 discitis. (*From* AR, Rooke R, Sivashankar S. Lumbar discitis. Arch Dis Child. 2006 Feb;91(2):116; with permission.)

more urgent evaluation. Treatment varies significantly and depends on tumor type and comorbidities.[1]

REFERENCES

1. Larson NA. Back pain, disk disease, spondylolysis and spondylolisthesis. In: Orthopedic knowledge update 5: pediatrics. 2016. p. 415–32.
2. Lawrence JP, Greene HS, Grauer JN. Back pain in athletes. J Am Acad Orthop Surg 2006;14(13):726–35.
3. Hu SS, Tribus CB, Diab M, et al. Spondylolisthesis and spondylolysis. J Bone Joint Surg Am 2008;90(3):656–71.

4. Hu SS, Tribus CB, Diab M, et al. Spondylolisthesis and spondylolysis. Instr Course Lect 2008;57:431–45.
5. Wenger DR, Frick SL. Scheuermann kyphosis. Spine (Phila Pa 1976) 1999; 24(24):2630–9.
6. Tribus CB. Scheuermann's kyphosis in adolescents and adults: diagnosis and management. J Am Acad Orthop Surg 1998;6(1):36–43.
7. Lee SS, Lenke LG, Kuklo TR, et al. Comparison of Scheuermann kyphosis correction by posterior-only thoracic pedicle screw fixation versus combined anterior/posterior fusion. Spine (Phila Pa 1976) 2006;31(20):2316–21.
8. Trobisch PD, Ducoffe AR, Lonner BS, et al. Choosing fusion levels in adolescent idiopathic scoliosis. J Am Acad Orthop Surg 2013;21(9):519–28.
9. Weinstein SL, Dolan LA, Wright JG, et al. Effects of bracing in adolescents with idiopathic scoliosis. N Engl J Med 2013;369(16):1512–21.
10. Sanders JO, Browne RH, McConnell SJ, et al. Maturity assessment and curve progression in girls with idiopathic scoliosis. J Bone Joint Surg Am 2007;89(1): 64–73.
11. Sanders JO, Khoury JG, Kishan S, et al. Predicting scoliosis progression from skeletal maturity: a simplified classification during adolescence. J Bone Joint Surg Am 2008;90(3):540–53.
12. Holte DC, Winter RB, Lonstein JE, et al. Excision of hemivertebrae and wedge resection in the treatment of congenital scoliosis. J Bone Joint Surg Am 1995; 77(2):159–71.
13. Glotzbecker MA. Early onset scoliosis and congenital spine disorders. In: Orthopedic knowledge update 5: pediatrics. 2016. p. 339–50.
14. Whitaker AT. Neuromuscular spine deformity. In: Orthopedic knowledge update 5: pediatrics. 2016. p. 365–84.

Pediatric Sports Injuries

Natasha Trentacosta, MD*

KEYWORDS

- Sports injuries • Overuse injuries • Pediatric injuries

KEY POINTS

- Sports injuries in youth athletics continue to increase with increased sports participation and competitiveness.
- Young athletes are susceptible to both acute, traumatic injuries leading to fractures and dislocations as well as chronic overuse injuries.
- Lower-extremity injuries are seen more commonly in pediatric and adolescent athletes than those of the upper extremity.

INTRODUCTION

Sports injuries in the athletic pediatric and adolescent population continue to increase as children increase their participation in organized sports, focus on single sports year round without cross-training, and achieve higher levels of competitive play. Although lower-extremity injuries are seen more commonly in athletics, children involved in such sports as baseball, judo, gymnastics, and snowboarding are more prone to upper-extremity injuries.[1]

HISTORY, PHYSICAL EXAMINATION, AND IMAGING

As with any injury presentation, a thorough history and physical examination are imperative to the diagnosis and treatment of sports injuries in the young athlete. The athlete's sport and position as well as mechanism of injury are important considerations.

Knowledge of an athlete's training is helpful as unsound practices and abrupt changes may lead to overuse injuries. Knowledge of the number and types of pitches per week for throwing athletes and weekly mileage for runners are examples as well as recent changes to their program. Growth history should be assessed, because peak growth velocity presents a risk factor for injury. The passive elongation of soft tissues over actively elongating bone leads to temporary inflexibility and muscle imbalance and an increased risk of injury.

No disclosures.
Cedars-Sinai Kerlan-Jobe Institute, Los Angeles, CA, USA
* 2020 Santa Monica Boulevard #400, Santa Monica, CA 90404.
E-mail address: natasha.trentacosta@cshs.org

Often neglected, nutrition and body image are vital components of an athlete's history. It is important to not only access how much energy is expended but also get an accurate assessment of the energy intake by an athlete. Particular attention should be given to those athletes who participate in high-risk sports, such as figure skating, cross-country running, and wrestling. Given the high demands athletes place on their bodies, sufficient energy intake is required to prevent stress and overuse injuries.

A focused musculoskeletal examination is integral to obtaining objective measures to aid in the diagnosis. The range of motion and muscle strength, especially compared with the contralateral side, should be assessed in the injured extremity. Stability of the joint should be assessed in both traumatic and atraumatic situations. Muscle atrophy may signal nerve impingement disorders. Provocative examination of the joint can provide further information to aid in the differential diagnosis.

Appropriate imaging is undertaken after obtaining a history and physical examination. When dealing with traumatic injuries, a radiograph is often all that is needed to reveal the pathologic condition. Pathologic bone lesions may be found incidentally in patients who have fractured through a weak bone lesion. Advanced imaging is usually reserved for those who fail nonoperative measures or those who have an abnormal physical examination or radiographic findings suggestive of internal derangement.

ACUTE SPORTS INJURIES

Traumatic injuries are very common injuries seen in the pediatric and adolescent athletic population. Patients presenting with a traumatic injury relay a story of a single event or an acute event superimposed on an overuse background. Often these occur in contact sports, such as football, basketball, hockey, and wrestling. Injuries may range from ligament sprains and muscle strains to fractures and dislocations.

CHRONIC OVERUSE INJURIES

Overuse injuries occur when training demands exceed the pediatric bodies' physiologic ability to mend itself, leading to repetitive submaximal forces causing microscopic damage tissues.[2] Children and adolescents are at particular risk given their weaker physes and muscle imbalance. The adolescent growth spurt is a unique time in development that can make them more susceptible to such injury. Bone and physeal cartilage tend to be weaker; the musculotendinous junction tightens as lengthening bones impart more tension, and coordination is lacking.[3–5]

UPPER-EXTREMITY INJURIES
Shoulder

The shoulder joint is particularly vulnerable in overhead pediatric athletes because they produce high levels of force throughout the upper extremity. These excessive forces may lead to overuse of the stabilizing structures. An increase in this force is seen during the mid to late teen years as the shoulder is subjected to progressively higher stresses with the increase in muscular development. Poor shoulder and core biomechanics as well as scapular dyskinesis along with excessive training contribute to the development of these common maladies in youth athletics.

Little League shoulder
Commonly seen in pediatric baseball pitchers, Little League shoulder is considered a chronic stress form of a nondisplaced Salter-Harris I fracture of the proximal

humerus. It is often seen in early male adolescents because at this time their physeal growth is at its maximal rate, and as a result, also weak. Pitchers who throw curve balls, continue to throw through fatigue, are overweight, lift weights, and play on multiple teams are at increased risk of this overuse condition.[6] Overhead athletes typically complain of insidious shoulder pain as well as limited range of motion in the shoulder. The repetitive stress of throwing produces radiographic physeal widening of the proximal humeral physis when compared with the contralateral side (**Fig. 1**). In severe cases, premature closure of the growth plate can be seen and can lead to angular deformity. The diagnosis relies mostly on clinical assessment and can be supported by radiographic widening. MRI, although rarely contributory to the diagnosis, may show widening and edema within the proximal humeral physis.

The treatment of Little League shoulder requires rest, followed by gradual rehabilitation of the shoulder, and return to play. This involves a program of progression from range of motion, through strengthening, endurance, and speed, while stressing control and proper biomechanics. Prevention of such an injury is paramount and requires adherence to recommendations on pitch count and rest days as well as maintenance of proper pitching biomechanics. Missed cases can lead to chronic pain with throwing, early shoulder instability, or degenerative arthritis.[7]

Glenohumeral internal rotation deficit
Glenohumeral internal rotation deficit (GIRD) is another shoulder syndrome commonly seen in overhead athletes. It is defined by the objective loss of internal rotation compared with the contralateral side as a result of derangements to the dynamic restraints in the shoulder. The posterior capsule becomes contracted, initially leading to a posterior superior migration of the humeral head on the glenoid. If continued, These adaptive changes can lead to bony adaptations, such as increased humeral head retroversion, and ultimately, alteration of the normal scapular and shoulder biomechanics.[8] GIRD can lead to internal impingement of the rotator cuff tendons and subsequent rotator cuff injury.

Integral to the treatment and prevention of GIRD is posterior capsular stretching to decrease pain and the adaptive changes seen in throwing. This along with a strengthening program helps treat and prevent shoulder pain in these throwing athletes.

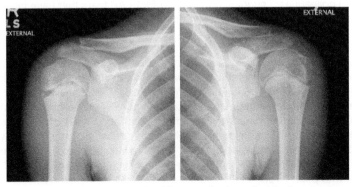

Fig. 1. External oblique images: right shoulder reveals physeal widening consistent with Little League shoulder; left shoulder normal. (*From* Anton C, Podberesky DJ. Little League shoulder: a growth plate injury. Pediatr Radiol (2010) 40(Suppl 1): 54. https://doi.org/10.1007/s00247-010-1868-3; with permission.)

Internal impingement and rotator cuff injury

Although rotator cuff injury tends to be rare in youth athletes when compared with adults, rotator cuff tendinitis has been increasingly described in the adolescent population, particularly swimmers, throwers, racquetball players, and tennis players, often occurring with other intraarticular pathologic condition, especially labral tears.[9–12] With internal impingement, the rotator cuff, labrum, and joint capsule are repetitively pinched between the greater tuberosity and superior glenoid rim at the extremes of abduction and external rotation, which can occur multiple times in overhead sports. Although frank tears of the rotator cuff were thought to only occur in the adult population, studies have shown they exist in the pediatric population as well.[13,14]

High-performance swimmers experience high repetitive forces across the shoulder as a result of the multiple revolutions their shoulders must undergo to propel their bodies long distances, and an increase in overuse shoulder injuries usually is seen after the age of 10. Swimmers often develop a condition dubbed "swimmer's shoulder," which is an ill-defined overuse injury of the shoulder synonymous with rotator cuff tendonitis and impingement syndrome that results in pain from impingement of the humeral head and rotator cuff on the coracoacromial ligament.

The treatment options for rotator cuff pathologic condition tend to involve nonoperative modalities, relying on a course of rest and physical therapy. Surgical intervention may be considered for those who fail conservative management with persistent symptoms and the presence of some degree of a rotator cuff tear and/or persistent impingement, but the results of surgical treatment are largely undetermined in the pediatric population.[12,15]

Superior labral tear from anterior to posterior tears

SLAP (superior labrum anterior to posterior) tears may be an uncommon cause of insidious shoulder pain in the pediatric or adolescent athlete, often felt while in the overhead position. The cause is thought to occur as a result of the peel-back phenomenon that results in a more vertical and posterior force vector on the biceps tendon in the abducted and externally rotated position. A high suspicion should be maintained in throwing athletes who have refractory pain because MRI may be necessary to aid in the diagnosis (**Fig. 2**).

Initial management should consist of nonoperative measures, including rest and physical therapy. The role for surgical treatment of SLAP tears remains controversial. Kocher and colleagues[16] suggest arthroscopy for SLAP tears that have failed nonoperative measures of rest, nonsteroidal anti-inflammatory drugs (NSAIDs), and physical therapy.

Elbow

The elbow is particularly vulnerable in throwing athletes and those involved in upper-extremity weight-bearing sports, such as gymnastics. Traumatic injuries in collision sports can lead to elbow fractures and dislocations. Repetitive overuse injuries can damage cartilage, subchondral bone, ligaments, and apophyses of the elbow.

With more than 5 million children participating in baseball, rates of elbow injuries seem to be increasing in throwing athletes.[17,18] Throwing curveballs has been associated with a 1.66 increased risk of pitching-related injuries in youth baseball players, and those who pitch through fatigue can have a 7-fold increased risk.[19]

Little League elbow

Although Little League elbow has been used to describe any elbow pain in the youth baseball player, it more commonly refers to medial epicondylar apophysitis, a traction

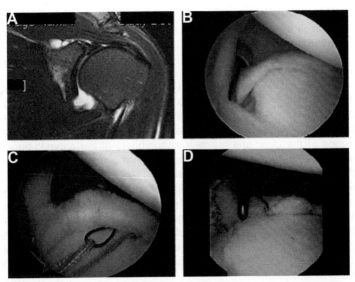

Fig. 2. (A) T2-weighted, coronal oblique MRI arthrogram of a left shoulder demonstrating branched linear high signal at superior labrum, suggestive of SLAP lesion, connecting with high-signal lobulated fluid outside the confines of the glenohumeral joint, suggestive of spinoglenoid cyst. (B) Unstable posterior SLAP tear of right shoulder in the lateral decubitus position. (C) A suture loop is used to pass suture through the unstable anterior portion of an SLAP tear in a right shoulder. (D) Completed suture anchor fixation of the labrum is probed for stability. (*From* Enad JG, Kurtz CA. Isolated and combined Type II SLAP repairs in a military population. Knee Surg Sports Traumatol Arthrosc. 2007 Nov;15(11):1382-9. Epub 2007 May 12; with permission.)

injury to the medial epicondyle in skeletally immature throwing athletes. Valgus extension overload occurs as a result of repetitive throwing, which places a tensile stress on the medial elbow. Throwing athletes experience gradual onset of pain in late cocking and early deceleration when valgus loads are maximal. Complaints of loss of throwing velocity as well as accuracy are also common. Imaging of the dominant throwing elbow as well as the contralateral elbow may show physeal widening in the affected elbow.

The mainstay of treatment involves strict cessation of throwing activities until symptoms have resolved, NSAIDs and icing, and occasionally, bracing. Appropriate treatment often involves education not only of the athlete but also the parents as well, in order to guide expectations. The key is preventing such injuries from occurring through education and adherence to proper pitch count guidelines and proper mechanics.

Medial epicondyle avulsion fracture

Avulsion of the medial epicondyle can result from either an acute trauma or an elbow dislocation, or from repetitive valgus extension overload forces in throwing athletes approaching skeletal maturity. It can be seen as a continuum of the injury spectrum of Little League elbow, where the forces result in fragmentation and avulsion of the medial epicondyle.

Although most agree that avulsion fractures with less than 5 mm of displacement can be treated with initial immobilization followed by early range-of-motion therapy, those with greater than 5 mm of displacement garner controversial recommendations. Treatment may include similar nonoperative measures, open reduction and internal fixation, or fragment excision with reattachment of ligamentous complex. Consideration of the displacement, fracture stability, age, and activity level can help guide treatment recommendations (**Fig. 3**).

Medial collateral ligament injury

With skeletal maturation, there is a shift from growth plate injuries to ligamentous injury. Although not the most common injury sustained by youth throwing athletes, medial collateral ligament (MCL) injuries are being seen with increasing frequency. Injury to the MCL can present as midsubtance, partial, or full-thickness tears. Complete avulsions of the ulnar and humeral attachments of the anterior bundle of the MCL have been reported.[20] It is often the result of an acute injury with reported "popping" sensation, swelling, and ecchymosis.

Initial treatment is with rest, bracing, NSAIDs, icing, and physical therapy. A gradual return to activities with a focus on core, hip, and lower-extremity strengthening, in addition to upper-extremity strengthening, is key. Proper kinetic chain activation and pitching mechanics will help prevent future injury. Should nonoperative measures fail, surgical intervention may be indicated to reconstruct the MCL in a similar fashion to adults or a primary repair. MCL reconstructions have doubled in high school baseball players in recent years.[21]

Osteochondritis dissecans

Osteochondritis dissecans (OCD) is a degeneration of subchondral bone and its overlying cartilage, which may be seen in the elbow of throwing athletes and gymnasts. It occurs commonly in the capitellum and rarely in the radial head. Repetitive

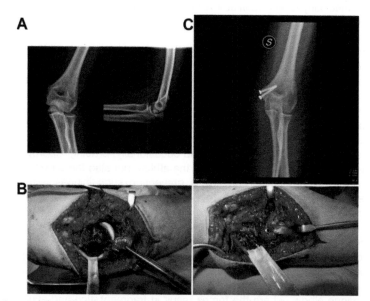

Fig. 3. Case 1. (*A*) Medial epicondyle fracture with intraarticular fragment incarceration. (*B*) Intraoperative view of ulnar nerve identification and protection followed by open reduction and internal fixation with 2 cannulated screws. (*C*) Radiograph at 3 months, showing complete healing of the fracture. (*From* Tarallo L., Mugnai R, Fiacchi F, et al. Pediatric medial epicondyle fractures with intra-articular elbow incarceration. J Orthop Traumatol 2015;16(2):117–23; with permission.)

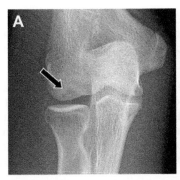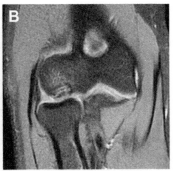

Fig. 4. OCD of the capitulum. (*A*) Anteroposterior radiograph of the elbow in a 16-year-old male pitcher with lateral elbow pain demonstrates a focal lucency in the subchondral bone (*arrow*) surrounded by a rim of sclerosis. (*B*) Coronal fat-suppressed proton density MRI demonstrates a high signal line along the margin of the lesion, indicating instability. (*From* Davis, KW. Imaging pediatric sports injuries: upper extremity. Radiologic clinics of North America 2010DOI:10.1016/j.rcl.2010.07.020; with permission.)

lateral compressive forces generated by throwing, axial compression in weight bearing, or racquet sports result in disruption of the local tenuous blood flow to the subchondral area. There are often activity-related pain and stiffness, and in more advanced disease, can lead to mechanical symptoms. Pain is usually felt in late cocking through acceleration when compressive forces are the greatest at the elbow (**Fig. 4**).

Management of elbow OCD lesions depends on the stability of the lesion. Intact and stable lesions are best treated nonoperatively with activity modification in order to reduce the axial load to the radiocapitellar joint and possible bracing. Surgery is recommended for cases not responding to nonoperative measures or unstable lesions. Surgical management typically consists of excision of the unstable lesion, followed by chondroplasty or drilling, or grafting for larger lesions. Variable results have been found with internal fixation of loose lesions.[22–25]

Olecranon apophyseal injury

Posterior elbow injuries are often the result of shear forces seen at the joint and repetitive abutment of the olecranon and the olecranon fossa, which can occur during the acceleration phase of throwing or tumbling exercises in gymnastics. In young children with open growth plates, the repetitive contraction of the triceps muscle on the olecranon as well as valgus extension overload can cause the physis to widen and fail to close. The spectrum of injury can range from apophysitis through avulsion fractures, or frank stress fractures in older adolescents. As high as 5.4% prevalence of olecranon stress fractures has been found among baseball-related elbow disorders.[26] Pain and tenderness are felt with elbow extension and may be associated with swelling.

Initial treatment is often nonoperative with activity modification, NSAIDs, icing, and physical therapy. Because stress fractures are the result of overuse and fatigue of the surrounding musculature, most heal with conservative measures. Physical therapy is focused on rotator cuff strength and scapular stabilization. Surgical intervention should be considered in those who do not heal with nonoperative measures and high-level competitive throwing athletes, such as baseball players and javelin throwers.

Hand and Wrist

Sports are a major cause of hand and wrist injuries in children and adolescents.[27–30] Injuries the hand and wrists of the pediatric athlete are frequently traumatic in nature.

Fractures

The distal radius is the most common site of fracture for the pediatric athlete. Soccer is the sport most frequently associated with these injuries.[31] In the metaphysis, both buckle fractures and complete fractures are commonly seen in children. The fracture commonly occurs at the transition of the dense lamellar bone of the diaphysis with the porous metaphyseal bone.[32] As children get older, this transition point moves distally, and fractures tend to occur closer to the physis in older children.

Gymnast wrist

Gymnast wrist is an overuse injury that primarily affects young gymnasts secondary to weight-bearing on the upper extremity necessary for the sport. The condition is common, seen in as many as 80% of elite gymnasts, but can occur in nonelite competitors as well.[33] The repetitive axial stress incurred by the wrist in extension causes inflammation at the physis, which can lead to microtrauma. This can result in slowed growth or complete cessation of the distal radius physis, which may lead to radial deformity or distal ulna overgrowth. Wrist pain and physeal tenderness on a competitive gymnast should prompt radiographs, which may show physeal widening or irregularity (**Fig. 5**).

Initial treatment consists of rest, NSAIDs, and immobilization for 3 to 6 months. Should a physeal bar develop, this may require resection, or ulnar epiphysiodesis with radial osteotomy as needed for large physeal closures.

Back

Low-back pain is estimated to occur in 10% to 15% of young athletes, although certain sports, such as football and gymnastics, show a higher prevalence than others.[34] Injuries to the back occur from either an acute traumatic injury or, more commonly, repetitive microtrauma.

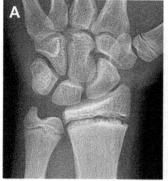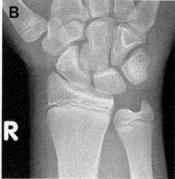

Fig. 5. Gymnast wrist. (*A*) Posteroanterior (PA) radiograph of the left wrist in a 14-year-old male weightlifter with 4 months of wrist pain reveals widening, sclerosis, and irregularity of the distal radial physis. (*B*) PA radiograph of the asymptomatic right wrist for comparison. (*From* Davis, KW. Imaging pediatric sports injuries: upper extremity. Radiologic clinics of North America 2010DOI:10.1016/j.rcl.2010.07.020; with permission.)

Spondylolysis

Repetitive hyperextension seen in such activities as gymnastics, weightlifting, and football linemen can place excessive stress on the posterior elements of the spine and create a stress fracture in the pars interarticularis with adjacent bone sclerosis. One study found that 47% of young athletes with back pain had spondylosis.[35] Athletes typically complain of insidious extension-based low-back pain, which may be associated with hamstring tightness.

Although most cases may be asymptomatic, activity-related low-back pain can occur and should be treated with physical therapy and activity restrictions. An exercise program, including core strengthening, hamstring stretches, and antilordotic exercises, for the lumbar spine should be prescribed. Bracing is controversial.[34,36–38]

LOWER-EXTREMITY INJURIES

Hip

Hip disorders in young athletes are increasingly recognized as a cause of dysfunction and disability in pediatric patients. Hip injuries account for approximately 5% to 9% of total athletic injuries in high school athletes.[39,40]

Femoroacetabular impingement and labral tears

Femoroacetabular impingement (FAI) is a painful and limiting hip pathologic condition that is thought to develop during the adolescent years in athletes who focus on early specialization. FAI describes the structural disorder of the hip that results in abnormal forces around the femoral neck and acetabulum that can lead to subsequent labral tearing and chondral damage. Evidence suggests that there is a distinct period during which the cam-type deformity occurs, because athletes with a history of participation in soccer, basketball, and ice hockey during periods of skeletal growth have an increased prevalence of cam lesion compared with their nonathletic counterparts.[41–43] It is thought that the repetitive stress seen in these sports may predispose individuals to develop a cam lesion because of the high shear forces applied to the femoral head.[44]

With increasing use of MRI and arthroscopic techniques, the diagnosis and treatment of FAI and hip labral tears have increased in the pediatric population. The simple presence of FAI deformity does not warrant surgical intervention in the setting of an asymptomatic athlete. Currently, there are no recommendations for prophylactic treatment of FAI. Even in symptomatic pediatric athletes found to have a labral tear, initial treatment is nonoperative with physical therapy, activity modification, and NSAIDs. Should young athletes fail conservative measures, arthroscopic treatment may be required for labral repair and/or chondroplasty.

Pelvic avulsion injuries

Often associated with sprinting activities and sports, avulsion fractures of the apophyses of the pelvis can occur given the high-impact forces on the tendon and muscles that attach to that bone and the relative weakness of the apophysis. It often is the result of an indirect trauma with forceful unbalanced contraction through the musculotendinous junction. Common locations include the anterior superior iliac spine, anterior inferior iliac spine (AIIS), and ischial tuberosity. Less commonly involved are the iliac crest, pubic rami, and pubic symphysis. Most pediatric athletes present with an acute or acute on chronic injury in which a pop or crack is felt about the hip. This may then be associated with immediate pain and weakness in the corresponding muscle.

Although most of these injuries do not require surgical treatment, the recovery can take several months. Early evaluation with activity restriction and protected weight-bearing as well as physical therapy can help return an athlete to their sport. Early weight-bearing and active stretching delay healing and increase the rate of associated complications, including nonunions.[45] Even though nonunions are generally well tolerated, they may lead to persistent pain, nerve entrapment, instability, weakness, and limitations in performing activities.[46–50]

Treatment is with initial rest and protected weight-bearing, followed by physical therapy and gradual return to activities. Controversy exists on which patients may benefit from early surgical intervention, but generally the grade of displacement, fracture site involved, and demands of the athlete should be taken into account.[46,51–57] Significantly displaced fragments greater than 1.5 to 2.0 cm may benefit from surgical intervention.[46,51,53,55,57] Extraarticular hip impingement may develop, particularly from displaced AIIS fragments, necessitating arthroscopic or open decompression.[58]

Knee

Knee pain is a common concern for which young athletes seek medical attention. Acute trauma to the knee, especially in contact or collision sports, is relatively less frequent than overuse injuries, which account for most knee pain in athletes.

Osteochondritis dissecans

OCD lesions are more commonly seen in the knee than any other location in the body. It is an idiopathic injury to the blood supply of the subchondral bone of the knee, which can lead to further damage of the overlying cartilage. One theory exists that the lesion is an overuse injury, given the most common location being in the weight-bearing medial femoral condyle. However, the lesion can be seen in sedentary individuals as well, suggesting a genetic component to its origin. The incidence of OCD of the knee in patients between 6 and 19 years of age was found to be 9.5 per 100,000 individuals overall.[59]

Patients may present with benign symptoms in the early stable period, but the pain may be associated with swelling, limping, and mechanical symptoms as the lesion advances. Radiographs are imperative in the evaluation of an OCD lesion because the physical examination may be noncontributory (**Fig. 6**). It is important to include sunrise and notch views in the radiographic series because lesions can otherwise be missed. For suspected OCD lesions, an MRI is imperative to assess chondral integrity, subchondral bone status, and OCD lesion stability.

Lesion size, location, stability, as well as age of the patient determine treatment measures as well as outcomes. Ultimately, the goal is to preserve the native osteochondral fragment when possible and prevent the development of early arthritis. Skeletally immature patients are more likely to heal without surgical intervention compared with adult counterparts. Healing may take 6 to 12 months with activity restrictions, bracing, and/or casting. However, should nonoperative measures fail or lesions present as unstable, surgical intervention is indicated. Many surgical techniques are available to stabilize OCD lesions of the knee, including drilling to stimulate a healing vascular response, fixation to stabilize the osteochondral fragment, or osteochondral resurfacing if the fragment is not salvageable.

Meniscus tears and discoid meniscus

Meniscal tears are another injury that are seen with greater frequency in children and adolescents as they increase their participation in sports. Acute meniscal tears are commonly seen in noncontact, twisting injuries while playing sports. They may present with mechanical symptoms, such as locking, catching, and giving way along with pain

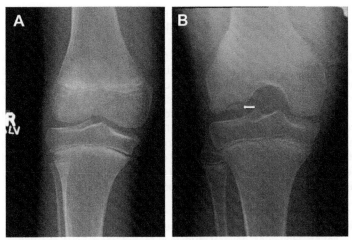

Fig. 6. A 14-year-old male patient with an OCD lesion on the lateral femoral condyle. (*A*) The abnormality of the articular surface is difficult to visualize on this view. The tunnel view (*B*) brings the posterior condyles into profile and clearly shows the lesion (*arrow*). (*From* Moktassi, Aiden & Popkin, Charles & M White, Lawrence & Murnaghan, Lucas. (2012). Imaging of Osteochondritis Dissecans. Orthopedic clinics of North America. 43. 201-11, v. 10.1016/j.ocl.2012.01.001.)

localized to the meniscus injured. In isolated meniscal tears, radiographs are negative, but advanced imaging with MRI will define the pathologic condition better.

The discoid meniscus is a variant that is often diagnosed in pediatric patients and may make the child more prone to tearing than a normal meniscus. It usually presents when symptomatic similar to other meniscal tears, but in younger discoid patients without tearing, presentation may be with audible snapping and locking. Incidence rates of discoid meniscus range from 0.4% to 17%, with higher reported rates in Asian countries.[60–62]

Treatment of meniscal tears is dictated by the size and morphology of the tear in the pediatric patient. Stable tears may be treated with nonoperative methods, whereas symptomatic and unstable meniscal tears require surgical intervention that includes arthroscopic evaluation of the knee and either debridement or repair of the meniscal tissue. Every attempt should be made to preserve as much meniscal tissue as possible through repair methods. Similar to adults, the red-red zone of the meniscus has a more robust blood supply with better healing rates. Surgical repair of more central zones of the meniscus should also be attempted in pediatric patients, because of the perceived healing potential in children and the importance of an intact meniscus for long-term knee health and avoidance of early arthritis development.

Treatment of symptomatic discoid menisci includes arthroscopic saucerization of the meniscus, with the goal of leaving a stable rim of approximately 6 to 8 mm of tissue. Saucerization involves the removal of the central abnormal and torn tissue. The remaining tissue is inspected for tearing and peripheral instability and repaired accordingly.

Tibial spine fracture
A tibial eminence fracture occurs in skeletally immature athletes who incur a twisting or hyperextension injury to the knee, similar to the mechanism that causes an anterior cruciate ligament (ACL) injury. Tibial eminence fractures are relatively uncommon

with an annual incidence estimated to be 3 per 100,000 children and adolescents.[63] Similar to an ACL injury, patients present with acute onset of knee pain and swelling with difficulty ambulating.

Radiographs often are able to identify and classify the fracture, but advanced imaging can help identify concurrent injuries and blocks to reduction. Recent studies have shown the rate of concomitant pathologic condition to be as high as 30%.[63,64]

The modified Myers and McKeever classification is often used to describe tibial spine fractures and helps in treatment decisions. A minimally displaced type I fracture can be treated with long leg casting. Type II fractures undergo an attempted closed reduction and casting, if reduction is adequate. Type II fractures that cannot be reduced by closed methods and completely displaced type III fractures require surgical intervention to reduce the displaced tibial spine fracture and stabilize the fragment. Various fixation methods have been described using screws and sutures.

Anterior cruciate ligament tears

Historically, it was thought that midsubstance ruptures of the ACL were rare in the pediatric population. However, several studies in recent years have showed a sharp increase in ACL injury and subsequent ACL reconstruction surgery in the pediatric and adolescent population.[65,66] ACL injuries often present as a noncontact twisting injury in a young athlete who recounts a popping sensation resulting in difficulty bearing weight and a large hemarthrosis. Radiographs are often negative, but confirmation and concomitant injuries can be evaluated with MRI (**Fig. 7**).

Partial tears of the ACL may occur in the pediatric patients, with data suggesting that nonoperative treatment may be successful in a certain subset of patients.[67,68] Those who required surgery for symptomatic ACL instability tended to have greater than 50% of the ACL fibers ruptured, to have the posterolateral bundle ruptured, to be older than 14 years of age, and to have a positive provocative testing on examination.

Given the high activity level of pediatric and adolescent athletes, surgical intervention to reconstruct the ACL is often indicated because historically nonsurgical measures with activity modification resulted in worse clinical outcomes in this patient population.[69] Delaying reconstruction as much as 3 months can lead to meniscal and chondral damage in pediatric patients.[70–73] The ACL reconstruction technique should be tailored to the level of skeletal and developmental maturity of the patient. Physeal-sparing techniques, in which no tunnels are drilled across the physis, have been developed for patients with significant growth remaining. Techniques include a

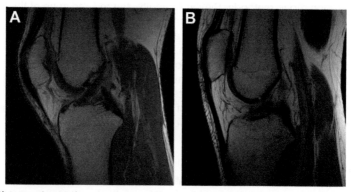

Fig. 7. (*A*) Normal MRI showing intact ACL. Arrow points to intact ACL. (*B*) MRI showing torn ACL. Arrow points to midsubstance rupture of ACL.

combined intraarticular and extraarticular technique in which the iliotibial band is used to re-create the torn ACL(**Fig. 8**) as well as an all-epiphyseal reconstruction technique in which tunnels are drilled through the epiphysis only (**Fig. 9**).[74–76] In older adolescents with a modest amount of growth remaining, various transphyseal techniques (**Fig. 10**) are used, including hybrid techniques in which a physeal-sparing technique is used on the femoral side, which is more vulnerable to growth disturbance, and a transphyseal technique on the tibial side. Physeal-respecting techniques have also been advocated to include the use of soft tissue grafts and metaphyseal fixation, avoidance of dissection about the perichondrial ring of LaCroix, optimization of tunnel size, and use of more vertical tunnels to minimize damage to the physis.

Given the frequency of ACL injuries in young athletes and the devastating consequences, various ACL injury prevention programs have been developed and implemented. A recently published study found that the introduction of neuromuscular prevention programs universally would be more cost-effective than simply screening for and training only at-risk athletes.[77]

Patellar instability

Patellar instability refers to the spectrum of injury seen at the patellofemoral joint that results in subluxation or dislocation of the patella out of the trochlear groove. An acute traumatic patellar dislocation is one of the most common acute knee disorders in adolescent athletes.[78]

Although plain radiographs should be obtained in suspected patellar instability cases, MRI helps to elucidate the anatomy of the knee and assess for concomitant injury. Important radiographic measures include sulcus angle, patellar tilt, and patellar height. MRI will help define medial patellofemoral ligament (MPFL) injury,

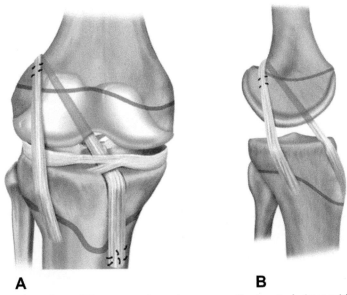

A   **B**

Fig. 8. Physeal-sparing ACL reconstruction using an over-the-top technique with iliotibial band. (*A*) Anterior view and (*B*) lateral view. (*From* Ardern CL, Ekås GR, Grindem H, et al 2018 International Olympic Committee consensus statement on prevention, diagnosis and management of paediatric anterior cruciate ligament (ACL) injuries British Journal of Sports Medicine 2018;52:422-438.)

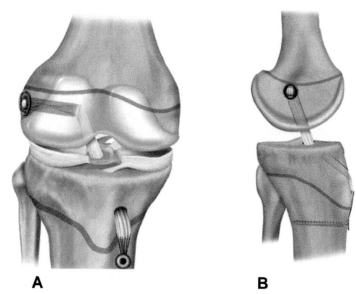

A   **B**

Fig. 9. Physeal-sparing ACL reconstruction using an all-epiphyseal technique. (*A*) Anterior view and (*B*) lateral view. (*From* Ardern CL, Ekås GR, Grindem H, et al 2018 International Olympic Committee consensus statement on prevention, diagnosis and management of paediatric anterior cruciate ligament (ACL) injuries British Journal of Sports Medicine 2018;52:422-438.)

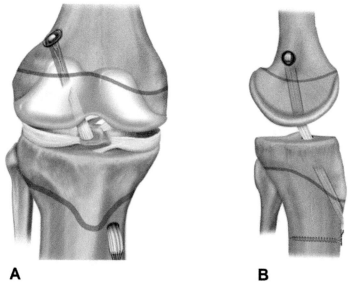

A   **B**

Fig. 10. Transphyseal ACL reconstruction. (*A*) Anterior view and (*B*) lateral view. (*From* Ardern CL, Ekås GR, Grindem H, et al 2018 International Olympic Committee consensus statement on prevention, diagnosis and management of paediatric anterior cruciate ligament (ACL) injuries British Journal of Sports Medicine 2018;52:422-438.)

osteochondral damage, and lower-extremity rotational alignment as defined by the tibial tubercle-trochlear groove distance.

There is no preferred method of treatment of patellar instability because the literature is lacking high-level data. Nonsurgical measures are often used, especially for first-time patellar dislocators and those with instability, but no frank dislocation. Therapy focuses on strengthening of the vastus medialis obliquus as well as the gluteal muscles. Bracing and taping of the patella may also provide assistance in rehabilitation. Surgical management is usually reserved for recurrent patellar dislocations with more than 100 procedures having been described to surgically correct and improve patellar stability. Similar to adults, surgical treatment is guided by the underlying pathoanatomy, condition of cartilage, and associated injuries. Compared with adult counterparts, surgery is dictated by the presence of growth plates in pediatric and adolescent patients. Possible procedures include lateral release, primary MPFL repair and medial reefing, tibial tubercle osteotomy, Roux-Goldthwait technique, MPFL reconstruction (**Fig. 11**), trochleoplasty, and guided growth.

Foot and Ankle

Ankle injuries are a leading cause of missed athletic participation in pediatric and adolescent athletes. They account for about 30% of visits to sports medicine clinics in the pediatric population.[79]

Ankle sprains
One of the most common injuries seen in young athletes is an ankle sprain, in which the ligamentous structures stabilizing the ankle joint are disrupted to varying degrees.

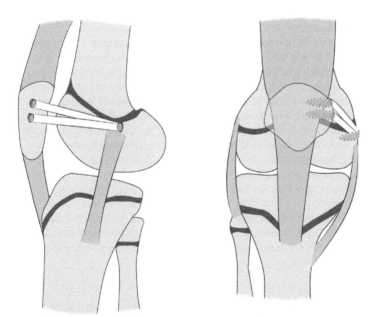

Fig. 11. Modified MPFL reconstruction technique. The 2 ends of the graft are docked in the superior-medial patella using partial socket tunnels, resulting in placement of the femoral attachment in a socket tunnel distal to the physis. (*From* Green, DW. Medial Patellofemoral Ligament Reconstruction Using Hamstring Autograft in Children and Adolescents. Arthroscopy Techniques, Vol 2, No 2 (May), 2013: pp e151-e154; with permission.)

It represents the most common reason for missed athletic participation in adolescent athletes and may result in long-term dysfunction if not treated appropriately. Most ankle sprains are low ankle sprains that are typically the result of an inversion injury that damages the lateral ligamentous structures of the ankle below the level of the distal tibiofibular syndesmosis. They typically present with lateral ankle swelling and pain as well as pain with weight-bearing.

High ankle sprains, which represent less than 10% of all ankle sprains, are an injury to the distal tibiofibular syndesmosis that results from a rotational injury. They are frequently unable to bear weight on the injured limb, a factor that distinguishes them from low ankle sprains.

The mainstay of treatment is nonoperative with initial rest, ice, compression, and elevation followed by rehabilitation and return to activities. Physical therapy is meant to focus on peroneal strengthening and proprioceptive training. Bracing is also used to prevent recurrent ligament sprains. Surgical measures are recommended when patients demonstrate persistent pain and instability despite aggressive nonsurgical treatment. Surgery may also be indicated in syndesmotic injuries that failed nonsurgical measures, have evidence of instability on stress radiographs, or are associated with a fracture.

In the skeletally immature patient, ankle sprain equivalents may occur given the weaker physes. Classically, the distal fibular physeal fracture has been considered the equivalent injury to the low ankle sprain, but recently evidence has shown that anterior talofibular ligament avulsion fractures are also common.[80–82] Ligamentous injuries of the ankle do occur in patients who are skeletally immature, despite the presence of open physes. Thus, the accurate diagnosis of ankle injuries can be challenging in the pediatric population.

Os trigonum syndrome

A separate ossification center is often seen along the posterior aspect of the talus that can form a large lateral talar process, known as a Stieda process, or remain unfused, forming an os trigonum. The os trigonum can become symptomatic in young athletes who actively plantar flex their ankle, which subsequently compresses the posterior talus between the posterior tibia and calcaneus. Repetitive impingement of the soft tissues in the interval can also result in capsulitis. This condition presents as posterolateral ankle pain and is seen in ballet dancers when they go into pointe, gymnastics, ice skaters, or soccer players. Lateral radiographs are helpful to initially evaluate the os trigonum or Stieda process. An MRI is useful to determine if the presence of these anatomic anomalies are the source of pain for the patient through abnormal bone edema. MRIs also are able to evaluate associated abnormalities within the flexor hal-luces longus tendon.

Initial treatment is through nonoperative measures, such as therapeutic injection, rest, NSAIDs, activity modification to avoid plantar flexion, and physical therapy. In recalcitrant cases in the completive athlete, resection of the os trigonum or Stieda process may be executed.

Calcaneal apophysitis

Sever's disease, or calcaneal apophysitis, refers osteochondrosis of the calcaneus from the repeated traction of the Achilles tendon at the secondary ossification center of the calcaneus (**Fig. 12**). It is the most common cause of heel pain in pediatric and adolescent athletes between the ages of 9 and 11 years of age. This is often seen in young athletes who participate in sports that require running and jumping, secondary to overuse, poor fitting shoes, and contractures of the Achilles tendon. Pain is often felt

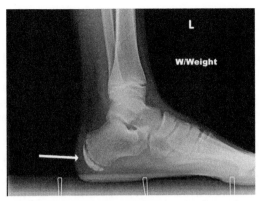

Fig. 12. Lateral radiograph of pediatric foot with (*arrow*) calcaneal apophysis.

with running and walking, with pain elicited on physical examination by palpation of the heel.

The mainstay of treatment is rest, NSAIDs, icing, plantar orthotic devices to provide cushioning, and physical therapy that focuses on stretching of the plantar flexors and Achilles tendon.

Stress fractures

Repetitive activities that outpace the capacity of bone to repair itself can lead to bony injury. Stress injury represents a spectrum of bone damage from stress reaction through overt fracture. In skeletally immature athletes, the rapid increase in muscle strength, presence of narrower bones with thinner cortices, low mineral density, and hormonal factors increase the susceptibility to stress injury.[83] In the foot and ankle, common locations for fractures are in the metatarsal or tarsal bones. Metatarsal stress fractures are commonly seen in runners, ballet dancers, and gymnasts. Conventional radiographs are relatively insensitive in the acute setting, and advanced imaging with an MRI is indicated in athletes with a high suspicion of stress injury to the foot or ankle.

SUMMARY

Pediatric and adolescent athletes may present with a unique set of injuries in sports and athletics that separate them from their adult counterparts. A thorough history and physical examination, along with corroborating imaging, can help define patho-logic condition and lead to an accurate diagnosis and appropriate treatment.

REFERENCES

1. Caine D, Caine C, Maffulli N. Incidence and distribution of pediatric sport-related injuries. Clin J Sport Med 2006;16(6):500–13.
2. Lord J, Winell JJ. Overuse injuries in pediatric athletes. Curr Opin Pediatr 2004; 16(1):47–50.
3. Bright RW, Burstein AH, Elmore SM. Epiphyseal-plate cartilage. A biomechanical and histological analysis of failure modes. J Bone Joint Surg Am 1974;56(4): 688–703.
4. Caine D, Maffulli N, Caine C. Epidemiology of injury in child and adolescent sports: injury rates, risk factors, and prevention. Clin Sports Med 2008;27(1): 19–50, vii.

5. Micheli LJ. Overuse injuries in children's sports: the growth factor. Orthop Clin North Am 1983;14(2):337–60.

6. Lyman S, Fleisig GS, Waterbor JW, et al. Longitudinal study of elbow and shoulder pain in youth baseball pitchers. Med Sci Sports Exerc 2001;33(11):1803–10.

7. Sabick MB, Kim YK, Torry MR, et al. Biomechanics of the shoulder in youth baseball pitchers: implications for the development of proximal humeral epiphysiolysis and humeral retrotorsion. Am J Sports Med 2005;33(11):1716–22.

8. Kurokawa D, Yamamoto N, Ishikawa H, et al. Differences in humeral retroversion in dominant and nondominant sides of young baseball players. J Shoulder Elbow Surg 2017;26(6):1083–7.

9. Drakos MC, Rudzki JR, Allen AA, et al. nternal impingement of the shoulder in the overhead athlete. J Bone Joint Surg Am 2009;91(11):2719–28.

10. Edmonds EW, Roocroft JH, Parikh SN. Spectrum of operative childhood intra-articular shoulder pathology. J Child Orthop 2014;8(4):337–40.

11. Eisner EA, Roocroft JH, Edmonds EW. Underestimation of labral pathology in adolescents with anterior shoulder instability. J Pediatr Orthop 2012;32(1):42–7.

12. Kibler WB, Dome D. Internal impingement: concurrent superior labral and rotator cuff injuries. Sports Med Arthrosc Rev 2012;20(1):30–3.

13. Ireland ML, Andrews JR. Shoulder and elbow injuries in the young athlete. Clin Sports Med 1988;7(3):473–94.

14. Ryu RK, Fan RS. Adolescent and pediatric sports injuries. Pediatr Clin North Am 1998;45(6):1601–35.

15. Kibler WB. Rehabilitation of rotator cuff tendinopathy. Clin Sports Med 2003;22(4):837–47.

16. Kocher MS, Waters PM, Micheli LJ. Upper extremity injuries in the paediatric athlete. Sports Med 2000;30(2):117–35.

17. Fleisig GS, Andrews JR. Prevention of elbow injuries in youth baseball pitchers. Sports Health 2012;4(5):419–24.

18. Popchak A, Burnett T, Weber N, et al. Factors related to injury in youth and adolescent baseball pitching, with an eye toward prevention. Am J Phys Med Rehabil 2015;94(5):395–409.

19. Yang J, Mann BJ, Guettler JH, et al. Risk-prone pitching activities and injuries in youth baseball: findings from a national sample. Am J Sports Med 2014;42(6):1456–63.

20. Salvo JP, Rizio L, Zvijac JE, et al. Avulsion fracture of the ulnar sublime tubercle in overhead throwing athletes. Am J Sports Med 2002;30(3):426–31.

21. Petty DH, Andrews JR, Fleisig GS, et al. Ulnar collateral ligament reconstruction in high school baseball players: clinical results and injury risk factors. Am J Sports Med 2004;32(5):1158–64.

22. Baumgarten TE, Andrews JR, Satterwhite YE. The arthroscopic classification and treatment of osteochondritis dissecans of the capitellum. Am J Sports Med 1998;26(4):520–3.

23. Peterson RK, Savoie FH, Field LD. Osteochondritis dissecans of the elbow. Instr Course Lect 1999;48:393–8.

24. Harada M, Ogino T, Takahara M, et al. Fragment fixation with a bone graft and dynamic staples for osteochondritis dissecans of the humeral capitellum. J Shoulder Elbow Surg 2002;11(4):368–72.

25. Takeda H, Waterai K, Matsushita T, et al. A surgical treatment for unstable osteochondritis dissecans lesions of the humeral capitellum in adolescent baseball players. Am J Sports Med 2002;30(5):713–7.

26. Furushima K, Itoh Y, Iwabu S, et al. Classification of olecranon stress fractures in baseball players. Am J Sports Med 2014;42(6):1343–51.

27. Landin LA. Fracture patterns in children. Analysis of 8,682 fractures with special reference to incidence, etiology and secular changes in a Swedish urban population 1950-1979. Acta Orthop Scand Suppl 1983;202:1–109.

28. Leininger RE, Knox CL, Comstock RD. Epidemiology of 1.6 million pediatric soccer-related injuries presenting to US emergency departments from 1990 to 2003. Am J Sports Med 2007;35(2):288–93.

29. Taylor BL, Attia MW. Sports-related injuries in children. Acad Emerg Med 2000; 7(12):1376–82.

30. Vadivelu R, Dias JJ, Burke FD, et al. Hand injuries in children: a prospective study. J Pediatr Orthop 2006;26(1):29–35.

31. Pannu GS, Herman M. Distal radius-ulna fractures in children. Orthop Clin North Am 2015;46(2):235–48.

32. Farr JN, Khosla S. Skeletal changes through the lifespan–from growth to senescence. Nat Rev Endocrinol 2015;11(9):513–21.

33. Soprano JV. Musculoskeletal injuries in the pediatric and adolescent athlete. Curr Sports Med Rep 2005;4(6):329–34.

34. d'Hemecourt PA, Gerbino PG, Micheli LJ. Back injuries in the young athlete. Clin Sports Med 2000;19(4):663–79.

35. Gregory PL, Batt ME, Kerslake RW, et al. Single photon emission computerized tomography and reverse gantry computerized tomography findings in patients with back pain investigated for spondylolysis. Clin J Sport Med 2005;15(2):79–86.

36. d'Hemecourt PA, Zurakowski D, Kriemler S, et al. Spondylolysis: returning the athlete to sports participation with brace treatment. Orthopedics 2002;25(6): 653–7.

37. Kraft DE. Low back pain in the adolescent athlete. Pediatr Clin North Am 2002; 49(3):643–53.

38. Standaert CJ, Herring SA. Spondylolysis: a critical review. Br J Sports Med 2000; 34(6):415–22.

39. DeLee JC, Farney WC. Incidence of injury in Texas high school football. Am J Sports Med 1992;20(5):575–80.

40. Gomez E, DeLee JC, Farney WC. Incidence of injury in Texas girls' high school basketball. Am J Sports Med 1996;24(5):684–7.

41. Agricola R, Heijboer MP, Ginai AZ, et al. A cam deformity is gradually acquired during skeletal maturation in adolescent and young male soccer players: a prospective study with minimum 2-year follow-up. Am J Sports Med 2014;42(4): 798–806.

42. Siebenrock KA, Ferner F, Noble PC, et al. The cam-type deformity of the proximal femur arises in childhood in response to vigorous sporting activity. Clin Orthop Relat Res 2011;469(11):3229–40.

43. Siebenrock KA, Kaschka I, Frauchiger L, et al. Prevalence of cam-type deformity and hip pain in elite ice hockey players before and after the end of growth. Am J Sports Med 2013;41(10):2308–13.

44. Morris WZ, Li RT, Liu RW, et al. Origin of cam morphology in femoroacetabular impingement. Am J Sports Med 2018;46(2):478–86.

45. Longo UG, Ciuffreda M, Locher J, et al. Apophyseal injuries in children's and youth sports. Br Med Bull 2016;120(1):139–59.

46. Schiller J, DeFroda S, Blood T. Lower extremity avulsion fractures in the pediatric and adolescent athlete. J Am Acad Orthop Surg 2017;5(4):251–9.

47. Moeller JL. Pelvic and hip apophyseal avulsion injuries in young athletes. Curr Sports Med Rep 2003;2(2):110–5.
48. Schoensee SK, Nilsson KJ. A novel approach to treatment for chronic avulsion fracture of the ischial tuberosity in three adolescent athletes: a case series. Int J Sports Phys Ther 2014;9(7):974–90.
49. Gidwani S, Jagiello J, Bircher M. Avulsion fracture of the ischial tuberosity in adolescents–an easily missed diagnosis. BMJ 2004;329(7457):99–100.
50. Hayashi S, Nishiyama T, Fujishiro T, et al. Avulsion-fracture of the anterior superior iliac spine with meralgia paresthetica: a case report. J Orthop Surg (Hong Kong) 2011;19(3):384–5.
51. Ali E, Khanduja V. Adolescent avulsion injuries of the pelvis: a case study and review of the literature. Orthop Nurs 2015;34(1):21–6 [quiz: 27–8].
52. Eberbach H, Hohloch L, Feucht MJ, et al. Operative versus conservative treatment of apophyseal avulsion fractures of the pelvis in the adolescents: a systematical review with meta-analysis of clinical outcome and return to sports. BMC Musculoskelet Disord 2017;18(1):162.
53. Ferlic PW, Sadoghi P, Singer G, et al. Treatment for ischial tuberosity avulsion fractures in adolescent athletes. Knee Surg Sports Traumatol Arthrosc 2014; 22(4):893–7.
54. Kautzner J, Trc T, Havlas V. Comparison of conservative against surgical treatment of anterior-superior iliac spine avulsion fractures in children and adolescents. Int Orthop 2014;38(7):1495–8.
55. Nguyen JC, Sheehan SE, Davis KW, et al. Sports and the growing musculoskeletal system: sports imaging series. Radiology 2017;284(1):25–42.
56. Pogliacomi F, Calderazzi F, Paterlini M, et al. Surgical treatment of anterior iliac spines fractures: our experience. Acta Biomed 2014;85(Suppl 2):52–8.
57. Singer G, Eberl R, Wegmann H, et al. Diagnosis and treatment of apophyseal injuries of the pelvis in adolescents. Semin Musculoskelet Radiol 2014;18(5): 498–504.
58. Novais EN, Riederer MF, Provance AJ. Anterior inferior iliac spine deformity as a cause for extra-articular hip impingement in young athletes after an avulsion fracture: a case report. Sports Health 2018;10(3):272–6.
59. Kessler JI, Nikizad H, Shea KG, et al. The demographics and epidemiology of osteochondritis dissecans of the knee in children and adolescents. Am J Sports Med 2014;42(2):320–6.
60. Francavilla ML, Restrepo R, Zamora KW, et al. Meniscal pathology in children: differences and similarities with the adult meniscus. Pediatr Radiol 2014;44(8): 910–25.
61. Kushare I, Klingele K, Samora W. Discoid meniscus: diagnosis and management. Orthop Clin North Am 2015;46(4):533–40.
62. McKay S, Checn C, Rosenfeld S. Orthopedic perspective on selected pediatric and adolescent knee conditions. Pediatr Radiol 2013;43(Suppl 1):S99–106.
63. Johnson AC, Wyat J,D, Treme G, et al. Incidence of associated knee injury in pediatric tibial eminence fractures. J Knee Surg 2014;27(3):215–9.
64. Anderson CN, Anderson AF. Tibial eminence fractures. Clin Sports Med 2011; 30(4):727–42.
65. Dodwell ER, Lamont LE, Green DW, et al. 20 years of pediatric anterior cruciate ligament reconstruction in New York State. Am J Sports Med 2014;42(3):675–80.
66. Werner BC, Yang S, Looney AM, et al. Trends in pediatric and adolescent anterior cruciate ligament injury and reconstruction. J Pediatr Orthop 2016;36(5):447–52.

67. Busch MT, Fernandez MD, Aarons C. Partial tears of the anterior cruciate ligament in children and adolescents. Clin Sports Med 2011;30(4):743–50.
68. Kocher MS, Micheli LJ, Zurakowski D, et al. Partial tears of the anterior cruciate ligament in children and adolescents. Am J Sports Med 2002;30(5):697–703.
69. Ramski DE, Kanj WW, Franklin CC, et al. Anterior cruciate ligament tears in children and adolescents: a meta-analysis of nonoperative versus operative treatment. Am J Sports Med 2014;42(11):2769–76.
70. Anderson AF, Anderson CN. Correlation of meniscal and articular cartilage injuries in children and adolescents with timing of anterior cruciate ligament reconstruction. Am J Sports Med 2015;43(2):275–81.
71. Dumont GD, Hogue GD, Padalecki JR, et al. Meniscal and chondral injuries associated with pediatric anterior cruciate ligament tears: relationship of treatment time and patient-specific factors. Am J Sports Med 2012;40(9):2128–33.
72. Lawrence JT, Argawal N, Ganley TJ. Degeneration of the knee joint in skeletally immature patients with a diagnosis of an anterior cruciate ligament tear: is there harm in delay of treatment? Am J Sports Med 2011;39(12):2582–7.
73. ewman JT, Carry PM, Terhune EB, et al. Factors predictive of concomitant injuries among children and adolescents undergoing anterior cruciate ligament surgery. Am J Sports Med 2015;43(2):282–8.
74. Anderson AF. Transepiphyseal replacement of the anterior cruciate ligament using quadruple hamstring grafts in skeletally immature patients. J Bone Joint Surg Am 2004;86-A:201–9. Suppl 1(Pt 2).
75. Kocher MS, Garg S, Micheli LJ. Physeal sparing reconstruction of the anterior cruciate ligament in skeletally immature prepubescent children and adolescents. J Bone Joint Surg Am 2005;87(11):2371–9.
76. Kocher MS, Garg S, Micheli LJ. Physeal sparing reconstruction of the anterior cruciate ligament in skeletally immature prepubescent children and adolescents. Surgical technique. J Bone Joint Surg Am 2006;88(Suppl 1 Pt 2):283–93.
77. Swart E, Redler L, Fabricant PD, et al. Prevention and screening programs for anterior cruciate ligament injuries in young athletes: a cost-effectiveness analysis. J Bone Joint Surg Am 2014;96(9):705–11.
78. Hennrikus W, Pylawka T. Patellofemoral instability in skeletally immature athletes. J Bone Joint Surg Am 2013;95(2):176–83.
79. Erickson JB, Samora WP, Klingele KE. Ankle injuries in the pediatric athlete. Sports Med Arthrosc Rev 2016;24(4):170–7.
80. Farley FA, Kuhns L, Jacobson JA, et al. Ultrasound examination of ankle injuries in children. J Pediatr Orthop 2001;21(5):604–7.
81. Kwak YH, Lim JY, Oh MK, et al. Radiographic diagnosis of occult distal fibular avulsion fracture in children with acute lateral ankle sprain. J Pediatr Orthop 2015;35(4):352–7.
82. Sankar WN, Chen J, Kay RM, et al. Incidence of occult fracture in children with acute ankle injuries. J Pediatr Orthop 2008;28(5):500–1.
83. Jones BH, Harris JM, Vinh TN, et al. Exercise-induced stress fractures and stress reactions of bone: epidemiology, etiology, and classification. Exerc Sport Sci Rev 1989;17:379–422.

Musculoskeletal Tumors

Amit Singla, MD*, David S. Geller, MD

KEYWORDS

- Soft tissue tumors • Bone tumors • Musculoskeletal tumors • Sarcoma • Biopsy
- Surgical margin • Translation research • Precision medicine

KEY POINTS

- Sarcoma treatment requires careful adherence to the well-described tenets of tumor management.
- Biopsy is a critical step in establishing the diagnosis, and its proper planning and execution are vital.
- Surgery is required for most bone and soft-tissue sarcomas treatment of soft tissue and bone sarcoma.
- Recent advances have helped to identify and classify tumors according to their molecular profile.
- Precision medicine describes treatment guided by a given tumor's molecular profile.

INTRODUCTION

Pediatric musculoskeletal tumors can arise in both bone and soft tissues. The overwhelming majority of these tumors are benign; however, rarely, malignant neoplasms do occur. These are collectively termed sarcomas, indicating mesenchymal origin. Sarcoma treatment requires careful adherence to the well-described tenets of tumor management. Unless the treating clinician and their institution are well versed in musculoskeletal tumor care and can safely and appropriately perform *both* the biopsy and the definitive surgery, referral to such a center is strongly recommended.

Benign bone tumors constitute a heterogenous mix of lesions, the most common of which include osteochondroma, nonossifying fibroma, Langerhans cell histiocytosis, unicameral or simple bone cyst (UBC), aneurysmal bone cyst (ABC), and osteoid osteoma. Benign bone tumors are most frequent in ages 5 to 25, and many of them are benign chondrogenic lesions[1] found incidentally following minor trauma. These, often times, do not require treatment. Alternatively, some lesions are symptomatic and may require surgical intervention. Some lesions require intermittent evaluation and imaging, recognizing that they may evolve or enlarge. For self-limited and asymptomatic

Department of Orthopaedic Surgery, Montefiore Medical Center, 3400 Bainbridge Avenue, 6th Floor, Bronx, NY 10467, USA
* Corresponding author. 3400 Bainbridge Avenue, Bronx NY 10467.
E-mail address: dgeller@montefiore.org

Pediatr Clin N Am 67 (2020) 227–245
https://doi.org/10.1016/j.pcl.2019.09.014
0031-3955/20/© 2019 Elsevier Inc. All rights reserved.

lesions, the clinician's role is largely one of observation and reassurance. In the setting of more aggressive or symptomatic tumors, goals of treatment include local disease control, restoration of skeletal integrity, and returning patients to their normal activities.

Malignant bone tumors constitute 6% of all childhood cancer in patients less than the age of 20 years. They are the seventh most common type of tumors in children,[2] with an incidence of approximately 650 to 700 cases. About two-thirds of these are osteosarcomas, with the remainder largely belonging to the Ewing sarcoma family of tumors. These generally occur during adolescence and young adulthood, roughly coinciding with skeletal growth. Male adolescents have a slightly higher incidence of bone sarcomas than do female adolescents. Ewing sarcoma has a 6-fold higher incidence in white children as compared with black children.[3,4] Patients with malignant bone tumors nearly always present with complains of pain and swelling. In the absence of extensive and aggressive multimodal treatment, these cancers are universally fatal. Following histologic diagnosis, the goals of surgical treatment are to completely excise the tumor and, whenever feasible, to reconstruct the defect. Limb-salvage surgery is generally preferred and usually achievable. Ablative surgery, such as amputations or disarticulations, are sometimes indicated in cases of advanced disease or in cases where alternative methods have failed. Although systemic therapy is essential, surgery remains a cornerstone of treatment and systemic therapy alone is currently inadequate to attain curative outcomes.

More than 500,000 benign soft tissue tumors are diagnosed in the United States annually.[5] Benign soft tissue tumors are a heterogenous group of lesions, the most common of which include lipomas, hemangiomas, peripheral nerve sheath tumors, and giant cell tumors of tendon sheath. Vascular lesions, generally considered hamartomas, represent the most common soft tissue masses in children.[6] Patients will often present with a bump or fullness, some of which can be symptomatic, whereas others may be entirely painless. Advanced imaging or even biopsy is often required for diagnosis; however, in broad terms, masses less than 4 cm are unlikely to be malignant.[7] Superficial lesions are also more likely to be benign and are often identified because they are either visible, palpable, or both. Goals of care for benign soft tissue lesions vary. Although simple reassurance is oftentimes appropriate, some patients prefer histologic confirmation and seek a biopsy or resection. In other cases, surgery is designed to realize pain relief, improve range of motion and function, curtail future extension or growth, and return patients to their normal activity levels.

Soft tissue sarcomas constitute 7% of all the childhood cancers in patients under the age the age of 20. They are collectively the sixth most common type of tumor in children.[2] Of approximately 11,000 children who will be diagnosed with cancer annually within the United states, 850 to 900 will develop a soft tissue sarcoma, the most common being rhabdomyosarcoma. Black and male children have a slightly higher incidence of soft tissue sarcoma as compared with white and female children.[3,4] Soft tissue sarcomas are a very heterogeneous group of malignant neoplasms, which despite being grouped together, have tremendous genetic disparities. They have historically been classified in accordance with their presumed tissue of origin. This, however, is a gross oversimplification, and increasingly, these tumors are being classified according to their genomic profile. Doing so is markedly more accurate and offers the prospect of improving prognostication, identifying relevant targets and treatments, and it is hoped, improving overall survival.

Despite the rarity of sarcomas, these tumors portend tremendous implications for both patients and their families. Realizing optimal outcomes depends on both proper timely diagnostic workup and a collaborative multidisciplinary treatment approach within an institution that has adequate clinical experience and available relevant resources. Broadly speaking, although recent advances in molecular biology have led to the development of prognostic markers and the identification of potential therapeutic targets, the most successful means of attaining a cure is usually through complete and total surgical resection of a localized tumor.

FUNDAMENTAL PRINCIPLES
Presentation

A complete medical history is an essential first step. The patient's age, presenting symptoms, and timecourse often provide important and relevant information. Although, generally, these tumors present in reproducible and characteristic ways, exceptions to the rule exist. It is important to be critical, cautious, and thorough, particularly during an initial evaluation. If something appears atypical, further investigation is advisable.

Benign bone tumors are often diagnosed incidentally. When patients are symptomatic, pain is the most common complaint. Its location, intensity, duration, and aggravating or relieving factors provide important insight. Pain that is mild, only activity-related, and non-progressive is usually indicative of a benign process. Pain can be due to structural bone weakness caused by tumor growth. In some instances, extensive growth or unrelated trauma can result in a pathologic fracture. This frequently occurs in the setting of a UBC but can also be secondary to another neoplasm, such as a non-ossifying fibroma. Pain can also be caused by mechanical irritation, such as in the case of exophytic lesions, most commonly osteochondromas (**Fig. 1**). In such instances, symptoms may be due to inflammation of overlying soft tissues or the development of a painful bursa. Less commonly, the pedunculated stalk of an osteochondroma can fracture. Nonprogressive nocturnal pain reliably relieved with aspirin or nonsteroidal anti-inflammatory drugs is typical of an osteoid osteoma, owing to its high local concentration of prostaglandins. In some instances, the presenting complaint may be swelling or loss of range of motion, rather than pain. For example, ABC can incite extensive bone remodeling,

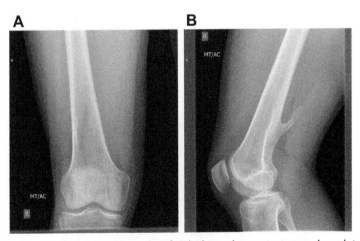

Fig. 1. AP (*A*) and lateral (*B*) radiographs of right knee demonstrate a pedunculated osteochondroma arising from the posterolateral metaphyseal region of the femur. The medullary canal of the femur is continuous with medullary canal of the osteochondroma.

resulting in "expansion" of the involved bone's width. This may have the effect of blocking or limiting motion across the adjacent joint.

Malignant bone tumors, conversely, often present with pain that is deep, achy, and unrelenting in nature. Patients often experience night pain or pain at rest. Both Ewing sarcoma and osteosarcoma generally develop an associated soft tissue mass (**Fig. 2**), prompting patients to report firmness, a bump, or warmth in the involved area. Pathologic fracture, although uncommon, can be a presenting feature in a minority of sarcomas (**Fig. 3**).

Soft tissue tumors usually present as a soft tissue fullness or mass. The presence of mass can vary from a few weeks to years, and its growth can be variable. Although the long-term presence can be generally reassuring, some soft tissue sarcomas remain static in size for years, providing a false sense of benignity. Unlike many bone tumors, pain is often minimal or absent. This can be particularly misleading in the case of malignant tumors. In the setting of peripheral nerve sheath tumors, pain can take on a radicular quality, termed a "Tinel's sign," which describes a sharp electrical discomfort following palpation. Late soft tissue sarcoma findings can include pain, skin discoloration, ulceration, bleeding, and neurologic changes. Constitutional symptoms like fever and weight loss are very infrequent and generally indicate very advanced disease and poor prognosis. Lymph node involvement is rare in sarcomas and is generally found in the setting of particular histologies, such as epithelioid sarcoma, synovial sarcoma, or rhabdomyosarcoma.

Physical Assessment

A complete physical examination should be performed, including generalized evaluation of head and neck, back and abdomen, and all extremities with the patient unclothed in a hospital gown. This can reveal potentially relevant findings. For example, patients with multiple hereditary osteochondroma can present with short stature and curved and shortened forearms. Proptosis and signs of refractory otitis media can suggest a diagnosis of Langerhans cell histiocytosis. Multiple café-au-lait spots in the setting of a soft tissue mass may suggest neurofibromatosis.

Focal inspection can help gauge tumor size, although admittedly deeply seated lesions are difficult to entirely appreciate. Palpation can, however, reveal overlying

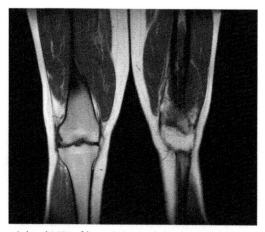

Fig. 2. Coronal T1-weighted MRI of knee joint and the distal femur demonstrate a marrow-replacing lesion in the left distal femur with associated soft-tissue extension.

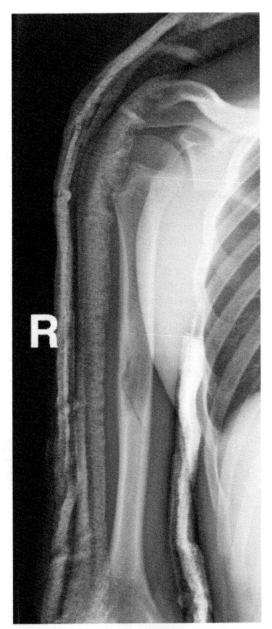

Fig. 3. AP radiograph of the right humerus in a plaster splint, demonstrate a non-displaced spiral pathological fracture through a diaphyseal lytic lesion. The lesion exhibits a permeative aggressive pattern of bone destruction.

temperature, tenderness, firmness, and mobility of the lesion relative to surrounding structures. High-flow vascular lesions can have a palpable thrill and/or an auscultable bruit. Tapping on the mass can elicit a Tinel's sign, indicating the lesion's proximity to or intimacy with a peripheral nerve. Successful transillumination can help differentiate a cystic lesion from a solid lesion.

Imaging Studies

Imaging studies provide essential information regarding the nature of the lesion, its size, anatomic location, effect on surrounding bone or soft tissue, and involvement of adjacent joints and neurovascular structures. It can aid in differentiating a benign from a malignant lesion and can help in planning the biopsy.

Plain radiographs should always be obtained before advanced imaging, because they offer a great deal of information, are relatively quick and inexpensive, and may avoid unnecessary expenditures associated with advanced imaging. Two orthogonal views, an anteroposterior view and a lateral view, are generally adequate and can provide information about the extent of the lesion and its location. Radiographs of the bone tumors are tremendously helpful in establishing a reasonable differential diagnosis. The lesion's anatomic location, its position within a given bone, and the patient's skeletal age all offer important clues (**Fig. 4**). Similarly, the lesion's relative radiolucency, radiodensity, or mixed appearance can provide tremendous insight (**Fig. 5**). Finally, it is important to consider the tumor's effect on the bone as well as the bone's effect on the tumor. Benign bone tumors often have sharply demarcated margins with a narrow transition zone (**Fig. 6**). They have a geographic pattern of bone destruction with smooth and uninterrupted periosteal reaction. Malignant bone tumors have poorly -defined margins with a wide zone of transition suggesting a fast-growing lesion. They have a permeative or a moth-eaten pattern of bone destruction (**Fig. 7**) and a malignant periosteal reaction that is usually described as sunburst or onionskin in appearance (**Fig. 8**). As a comparison, consider a nonossifying fibroma and a conventional osteosarcoma. The former is benign and will generally appear as an eccentric bubbly metaphyseal lesion with radiodense borders. It does not demonstrate matrix formation, periosteal reaction, or soft tissue extension.

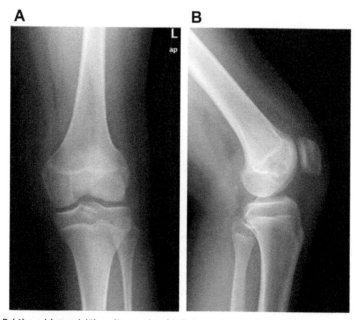

Fig. 4. AP (*A*) and lateral (*B*) radiograph of left knee demonstrate a lytic lesion within the epiphyseal area of the lateral femur condyle in a skeletally immature patient. A radio-dense border is visible, suggesting benign etiology.

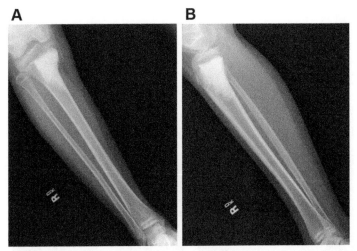

Fig. 5. AP (*A*) and lateral (*B*) radiographs of the right leg demonstrate a radio-dense lesion within the proximal tibial metaphysis, consistent with a high-grade osteoblastic osteosarcoma.

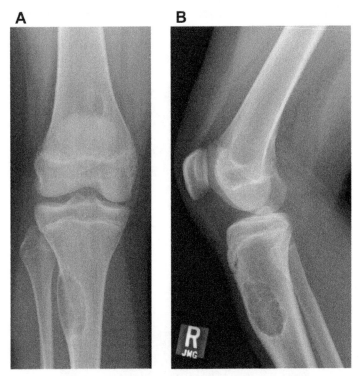

Fig. 6. AP (*A*) and lateral (*B*) radiographs of the right knee demonstrate an eccentric bubbly radiolucent lesion involving metadiaphyseal tibia. Another smaller but similar lesion is seen in distal femur. Both exhibit a narrow zone of transition and a sharply demarcated sclerotic rim. These features are suggestive of a benign entity and most consistent with a non-ossifying fibroma or its smaller counterpart, a fibrous cortical defect.

A

B

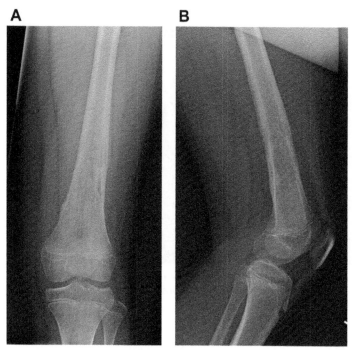

Fig. 7. AP (*A*) and lateral (*B*) radiographs of the distal femur demonstrating a permeative moth-eaten pattern of destruction with a wide zone of transition suggestive of a malignant process. Subtle periosteal reaction is noted laterally.

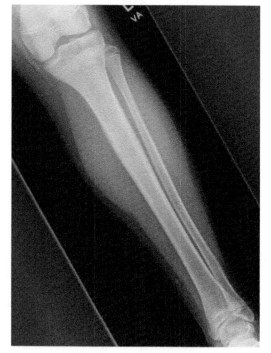

Fig. 8. AP radiograph of left leg showing subtle "onionskin" periosteal reaction along the lateral aspect of the proximal tibia diaphysis.

Conversely, the latter is a high-grade malignancy and will generally appear as a large metaphyseal or metadiaphyseal lesion, with a mixed radiodense and radiolucent pattern. It will exhibit a characteristic sunburst malignant periosteal reaction and usually a large adjacent soft tissue mass (**Fig. 9**).

Plain radiographs can also provide information regarding soft tissue tumors. For example, stippled calcification within a soft tissue mass may suggest synovial sarcoma; phleboliths are suggestive of vascular malformation, and peripheral ossification is most characteristic of myositis ossificans. In addition, a soft tissue mass may exert pressure on an adjacent bone over time, resulting in its scalloping or erosion. This is generally a sign of long-term remodeling and suggestive of a benign entity. Conversely, a more destructive or invasive appearance can suggest malignancy.

MRI provides additional useful information, such as the relative makeup of the involved tumor, its extent and size, and its intimacy with adjacent or proximate anatomic structures. In the case of bone tumors, it can detect the local extension of disease (**Fig. 10**), both within and beyond the bone. It can also diagnose skip metastasis, which is essential for surgical planning. In the setting of soft tissue tumors, MRI can reliably distinguish fat from nonadipose tissues, and with contrast administration, can differentiate cystic from solid tumors. It can clearly depict tumor heterogeneity, often suggestive of malignancy. MRI should ideally be obtained before a biopsy

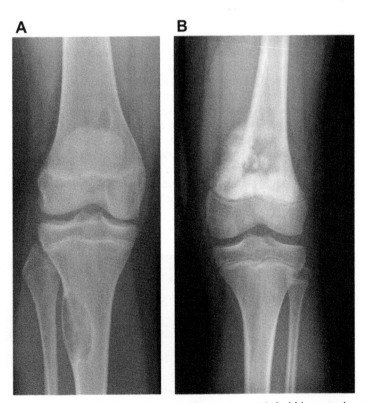

Fig. 9. (*A*) AP radiograph of a knee demonstrating an eccentric bubbly metaphyseal lesion within the proximal tibia with no matrix formation, periosteal reaction or soft tissue extension. (*B*) AP radiograph of a knee demonstrating a mixed radiodense and radiolucent lesion within the distal femur with "sunburst" periosteal reaction most consistent with a conventional high-grade osteosarcoma.

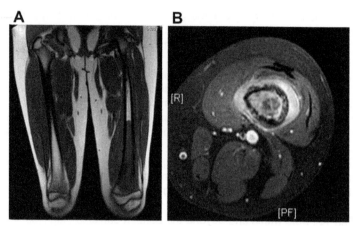

Fig. 10. (*A*) A coronal T-1 weighted MRI demonstrating a marrow-replacing lesion within the left distal femur extending from the middle of the diaphysis distally to the level of the physis. (*B*) An axial T-1 weighted fat suppressed post-contrast MRI demonstrating an aggressive intramedullary lesion with extension through the cortex and into the surrounding circumferential soft-tissue.

because even a needle biopsy can induce edema and bleeding, which will impact image quality. It may also prove useful in guiding the biopsy and ensuring that representative and diagnostic material is sampled (**Fig. 11**).

Computed tomographic (CT) scan is useful for detailed evaluation of the bone (**Fig. 12**). CT is helpful in identifying cortical breaches not clear on radiographs, and 3-dimensional (3D) images can be reconstructed to help in surgical planning. CT-guidance can ensure both proper biopsy location and avoidance of adjacent structures. CT-guided radiofrequency ablation similarly confirms proper probe positioning, ensuring adequate therapy and mitigating collateral injury.

Bone scan is an imaging technique used to screen for bone-forming lesions elsewhere in the skeletal body. The radiotracer substance, ^{99m}Tc- methylene diphosphonate (^{99m}Tc-MDP), is administered intravenously and taken up in active bone-forming

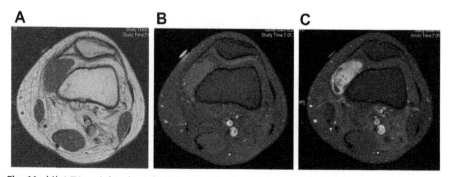

Fig. 11. (*A*) A T1-weighted axial MR image of a distal femur demonstrating a soft-tissue mass adjacent to the medial femur, abutting the medial femoral condyle. (*B*) A T2-weighted axial MR image at the same level demonstrating the soft-tissue lesion mildly hyperintense to muscle. (*C*) A T-1 weighted fat suppressed post-contrast image demonstrating heterogeneous contrast uptake within the lesion.

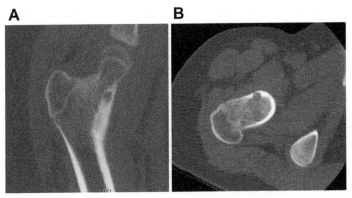

Fig. 12. Coronal (*A*) and axial (*B*) CT images demonstrating an oval radiolucent nidus with surrounding sclerotic bone within the anteromedial femoral neck most consistent with an osteoid osteoma.

lesions after which it can be imaged. It is useful in detecting benign and malignant bone-forming lesions or lesions inciting reactive bone formation (**Fig. 13**). Purely lytic lesions, such as eosinophilic granuloma, often go undetected and are best imaged using other modalities.

^{18}F-2-Fluoro-2-deoxy-D-glucose (^{18}F-FDG)-PET uses a glucose analogue, ^{18}F-FDG, which is retained by tissues with higher metabolic activity. ^{18}F-FDG-PET is used to either stage newly diagnosed patients or, in some cases, assess patients' response to treatment. Compared with ^{99m}Tc-MDP bone scan, it has been reported to be more sensitive and specific for the detection of metastasis in osteosarcoma.[8]

Biopsy

In most instances, a diagnosis is based on histologic features, and therefore, a biopsy remains a critically important step in the process. Its proper planning and execution are vital. It should be performed by the team who will ultimately render definitive

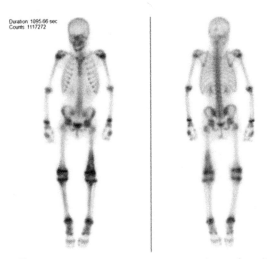

Fig. 13. A technetium[99] Bone scan demonstrating asymmetric uptake within the left distal femur suggestive of a bone forming lesion.

care within an environment equipped to manage complex musculoskeletal tumors. If a tourniquet is used, it should be let down before closure to ensure hemostasis. Hemostasis is essential to limit tumor spillage into or seeding of the surrounding tissue. If a drain needs to be placed, it should be done so in line with the incision. A cortical window or drill hole can be sealed with bone cement, thereby limiting bleeding and minimizing the risk of local contamination. An Esmark bandage should not be used, because its pressure may artificially disrupt the tumor and cause local spread. The biopsy should be obtained via a longitudinal incision centered in line with the anticipated future resection incision. This will permit for excision of the biopsy tract. Generally, the biopsy should be obtained in as direct a manner as possible, should avoid intermuscular planes, and should traverse only a single compartment. The most representative tissue is usually the advancing edge or the periphery of the tumor and not the central area, which is more likely necrotic and less revealing. An adequate amount of sample should be obtained to permit for all necessary studies, which in addition to hematoxylin and eosin stains may also include immunohistochemistry, cytogenetics, fluorescence in situ hybridization, and flow cytometry. The sutures should be placed close to the skin edges to minimize the amount of skin to be resected at the time of definitive surgery.[9]

Staging

Staging is a method of communicating the extent of disease burden in a consistent histology-specific manner and is the most reliable determinant of overall survival.[10] It is largely based on histologic grade, tumor size, nodal dissemination, and distant metastasis. The histology is determined by microscopic appearance, immunohistochemical staining, and cytogenetic aberrations, such as translocations. The tumor grade is based on tumor differentiation, mitotic activity, and necrosis, which is determined by a pathologist. Tumor grade determines the likelihood of subsequent metastasis, making it an important prognostic parameter. The dissemination of tumor to either adjacent lymph nodes or distant sites represents the extent of the disease beyond the primary tumor. The tumor dissemination is a compilation of radiographic imaging and clinical examination. Sarcoma metastasis generally occurs hematogenously, with the lungs being the most commonly involved location. A chest CT can often detect most lung lesions once they reach a few millimeters in size (**Fig. 14**). PET scan is used to screen the whole body for metastatic disease,

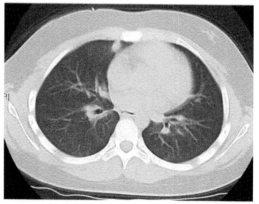

Fig. 14. An axial CT image of the chest demonstrating a pulmonary nodule within the anterior aspect of the left lung consistent with metastatic disease.

but generally cannot identify lesions less than 1 cm in size. Sentinel node biopsy is relevant in histologies that have a greater propensity for lymphatic spread, such as epithelioid sarcoma, rhabdomyosarcoma, and synovial sarcoma.

Surgical Treatment: General Principles

Benign bone and soft tissue tumors are generally managed with surgery alone. Surgery is also the mainstay of treatment of soft tissue sarcomas and a cornerstone of treatment of bone malignancies. Surgery can be categorized as being either intralesional, marginal, wide, or radical. An intralesional procedure implies that the plane of dissection is through or within the tumor. It describes a curettage, which is commonly used to manage benign bone tumors. A marginal resection implies that the plane of dissection is through the surrounding reactive tissue but not within the actual tumor. It is often commonly used for the removal of benign soft tissue tumors. Wide resections imply that the tumor is removed together with a normal surrounding cuff of tissue, maintaining the tumor entirely encased and ensuring its complete extirpation. It is used in the management of malignant bone and soft tissue sarcomas, where complete resection is essential for cure. Historically, amputations and disarticulations were the preferred surgical treatments; however, advances in imaging, implant manufacturing, and chemotherapy have allowed for a much higher rate of limb-salvage surgery (**Fig. 15**A, B). Wide resection has resulted in survival outcomes equivalent to amputation, albeit with slightly higher local recurrence rates.[11] Radical resection is a procedure that implies complete removal of an anatomic compartment. It is a somewhat dated concept and rarely applicable. As a general rule, functional outcomes remain secondary to oncologic considerations, with life generally prioritized over limb.

Margin assessment is performed on the tumor resection by a bone and soft tissue pathologist, who quantitatively measures the tumor margin from the resection surface or edge. There remains ongoing controversy as to what constitutes an adequate negative margin.[12] Within the context of many malignant tumors, a positive margin or "tumor on ink" is associated with an increase in local recurrence. The local recurrence is a poor prognostic sign and is shown to be strongly associated with subsequent metastasis and tumor-related mortality.[13,14]

Adjuvant Therapy

Adjuvant therapy describes the addition of either chemotherapy or radiation therapy to augment surgical management. Its utility and application require careful weighing of its risks and benefits. Toward that end, conditions that are unlikely to recur or

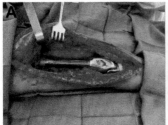 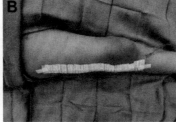

Fig. 15. An intraoperative photograph of a limb -salvage reconstruction with a non-invasive growing distal femoral replacing endoprosthesis (*A*) and the limb immediately following closure (*B*).

metastasize rarely require adjuvant treatments. Alternatively, high-grade tumors that are likely to disseminate or recur often benefit from added therapy.

Systemic chemotherapy is essential for the treatment of malignant bone tumors, such as osteosarcoma. Without it, surgery will cure only a minority of patients with truly localized disease. In the setting of large high-grade soft tissue sarcomas, the addition of adjuvant chemotherapy is often considered because it has historically yielded a modest increase in overall survival.[15,16] Intermediate-sized tumors or tumors that are chemo-resistant lack a consensus and require a patient-tailored approach. In patients who present with overtly metastatic disease, chemotherapy may slow disease progression; however, cure becomes much less realistic.

Adjuvant radiation is generally used to improve the local control of high-grade soft tissue sarcomas greater than 5 cm in size. Both preoperative and postoperative radiation can aid in this endeavor, both having respective benefits and risks. In addition, radiation can augment local control in the context of positive margins and can decrease the likelihood of local recurrence.[17,18] The use of additional postoperative radiation or a radiation "boost" following preoperative radiation has not improved the rate of local recurrence and has largely fallen out of favor.[19]

Recent Advances in Translational Research

Tumors are increasingly being identified and classified according to their molecular profile. For example, sarcomas are being considered as either having a chromosomal translocation and specific gene rearrangement or having complex genetic mutations dominated by copy number alterations.[20]

In addition to broadly classifying tumors, molecular profiling may help accurately diagnose entities in which conventional histology alone cannot confirm a diagnosis. For example, a driver mutation in histone H3F3A is specific for giant cell tumor of bone, and a mutation in H3F3B is supportive of chondroblastoma.[21] Amplification of MDM2 (murine double minutes) is associated with well-differentiated liposarcoma but absent in lipoma. DNA DDIT3 (damage inducible transcript 3) rearrangement is specific for myxoliposarcoma and can help in differentiating it from the other subtypes.[22] Genomic rearrangement of USP6 (ubiquitin-specific protease 6) is seen in primary ABC and is used as a diagnostic tool to differentiate from secondary ABC.[23]

Molecular profiling has also been shown to be useful in prognostication. The French Sarcoma Group has described a CINSARC (complexity index in sarcomas), which is a prognostic expression profile signature. It can predict tumor aggressiveness and metastatic ability in non-translocation-associated sarcomas.[24] In translocation-associated sarcomas, prognosis can also be predicted by expression profiling. Expression profiling has helped to reclassify certain tumors classified earlier as not-otherwise-specified or malignant fibrous histiocytoma as leiomyosarcomas, liposarcomas, and fibrosarcomas.[25]

Genomic index (GI) is a measure of genomic complexity, measured as A^2/C, where A is total number of genetic alterations and C is number of involved chromosomes. GI can reveal intrinsic biological characteristics of tumor and could be used to stratify the patients according to their risk of future metastasis, which can point to the need of more intensive therapy in some cases. For example, GI has emerged as a prognostic tool in synovial sarcoma.[26]

Recently, osteosarcoma has been characterized on the basis of somatic copy number alterations and structural rearrangements. It has been shown that somatic copy number alterations represent a novel target for patient-specific targeted therapy.[27]

Recent Advances in Imaging

Recent reports have demonstrated the use of PET/CT as a surrogate biomarker of chemotherapy response in osteosarcoma and Ewing sarcoma.[28,29] Measurements can be made both before and following chemotherapy administration and differences between metabolic activities used as a proxy for outcome. For example, the difference between standard uptake values (SUVs) obtained at time of diagnosis and again following neoadjuvant chemotherapy is reflective of chemotherapy response. Persistently high SUV measurements are associated with worse progression-free survival. Similarly, elevated total lesion glycolysis, defined as mean SUV multiplied by metabolic tumor volume, is also associated with poor overall survival. Conversely, a decrease in SUV is associated with tumor necrosis greater than 90%.[29] The predictive value has been further improved using dual time point PET/CT techniques. Pretreatment dual-phase PET/CT can predict histologic response in osteosarcoma.[30] Recently, PET/CT has been shown to be useful for the detection of both distant and local relapse in osteosarcoma.[31]

Recent Advances in Surgical Techniques and Technology

Navigation-guided or computer-assisted surgery (CAS) has been increasingly used in the setting of geometrically complex sarcoma surgery, such as in the pelvis and in the sacrum. The theoretic benefits have been demonstrated in several saw-bone models.[32,33] A negative margin was reproducibly obtained using CAS, using 5 mm as a planned or anticipated margin (**Fig. 16**).[32]

Robotic technology can increase cutting instruments' accuracy, but giving control of these instruments to a robot can introduce potential serious complications. Haptic robotic-assisted surgery is passive robotic-assisted resection technique for bone sarcoma, which takes advantage of robotic accuracy, while the surgeon still controls the cutting instruments. Haptic robotic-assisted technique has been shown to improve accuracy of wide resection of bone tumors as compared with standard manual technique.[34]

3D printed technology can be used preoperatively for surgical planning and intraoperatively for patient-specific instrumentation and custom-made prostheses. 3D-printed resection guides, which are personalized or tailored to match patient-

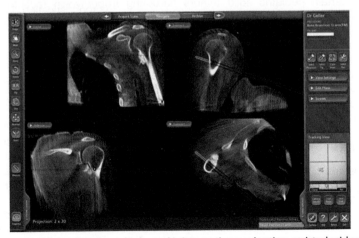

Fig. 16. Images obtained during a limb- and joint-sparing navigation-assisted wide resection of a proximal humeral parosteal osteosarcoma.

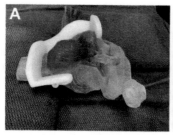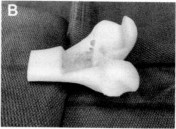

Fig. 17. A 3-D printed patient-specific resection guide (*A*) created for resection of a parosteal osteosarcoma of the posterior femur. A 3-d printed model of the post-resected bone and anticipated osseous defect (*B*). A similar guide (not shown) was also created for the structural allograft used for reconstruction, thereby creating a more accurate allograft osteotomy and a better allograft fit.

specific anatomy, have been used to guide the resection and the allograft preparation, as well as to reduce operative time (**Fig. 17**A, B).[35,36]

There is increasing interest in augmenting a surgeon's ability to intraoperatively visualize tumor margins. Recently, intraoperative indocyanine green guidance in preclinical models has yielded negative surgical margins and diminished local recurrence rates.[37]

Recent Advances in Adjuvant Therapy

The EURAMOS-1 osteosarcoma trial, which spanned a decade and included greater than 2000 patients, sought to answer whether the addition of adjuvant therapy to the standard 3-drug chemotherapy backbone could improve survival outcomes. Unfortunately, negative results were recently reported. Neither the addition of ifosfamide and etoposide to the poor responder group nor the addition of interferon-alpha to the good responder group yielded improved survival, and at this time, standard of care for newly diagnosed osteosarcoma patients remains unchanged.[38,39]

There is increasing interest in precision medicine, which generally describes treatment guided by a given tumor's molecular profiling. Targetable mutations have been reported in up to 60% of soft tissue sarcoma using next-generation sequencing, and there is growing use of such actionable findings in the clinical arena.[40] For example, certain pediatric solid tumors harboring tropomyosin receptor kinase (TRK) gene fusions like infantile fibrosarcoma are now being treated with a highly selective TRK inhibitor, larotrectinib.[41]

Immunotherapy is currently of tremendous interest. To date, numerous checkpoint inhibitors have entered various clinical trials,[42] including those targeting programmed cell death receptor-1 (PD-1), its associate ligand (PD-L1), and cytotoxic T-lymphocyte–associated protein 4. Agents, such as anti PD-1/PD-L1 antibodies, nivolumab and pembrolizumab, are being evaluated in several ongoing clinical trials for use in bone and soft tissue sarcoma treatment.

DISCLOSURES

No disclosures.

REFERENCES

1. Sugiyama H, Omonishi K, Yonehara S, et al. Characteristics of benign and malignant bone tumors registered in the Hiroshima Tumor Tissue Registry, 1973-2012. JB JS Open Access 2018;3(2):e0064.

2. Hewitt M, Weiner SL, Simone JV, editors. Childhood cancer survivorship: improving care and quality of life. Washington, DC: the National Academy of Sciences; 2003.
3. Gurney JG, Swensen AR, Bulterys M. Malignant bone tumors. In: Ries LA, Smith MA, Gurney JG, et al, editors. Cancer incidence and survival among children and adolescents: United States SEER program 1975-1995. Bethesda (MD): National institutes of Health; 1999. p. 99–110.
4. Gurney JG, Young JL Jr, Roffers SD, et al. Soft tissue sarcomas. In: Ries LA, Smith MA, Gurney JG, et al, editors. Cancer incidence and survival among children and adolescents: United States SEER program 1975-1995. Bethesda (MD): National Cancer Institute; 1999. p. 111–25. SEER Program.
5. Hajdu SI. Benign soft tissue tumors: classification and natural history. CA Cancer J Clin 1987;37(2):66–76.
6. Thacker MM. Benign soft tissue tumors in children. Orthop Clin North Am 2013; 44(3):433–44, xi.
7. Grimer RJ. Size matters for sarcomas! Ann R Coll Surg Engl 2006;88(6):519–24.
8. Hurley C, McCarville MB, Shulkin BL, et al. Comparison of (18) F-FDG-PET-CT and bone scintigraphy for evaluation of osseous metastases in newly diagnosed and recurrent osteosarcoma. Pediatr Blood Cancer 2016;63(8):1381–6.
9. Thacker MM. Malignant soft tissue tumors in children. Orthop Clin North Am 2013; 44(4):657–67.
10. Tanaka K, Ozaki T. New TNM classification (AJCC eighth edition) of bone and soft tissue sarcomas: JCOG Bone and Soft Tissue Tumor Study Group. Jpn J Clin Oncol 2019;49(2):103–7.
11. Williard WC, Hajdu SI, Casper ES, et al. Comparison of amputation with limb-sparing operations for adult soft tissue sarcoma of the extremity. Ann Surg 1992;215(3):269–75.
12. King DM, Hackbarth DA, Kirkpatrick A. Extremity soft tissue sarcoma resections: how wide do you need to be? Clin Orthop Relat Res 2012;470(3):692–9.
13. Lewis JJ, Leung D, Heslin M, et al. Association of local recurrence with subsequent survival in extremity soft tissue sarcoma. J Clin Oncol 1997;15(2):646–52.
14. Gronchi A, Lo Vullo S, Colombo C, et al. Extremity soft tissue sarcoma in a series of patients treated at a single institution: local control directly impacts survival. Ann Surg 2010;251(3):506–11.
15. Mahmoud O, Tunceroglu A, Chokshi R, et al. Overall survival advantage of chemotherapy and radiotherapy in the perioperative management of large extremity and trunk soft tissue sarcoma; a large database analysis. Radiother Oncol 2017;124(2):277–84.
16. Pasquali S, Pizzamiglio S, Touati N, et al. The impact of chemotherapy on survival of patients with extremity and trunk wall soft tissue sarcoma: revisiting the results of the EORTC-STBSG 62931 randomised trial. Eur J Cancer 2019;109:51–60.
17. Yang JC, Chang AE, Baker AR, et al. Randomized prospective study of the benefit of adjuvant radiation therapy in the treatment of soft tissue sarcomas of the extremity. J Clin Oncol 1998;16(1):197–203.
18. Pisters PW, Harrison LB, Leung DH, et al. Long-term results of a prospective randomized trial of adjuvant brachytherapy in soft tissue sarcoma. J Clin Oncol 1996;14(3):859–68.
19. Al Yami A, Griffin AM, Ferguson PC, et al. Positive surgical margins in soft tissue sarcoma treated with preoperative radiation: is a postoperative boost necessary? Int J Radiat Oncol Biol Phys 2010;77(4):1191–7.

20. Yazawa Y. Recent impacts of cytogenetic studies in musculoskeletal oncology. J Orthop Sci 2019;24(3):385–6.
21. Behjati S, Tarpey PS, Presneau N, et al. Distinct H3F3A and H3F3B driver mutations define chondroblastoma and giant cell tumor of bone. Nat Genet 2013; 45(12):1479–82.
22. Cho J, Lee SE, Choi YL. Diagnostic value of MDM2 and DDIT3 fluorescence in situ hybridization in liposarcoma classification: a single-institution experience. Korean J Pathol 2012;46(2):115–22.
23. Oliveira AM, Chou MM. USP6-induced neoplasms: the biologic spectrum of aneurysmal bone cyst and nodular fasciitis. Hum Pathol 2014;45(1):1–11.
24. Chibon F, Lagarde P, Salas S, et al. Validated prediction of clinical outcome in sarcomas and multiple types of cancer on the basis of a gene expression signature related to genome complexity. Nat Med 2010;16(7):781–7.
25. Konstantinopoulos PA, Fountzilas E, Goldsmith JD, et al. Analysis of multiple sarcoma expression datasets: implications for classification, oncogenic pathway activation and chemotherapy resistance. PLoS One 2010;5(4):e9747.
26. Orbach D, Mosseri V, Pissaloux D, et al. Genomic complexity in pediatric synovial sarcomas (Synobio study): the European Pediatric Soft Tissue Sarcoma Group (EpSSG) experience. Cancer Med 2018;7(4):1384–93.
27. Sayles LC, Breese MR, Koehne AL, et al. Genome-informed targeted therapy for osteosarcoma. Cancer Discov 2019;9(1):46–63.
28. Salem U, Amini B, Chuang HH, et al. (18)F-FDG PET/CT as an indicator of survival in Ewing sarcoma of bone. J Cancer 2017;8(15):2892–8.
29. Costelloe CM, Macapinlac HA, Madewell JE, et al. 18F-FDG PET/CT as an indicator of progression-free and overall survival in osteosarcoma. J Nucl Med 2009; 50(3):340–7.
30. Byun BH, Kim SH, Lim SM, et al. Prediction of response to neoadjuvant chemotherapy in osteosarcoma using dual-phase (18)F-FDG PET/CT. Eur Radiol 2015; 25(7):2015–24.
31. Angelini A, Ceci F, Castellucci P, et al. The role of (18)F-FDG PET/CT in the detection of osteosarcoma recurrence. Eur J Nucl Med Mol Imaging 2017;44(10): 1712–20.
32. Sternheim A, Daly M, Qiu J, et al. Navigated pelvic osteotomy and tumor resection: a study assessing the accuracy and reproducibility of resection planes in sawbones and cadavers. J Bone Joint Surg Am 2015;97(1):40–6.
33. Sternheim A, Kashigar A, Daly M, et al. Cone-beam computed tomography-guided navigation in complex osteotomies improves accuracy at all competence levels: a study assessing accuracy and reproducibility of joint-sparing bone cuts. J Bone Joint Surg Am 2018;100(10):e67.
34. Khan F, Pearle A, Lightcap C, et al. Haptic robot-assisted surgery improves accuracy of wide resection of bone tumors: a pilot study. Clin Orthop Relat Res 2013;471(3):851–9.
35. Park JW, Kang HG, Lim KM, et al. Bone tumor resection guide using three-dimensional printing for limb salvage surgery. J Surg Oncol 2018;118(6): 898–905.
36. Wong KC, Sze KY, Wong IO, et al. Patient-specific instrument can achieve same accuracy with less resection time than navigation assistance in periacetabular pelvic tumor surgery: a cadaveric study. Int J Comput Assist Radiol Surg 2016; 11(2):307–16.
37. Mahjoub A, Morales-Restrepo A, Fourman MS, et al. Tumor resection guided by intraoperative indocyanine green dye fluorescence angiography results in

negative surgical margins and decreased local recurrence in an orthotopic mouse model of osteosarcoma. Ann Surg Oncol 2019;26(3):894–8.

38. Bielack SS, Smeland S, Whelan JS, et al. Methotrexate, doxorubicin, and cisplatin (MAP) plus maintenance pegylated interferon Alfa-2b versus MAP alone in patients with resectable high-grade osteosarcoma and good histologic response to preoperative map: first results of the EURAMOS-1 good response randomized controlled trial. J Clin Oncol 2015;33(20):2279–87.

39. Marina NM, Smeland S, Bielack SS, et al. Comparison of MAPIE versus MAP in patients with a poor response to preoperative chemotherapy for newly diagnosed high-grade osteosarcoma (EURAMOS-1): an open-label, international, randomised controlled trial. Lancet Oncol 2016;17(10):1396–408.

40. Jour G, Scarborough JD, Jones RL, et al. Molecular profiling of soft tissue sarcomas using next-generation sequencing: a pilot study toward precision therapeutics. Hum Pathol 2014;45(8):1563–71.

41. Drilon A, Laetsch TW, Kummar S, et al. Efficacy of larotrectinib in TRK fusion-positive cancers in adults and children. N Engl J Med 2018;378(8):731–9.

42. Dancsok AR, Asleh-Aburaya K, Nielsen TO. Advances in sarcoma diagnostics and treatment. Oncotarget 2017;8(4):7068–93.

Printed and bound by CPI Group (UK) Ltd, Croydon, CR0 4YY

03/10/2024

01040484-0009